THE
HUMAN
BODY

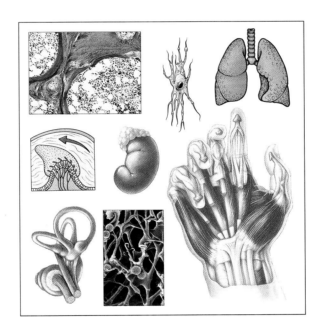

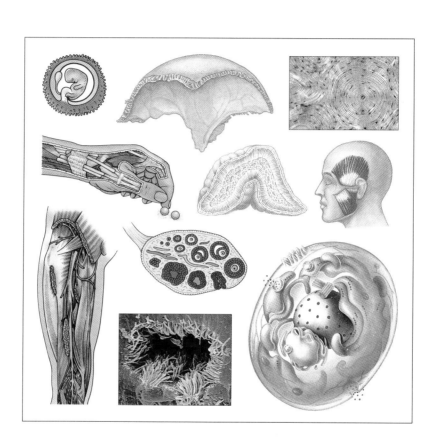

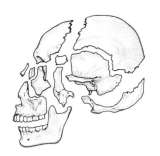
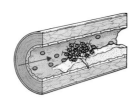
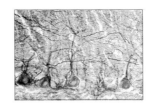
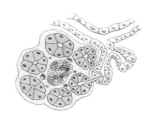
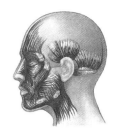

THE
HUMAN
BODY

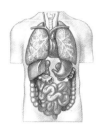
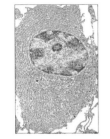
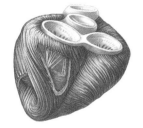
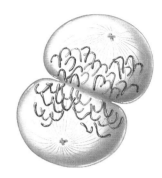
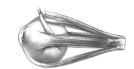
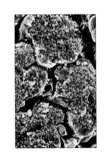

AN ILLUSTRATED GUIDE TO
ITS STRUCTURE, FUNCTION,
AND DISORDERS

Editor-in-Chief Dr Tony Smith

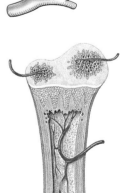
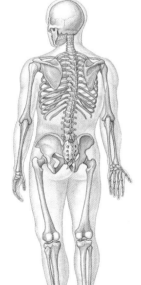

DK

DORLING KINDERSLEY
LONDON · NEW YORK · MUNICH · MELBOURNE · DELHI

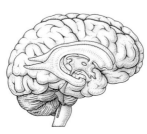
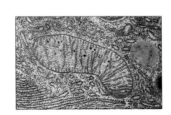
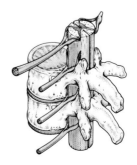

A DORLING KINDERSLEY BOOK
CONCEIVED, EDITED, AND DESIGNED BY DK DIRECT LIMITED

Editor-in-Chief Dr Tony Smith

Senior Editor Andrea Bagg

Art Editor Marianne Markham

Project Editors Christine Murdock, Nance Fyson

Designers Poppy Jenkins, Donna Askem, Tim Mann, Stephen Cummiskey

Commissioning Designer Jenny Hobson

Visualizers Lydia Umney, Joanna Cameron, Peter Dawson

Illustrators Joanna Cameron, Halli Verrinder, Tony Graham, Philip Wilson,
Sandie Hill, Janos Marffy, Andrew Green, Deborah Maizels

Picture Researchers Sharon Southren, Christina Bankes, Christine Murdock

Text Contributors Dr Frances Williams, Duncan Brewer, Dr Tony Smith,
Dr Robert M. Youngson, Dr Amanda Jackson,
Dr Fiona Payne, Dr Pinkinder Sahota

Indexer Sue Bosanko

Production Manager Ian Paton

Design Director Ed Day

Publisher Jonathan Reed

First published in Great Britain in 1995
by Dorling Kindersley Limited
80 Strand, London WC2 ORL
A Penguin Company

2 4 6 8 10 9 7 5 3 1

Copyright © 1995, 2006 Dorling Kindersley Limited, London

A CIP catalogue record for this book is available
from the British Library

ISBN-10: 1-4053-1466-4

ISBN-13: 978-1-4053-1466-4

Reproduced by Colourscan, Singapore
Printed and bound in Slovakia by TBB

PREFACE

Throughout history, surgeons and scientists have relied on pictures of the human body to understand its structures and teach their students. Early anatomical investigations by artists such as Leonardo da Vinci are recognized as aesthetic masterpieces, but they are also amazingly accurate. Drawing the body from living models and post-mortem specimens has largely been replaced by technological innovation: the inner organs and structures can now be portrayed with astonishing clarity by the computer analysis of X-ray, magnetic resonance, ultrasound, and other data, often producing images of stunning beauty.

The great advances in medical imaging techniques of the past two decades form the background to our unique project: a visual exploration of the human body that takes into full account the extended boundaries of current scientific knowledge. *The Human Body* features beautiful illustrations produced by medical artists who, having benefited from this knowledge, can now render details of human anatomy with greater accuracy than ever before. Complementing the drawings are vivid computer and microscope images created with today's advanced technology.

The Human Body is the most ambitious and detailed presentation of anatomy and function yet offered to the general reader. It contains over 1000 images, which reveal the body's structures and illustrate the seemingly simple processes we take for granted, such as breathing and heartbeat. In addition to normal anatomy and function, we illustrate and describe the causes, symptoms, diagnosis, and treatment – including many common surgical procedures – of a wide range of diseases and disorders.

As medical science advances, pictures still remain the easiest way to show how the body is constructed, and how it is affected by disease. We believe the illustrations in *The Human Body* will, like the compelling works of earlier artists, stand the test of time.

Dr Tony Smith

CONTENTS

ILLUSTRATING *the* HUMAN BODY

TO REVEAL THE INTRICATE STRUCTURES of the human body, this book uses many types of illustration. Some show whole areas, such as the nervous system at right, with its complex branching system of nerve trunks, while others concentrate on smaller parts. Also incorporated are microscope and computer-generated images produced using the latest techniques; most of these are colour-enhanced.

THE NERVOUS
SYSTEM

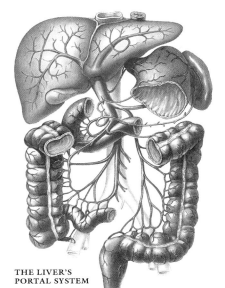

THE LIVER'S
PORTAL SYSTEM

BODY PARTS

After an initial overview, each body system is explored in greater depth by illustrating smaller sections or individual organs. Shown at left is the portal system, the special blood supply to the liver (which processes nutrients from the intestinal tract). Illustrations peel back layers or use cutaways to expose deeper tissues and structures in more detail.

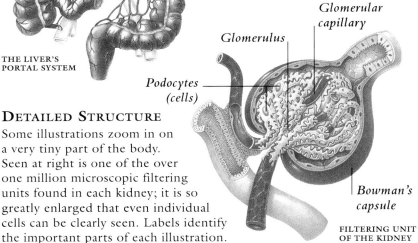

Glomerular
capillary

Glomerulus

Podocytes
(cells)

Bowman's
capsule

FILTERING UNIT
OF THE KIDNEY

DETAILED STRUCTURE

Some illustrations zoom in on a very tiny part of the body. Seen at right is one of the over one million microscopic filtering units found in each kidney; it is so greatly enlarged that even individual cells can be clearly seen. Labels identify the important parts of each illustration.

DYNAMIC PROCESSES

A diagrammatic approach helps clarify the many complex processes that take place inside the body. These may be normal functions, such as digestion, or disease processes, such as how tobacco smoking causes cancer. In some cases, the text and illustrations are organized into "steps". Those at right show how blood clots can form in an artery that has been damaged by the accumulation of fatty deposits (atheroma).

1 If the inner wall of an artery is damaged by deposits of atheroma, platelets in the blood may release chemicals.

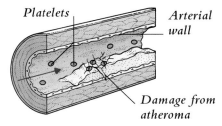

Fibrin strands

Platelets

Arterial
wall

Platelets

Damage from
atheroma

2 These chemicals convert a blood protein into fibrin strands that trap blood cells and form a clot, blocking the artery.

The BODY SYSTEMS

THE HUMAN BODY, LIKE THAT OF EVERY OTHER LIVING CREATURE, has one prime biological function – to reproduce itself and ensure the survival of its offspring. However, this is possible only when all the body systems work together efficiently to maintain health. In this book, we describe how every system works as a separate entity, and also how each system is dependent on the others for physical and biochemical support, a true functioning cooperative.

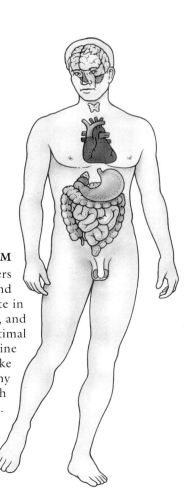

SKELETAL SYSTEM

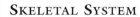

The skeleton is the framework on which the rest of the body is built. Bones also play a role in the other body systems: red and white blood cells grow and develop in fatty inner tissue known as red marrow. The minerals stored in the bones, especially calcium, are released when the body needs them.

CARDIOVASCULAR SYSTEM

The cardiovascular system's most basic function is to pump blood around the body, and a pause of more than just a few seconds will result in loss of consciousness. All body organs and tissues need a supply of oxygenated blood and the removal of waste products. This delivery system can adapt swiftly to changes in demand.

NERVOUS SYSTEM

The brain is the seat of both consciousness and creativity. Through the spinal cord and nerve branches, the brain also controls all body movement. The nervous system works with endocrine glands to monitor and maintain other systems.

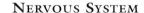

MUSCULAR SYSTEM

Muscles make up about half the body's bulk. Working with the skeleton, they generate the energy to move, make precise and intricate hand movements, lift objects, and even speak. Involuntary muscles, including the specialized cardiac muscle and all smooth muscles, provide the essential power for the respiratory, cardiovascular, and digestive systems. Muscles are dependent on a healthy nerve and blood supply.

ENDOCRINE SYSTEM

Hormones are chemical messengers secreted by the endocrine glands and some other organs. They circulate in the blood and other body fluids, and help the body to maintain an optimal internal environment. The endocrine system initiates the changes that take place at puberty, and governs many of those that are associated with ageing, including the menopause.

TISSUES: *The* FABRIC *of the* BODY

THE BODY IS MADE UP OF TISSUES – collections of similar cells that are specialized to perform a particular function. Tissues fall into five main categories: muscle; nervous tissue; blood; epithelial tissue, which covers or lines surfaces and forms glands; and connective tissue (including bone), which supports or binds organs. All categories subdivide into a variety of individual types, with their own specialized functions. The microscopic study of tissues is called histology.

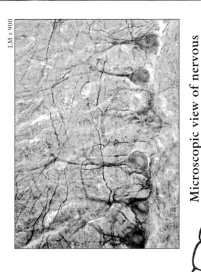

LM x 900

Microscopic view of nervous tissue from the cerebellum

In this sample taken from the cerebellum, a number of flask-shaped nerve cells (Purkinje cells) are seen. Thin projecting fibres extend through the cerebellum from the Purkinje cell bodies.

Nervous tissue

Nervous tissue consists of a network made up of two basic types of cell. Neurons transmit and receive electrical impulses via fibres that project from the cell body. Glial cells play a supporting role. The grey matter of the brain and spinal cord consists mainly of neuron bodies; the white matter is mainly nerve fibres.

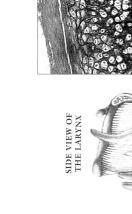

LM x 90

SIDE VIEW OF
THE LARYNX

CROSS-SECTION
OF THE BRAIN

White matter

Grey matter

Cerebellum

Brain stem

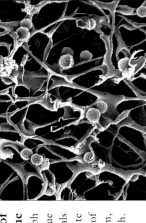

SEM x 1250

Microscopic view of lymphatic tissue

This is an electron micrograph of a piece of lymphatic tissue inside a lymph node. It reveals a fine, fibrous network. White blood cells, a key feature of the body's immune system, are entangled within its mesh.

Lymphatic tissue

This type of tissue has features of both connective tissue and blood. It forms part of the immune system – the body's defence against infection. It occurs in lymph nodes, the spleen, the thymus, and in the walls of the digestive and respiratory tracts.

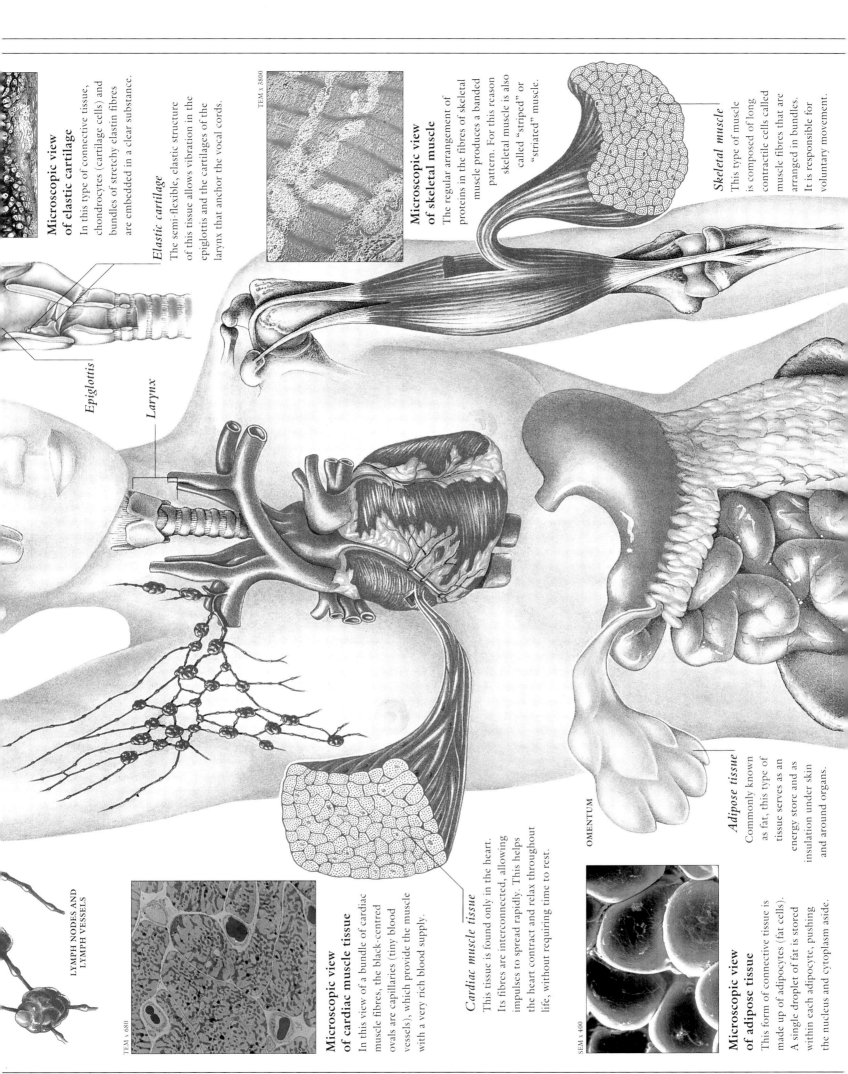

Microscopic view of elastic cartilage

In this type of connective tissue, chondrocytes (cartilage cells) and bundles of stretchy elastin fibres are embedded in a clear substance.

Elastic cartilage

The semi-flexible, elastic structure of this tissue allows vibration in the epiglottis and the cartilages of the larynx that anchor the vocal cords.

TEM x 3800

Microscopic view of skeletal muscle

The regular arrangement of proteins in the fibres of skeletal muscle produces a banded pattern. For this reason skeletal muscle is also called "striped" or "striated" muscle.

Skeletal muscle

This type of muscle is composed of long contractile cells called muscle fibres that are arranged in bundles. It is responsible for voluntary movement.

Epiglottis

Larynx

LYMPH NODES AND LYMPH VESSELS

TEM x 680

Microscopic view of cardiac muscle tissue

In this view of a bundle of cardiac muscle fibres, the black-centred ovals are capillaries (tiny blood vessels), which provide the muscle with a very rich blood supply.

Cardiac muscle tissue

This tissue is found only in the heart. Its fibres are interconnected, allowing impulses to spread rapidly. This helps the heart contract and relax throughout life, without requiring time to rest.

OMENTUM

Adipose tissue

Commonly known as fat, this type of tissue serves as an energy store and as insulation under skin and around organs.

SEM x 400

Microscopic view of adipose tissue

This form of connective tissue is made up of adipocytes (fat cells). A single droplet of fat is stored within each adipocyte, pushing the nucleus and cytoplasm aside.

MICROSCOPY

The simplest microscopic technique uses focused light rays and magnifying lenses. Specimens viewed through a light microscope – labelled in this book as LM – can be enlarged about 1500 times. Higher magnifications can be achieved with techniques that use beams of electrons rather than light, either transmission electron microscopy (TEM) or scanning electron microscopy (SEM).

TEM of skin section

For transmission electron microscopy, the specimen is sliced extremely thinly. An electron beam focused by electromagnets is passed through the specimen and onto a photographic plate or fluorescent screen. The images can be magnified up to five million times.

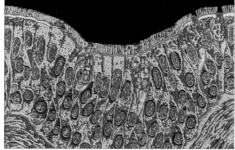
TEM x 700

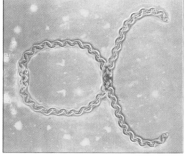
SEM x 33,000

SEM of *Leptospira* bacterium

For scanning electron microscopy, the surface of the specimen is coated with a very thin gold film, over which an electron beam is scanned. Secondary electrons, whose intensity varies with the surface contours, bounce off. The emission patterns create a 3-D image, magnified up to 100,000 times.

PLAIN X-RAYS

X-rays are short electromagnetic waves. When passed through the body to strike photographic film, they create shadow images. Dense structures such as bone absorb more X-rays and show up white, while soft tissues such as muscle appear as shades of grey.

X-ray of deformed spine

This colour-enhanced X-ray of the thoracic spine shows severe deformity due to osteoporosis.

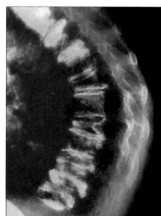
X-RAY

CONTRAST X-RAYS

To view hollow or fluid-filled structures clearly, they must first be filled with a contrast medium, a substance that is opaque to X-rays. Angiography involves injecting contrast into blood vessels. For examining the digestive tract, a barium sulphate mixture is swallowed, or is passed into the rectum via a tube (barium enema).

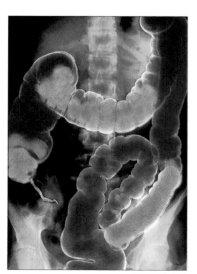

Barium X-ray of colon

The image at left of a healthy colon was taken after a barium enema.

BARIUM X-RAY

CT SCANNING

Computerized tomography (CT) scanning uses an X-ray scanner that rotates around the patient, and a computer that records the varying proportions of X-rays absorbed by tissues of different densities. This information is used to construct cross-sectional images ("slices") of the body.

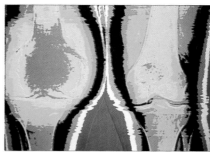

CT scan of sarcoma

CT scans are an especially useful means of investigating bleeding, assessing injuries, or diagnosing the cause of abnormal swellings. The image shows a soft-tissue tumour, called a sarcoma, in the right knee (left of image).

CT SCAN

PET SCANNING

The technique of positron emission tomography (PET) scanning relies on chemical tracers that emit radioactive particles called positrons. It can provide data about the function as well as structure of organs such as the brain.

PET scan of the brain

A radioactive tracer reveals areas of brain activity from high (yellow) to low (blue).

PET SCAN

ULTRASOUND SCANNING

Sound waves of an extremely high frequency are emitted by a device called a transducer as it is passed back and forth over the part of the body being examined, such as the uterus. The sound waves echo back to the transducer and are analyzed by a computer; it creates an image that is displayed on a screen.

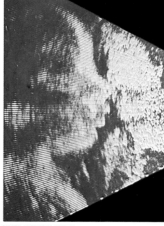

Ultrasound scan of a fetus

Because no radiation is used, this technique is a safe and reliable method for examining the fetus.

ULTRASOUND SCAN

MRI

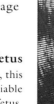

In magnetic resonance imaging (MRI), the person lies inside a magnetic chamber, which causes the nuclei of hydrogen atoms in the body to line up. A pulse of radio waves is released, throwing the atoms out of alignment. As they realign, they produce radio signals, which are analyzed by a computer to create an image.

MRI scan of the brain

MRI scans are particularly useful for studying the brain and spinal cord.

MRI SCAN

IMMUNE SYSTEM

The immune system defences help to provide vital protection against infectious disease and malfunctions of the internal body systems. In a healthy person, the intricate inter-relationship of physical, cellular, and chemical defences can help protect against many threats. Poor general health lowers the body's resistance.

RESPIRATORY SYSTEM

The respiratory tract, working together with breathing muscles, carries air into and out of the lungs, where gases are exchanged. The cardiovascular system transports these gases to and from all body tissues, supplying vital oxygen and removing waste carbon dioxide. A variety of viruses, bacteria, and chemicals contaminate most of the air we breathe; overcoming these threats to our health is a vital role played by the immune system.

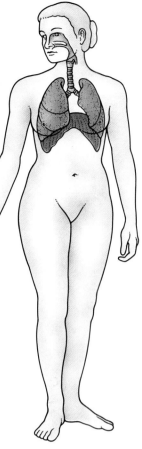

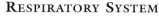

DIGESTIVE SYSTEM

The 9m (30ft) of tubing between the mouth and anus has a complex range of functions. It is needed to store food, digest it, eliminate the wastes, and make optimal use of nutrients. A healthy digestion depends on the proper functioning of the immune and nervous systems. Psychological health is also essential to efficient digestion.

REPRODUCTIVE SYSTEM

Although small when compared to other body systems, the reproductive system is without doubt the body's biological centrepiece. Unlike other systems, it functions only for part of the human lifespan. It is also the only system that can be surgically removed without threatening a person's life.

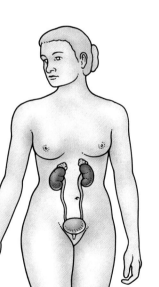

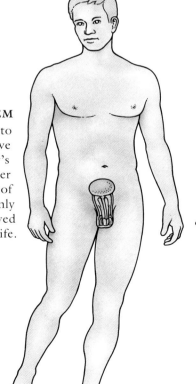

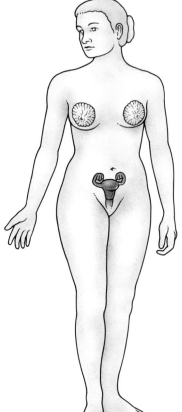

URINARY SYSTEM

The formation of urine by the kidneys eliminates wastes and helps to maintain the body's chemical balance. Production of urine is influenced by blood flow and blood pressure, hormones, and various general rhythms and cycles of the body, such as sleeping and waking.

Microscopic view of hyaline cartilage

The cartilage cells (chondrocytes) are seen here as clear spaces with pink nuclei in the centres. In this type of cartilage – named for the Greek word *hyalos*, which means "glass" – the chondrocytes are embedded in a smooth, featureless, glassy background substance that is secreted by the cells themselves.

LM x 310

Hyaline cartilage

This is the commonest cartilage in the body. It covers the ends of bones in movable joints, and the ends of ribs where they join the sternum. It is also found in the nose and the trachea. Most bones in the body start out as hyaline cartilage and gradually turn into bone.

Tendon

Tendons are strong but flexible cords made of dense connective tissue that join a muscle to a bone or to other muscles.

Muscle

STRUCTURE OF THE FOOT

Microscopic view of dense connective tissue

Tightly grouped bundles of collagen fibres provide this tissue with great strength, especially where fibres are arranged regularly, as here. Dense connective tissue is present in tendons, ligaments, and the dermis of the skin.

SEM x 1600

Microscopic view of loose connective tissue

Wavy, interlacing bundles of collagen and elastin fibres are loosely embedded in a transparent material called ground substance. Collagen fibres provide strength; elastin fibres give elasticity.

SEM x 1500

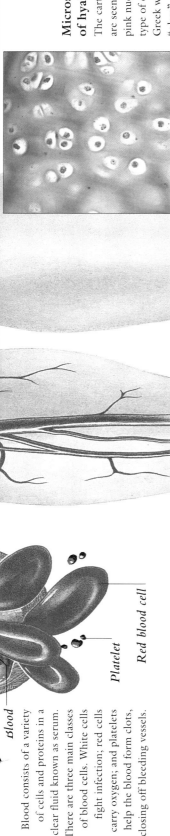

Blood

Blood consists of a variety of cells and proteins in a clear fluid known as serum. There are three main classes of blood cells. White cells fight infection; red cells carry oxygen; and platelets help the blood form clots, closing off bleeding vessels.

Platelet

Red blood cell

Microscopic view of epithelial tissue

This view shows a type known as stratified squamous epithelial tissue, which is mainly protective in function. Cells at the base are cube-like, but become flat when pushed to the surface.

LM x 200

Epithelial tissue

The epidermis is composed of stratified squamous epithelium that functions primarily as a protective outer layer for the body. Various other types of epithelium exist, specialized to perform particular functions such as sensory reception, secretion, or absorption.

Epidermis

Dermis

Fat

Blood vessels

Muscle

SKIN SECTION

Loose connective tissue

This tissue packs and binds tissues and organs, supports the linings of tubes, and is present beneath the skin. Loose connective tissue carries blood vessels and nerves.

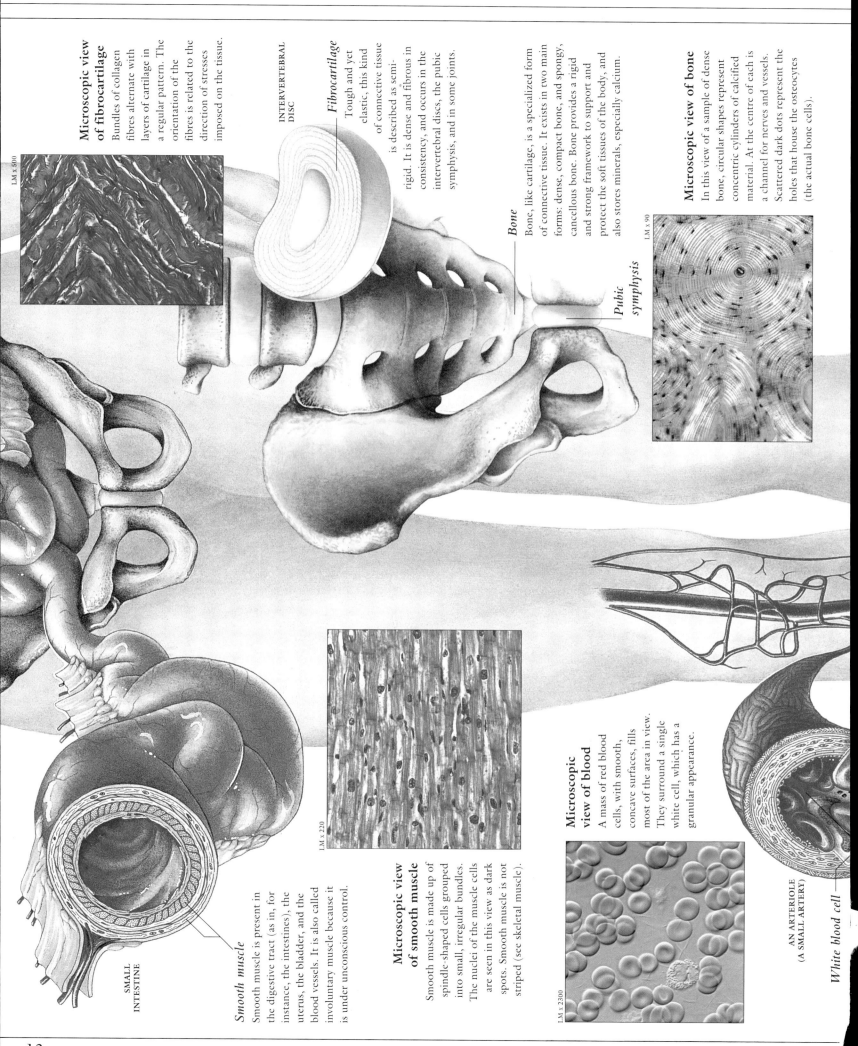

Microscopic view of fibrocartilage

Bundles of collagen fibres alternate with layers of cartilage in a regular pattern. The orientation of the fibres is related to the direction of stresses imposed on the tissue.

LM x 500

INTERVERTEBRAL DISC

Fibrocartilage

Tough and yet elastic, this kind of connective tissue is described as semi-rigid. It is dense and fibrous in consistency, and occurs in the intervertebral discs, the pubic symphysis, and in some joints.

Bone

Bone, like cartilage, is a specialized form of connective tissue. It exists in two main forms: dense, compact bone, and spongy, cancellous bone. Bone provides a rigid and strong framework to support and protect the soft tissues of the body, and also stores minerals, especially calcium.

Pubic symphysis

Microscopic view of bone

In this view of a sample of dense bone, circular shapes represent concentric cylinders of calcified material. At the centre of each is a channel for nerves and vessels. Scattered dark dots represent the holes that house the osteocytes (the actual bone cells).

LM x 90

SMALL INTESTINE

Smooth muscle

Smooth muscle is present in the digestive tract (as in, for instance, the intestines), the uterus, the bladder, and the blood vessels. It is also called involuntary muscle because it is under unconscious control.

Microscopic view of smooth muscle

Smooth muscle is made up of spindle-shaped cells grouped into small, irregular bundles. The nuclei of the muscle cells are seen in this view as dark spots. Smooth muscle is not striped (see skeletal muscle).

LM x 220

Microscopic view of blood

A mass of red blood cells, with smooth, concave surfaces, fills most of the area in view. They surround a single white cell, which has a granular appearance.

LM x 2300

AN ARTERIOLE
(A SMALL ARTERY)

White blood cell

13

CHAPTER 1

CELLS, SKIN,
and
EPITHELIUM

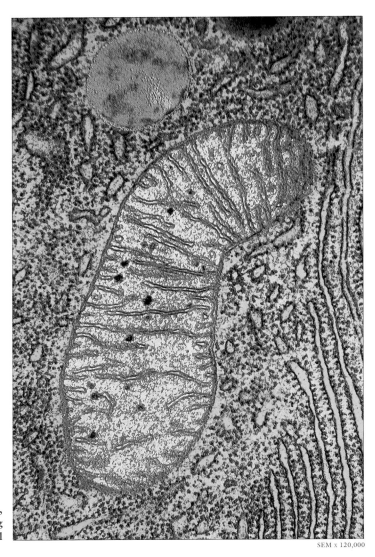

A mitochondrion,
an energy-producing
unit in the cell

SEM x 120,000

INTRODUCTION

Human beings begin life as a single, newly fertilized cell. Like every cell that contains a nucleus, the fertilized cell holds all the instructions for its future growth and development. The term "cell" was first applied by Robert Hooke, a seventeenth-century English scientist, who compared the internal structure of a piece of cork to the "cells" inhabited by monks in a monastery. The characteristics common to all living cells include the ability to reproduce, breathe, move, react to external stimuli, and create or utilize energy to perform their tasks. During the course of human evolution, the cells of the body have become ever more specialized. One example is in the retina of the eye, where there are two kinds of cone cell, some reacting to red light and some to blue or green. When similar cells are grouped together, they form tissues, such as the epithelial cells that make up the protective coverings of body surfaces and the linings of the lungs and the intestines. The outer layer of the skin (the epidermis) is another type of epithelial tissue. This is subjected to continuous wear and tear: though it is capable of a fair amount of self-repair, it is also vulnerable to a wide range of disorders, from minor rashes to cancer.

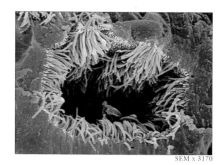

Epithelial tissue lining the trachea

SEM x 3170

A boil – a common disorder of the skin

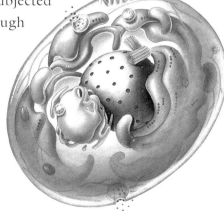

Features of a human cell

CELL STRUCTURE

THE CELL IS THE FUNDAMENTAL UNIT OF LIFE. It is the smallest structure of the body capable of performing all the processes that define life, including respiration, movement, digestion, and reproduction – although not every cell can perform all these functions. Most cells are invisible to the naked eye. Even the female sex cell, the largest in the body, is only as large as the full stop at the end of this sentence. Size and shape vary with cell functions.

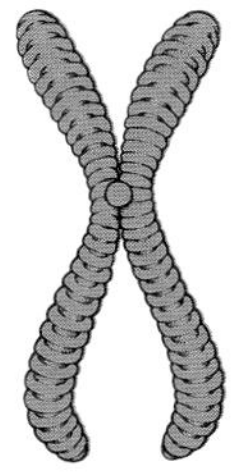

Chromosome
Just before dividing, a cell's genetic material, chromatin, duplicates and coils into rod-like bodies; these link to form X-shaped chromosomes.

FEATURES OF CELLS

Most human cells contain smaller substructures known as organelles ("little organs"); each of these performs a highly specialized task, and most are surrounded by a membrane. Organelles float in cytoplasm, a jelly-like substance, 90 per cent of which is water. It also contains enzymes, amino acids, and other molecules needed for cell functions.

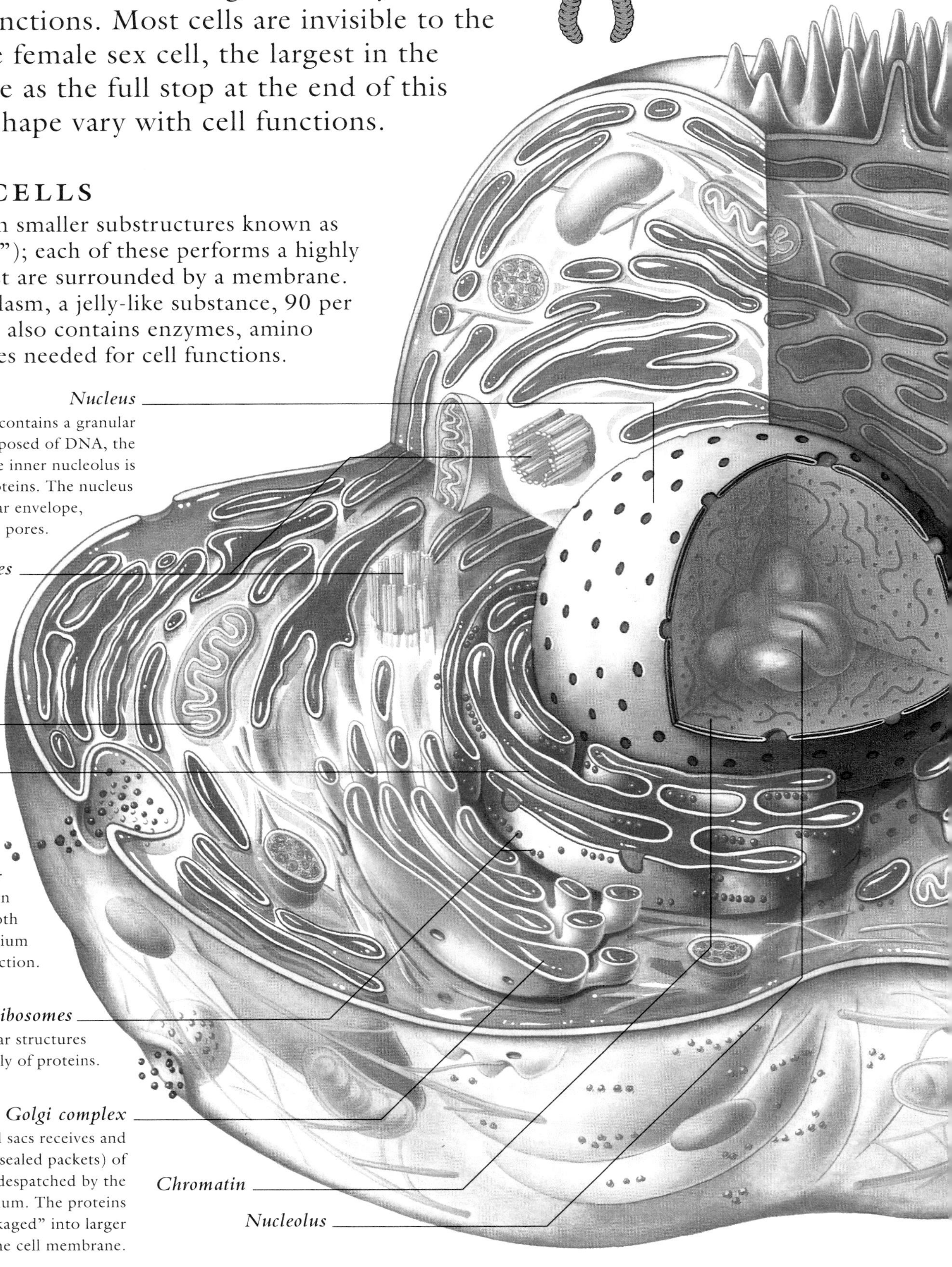

Nucleus
The cell's control centre contains a granular material – chromatin – composed of DNA, the cell's genetic material. The inner nucleolus is made up of RNA and proteins. The nucleus is surrounded by the nuclear envelope, a two-layered membrane with pores.

Centrioles
Located near the centre of the cell are these two structures; each is made up of nine pairs of hollow tubules. The centrioles play an important role in cell division.

Mitochondrion

Endoplasmic reticulum
This network of tubules and flat, curved sacs helps transport materials through the cell. Rough reticulum is the site of attachment for ribosomes, which play a role in protein manufacture; smooth reticulum is the site of calcium storage and of fat production.

Ribosomes
These small, granular structures function in the assembly of proteins.

Golgi complex
A stack of flattened sacs receives and processes small vesicles (sealed packets) of protein that have been despatched by the rough endoplasmic reticulum. The proteins are modified and "repackaged" into larger vesicles and released at the cell membrane.

Chromatin

Nucleolus

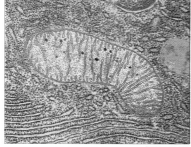

Mitochondrion
Known as the cell's powerhouse, this organelle is the site of respiration and the breakdown of fats and sugars in order to produce energy. The inner folds contain enzymes that produce an energizing chemical called adenosine triphosphate (ATP). It provides the energy needed for many cell functions.

TEM x 12,000

Microvilli
Some cells, such as those lining the small intestine, have projections that increase their surface area to facilitate absorption.

Lysosome
The powerful enzymes of this organelle degrade dangerous materials taken into the cell, such as bacteria, and also dispose of other unwanted substances and any worn-out organelles. These degraded products may be expelled at the cell membrane.

Cell membrane
The membrane encloses the contents of the cell, and regulates the flow of substances into and out of the cell.

Vacuole
This sac transports and stores ingested materials, waste products, and water.

Vesicle
These sacs contain various substances, such as enzymes, produced by the cell; they secrete them at the cell membrane.

Peroxisome
Enzymes that are made here oxidize some cell substances.

Cytoskeleton
The internal framework of the cell is made up of two main types of structure. Prominent in all cells are filaments, which are thought to provide support for the cell and are sometimes associated with the plasma membrane. Hollow microtubules are thought to aid movement of substances through the cell's watery cytoplasm.

TRANSPORT MECHANISMS

The cell membrane regulates the substances that flow in and out of the cell. Because cell membranes allow only certain substances to pass through, determined in part by the cell's role in the body, they are called selectively permeable. Cell membranes may contain several types of receptor protein, each responding to a specific molecule. Some membrane proteins bind to each other, forming connections between cells.

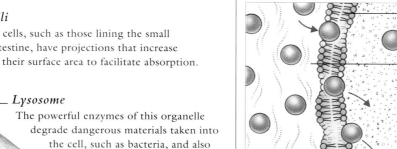

Cell membrane

Cell interior

Fluid outside cell

Diffusion
Diffusion describes the random movement of molecules from areas of high concentration to areas of low concentration. Most movement of liquids or gases occurs by diffusion.

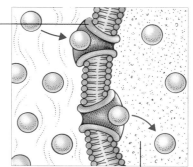

Carrier protein

Facilitated diffusion
A carrier protein temporarily binds with large molecules, such as glucose, outside of the cell membrane. It then changes its shape, opening up to the interior of the cell. Every substance will be carried by a specific protein.

Cell interior

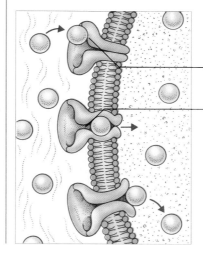

Molecule at receptor site

Protein forms channel

Active transport
If substances must be moved from areas of low to high concentration, energy is supplied by ATP. Molecules bind to a receptor site on the cell membrane, triggering a protein to change into a channel through which molecules are squeezed and ejected.

TYPES OF CELL

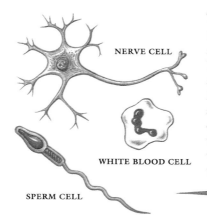

NERVE CELL

WHITE BLOOD CELL

SPERM CELL

SMOOTH MUSCLE CELL

Each human cell has a characteristic shape, size, and lifespan adapted for its function. Nerve cells have axons along which nerve signals are despatched. White blood cells have a flexible membrane so that they can squeeze through the tiny spaces between capillaries. Sperm have whip-like tails so that they can propel themselves up into the genital tract. Muscle cells can change their length, which varies contractile force.

DNA: CONTROLLER *of* CELL ACTIVITY

DNA (DEOXYRIBONUCLEIC ACID), the material from which the chromosomes of a cell's nucleus are formed, governs cell growth and inheritance. Shown on these pages is the process by which DNA instructs chemical compounds to form, or synthesize, the proteins that control specific cell functions. Protein synthesis starts when DNA temporarily unwinds at specific points.

Cell nucleus

Cell membrane

Cytoplasm

Mitochondrion

Endoplasmic reticulum studded with ribosomes

1 The nucleus of every human cell contains 46 chromosomes; each is a long, coiled molecule of DNA, and together they contain about 100,000 genes. Every gene is a tiny segment of DNA that controls a specific cell function by governing the synthesis, or manufacture, of a specific protein.

2 When the thread-like chromosome is unravelled, DNA structure is seen to be two intertwined strands: a double helix. Each strand is composed of four types of subunits called nucleotide bases projecting from a backbone of sugar and phosphate.

The DNA molecule
Seen at left is *Escherichia coli*, a normally harmless bacterium found in the intestinal tract. It is surrounded by its DNA, whose total length is 1000 times that of the bacterium. In humans, a DNA molecule is longer than the body itself.

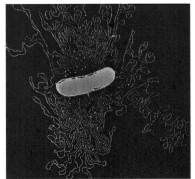

TEM x 15,000

Nucleotide bases
The large DNA molecule is classed as a polymer because it comprises several smaller molecules. These subunits, known as nucleotide bases, always pair in specific ways: adenine with thymine and cytosine with guanine.

Paired nucleotide bases

Nucleosome
DNA wraps around a core of binding proteins in bead-like bodies seen when the chromosomes unwind.

Base triplet

DNA double helix unwinds

3 A unit of three successive pairs of nucleotide bases is called a triplet. Each triplet carries the code for one of the 20 amino acids, the building blocks that form proteins. The sequence of the pairs in each segment of DNA – or gene – determines which protein is synthesized under the control of that particular gene.

Sugar-phosphate backbone

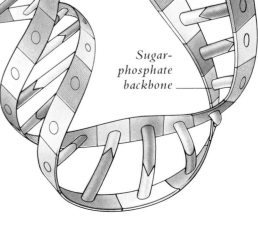

THE MANY ROLES OF PROTEINS

Proteins are needed for development and growth as well as for carrying out vital chemical functions in the body. Some proteins form structures such as hair and muscle. Others serve as antibodies, hormones, or enzymes, or, like oxygen-carrying haemoglobin, transport substances in the body.

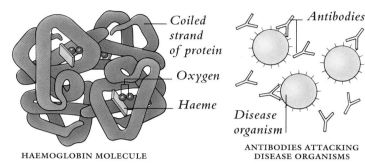

Coiled strand of protein

Oxygen

Haeme

Antibodies

Disease organism

HAEMOGLOBIN MOLECULE

ANTIBODIES ATTACKING DISEASE ORGANISMS

4 For protein synthesis, the DNA strands temporarily separate along the length of the gene that governs the production of that protein. Only one strand carries the genetic code and acts as a template for the formation of messenger ribonucleic acid (mRNA). The process of creating a molecule of mRNA from DNA is known as transcription.

Molecule of messenger RNA (shown here as a 6-based strand)

Pore in nuclear membrane

5 Once the mRNA has formed, the strands of DNA reunite and mRNA leaves the cell nucleus and enters the cytoplasm. Here it attaches to structures known as ribosomes; using raw materials of the cell, ribosomes produce the protein by following the sequence of nucleotide bases in the mRNA.

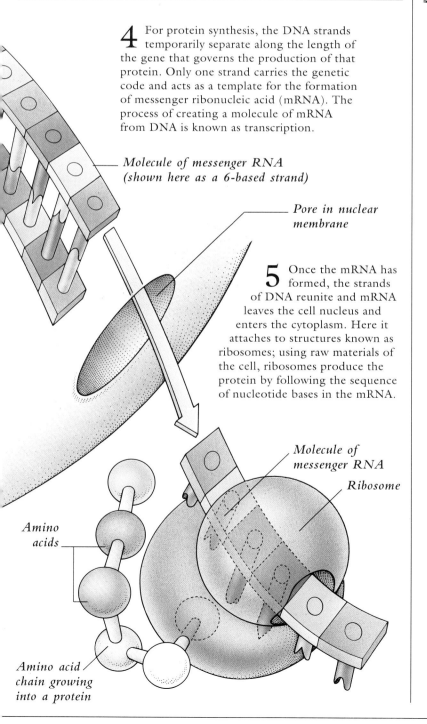

Molecule of messenger RNA

Ribosome

Amino acids

Amino acid chain growing into a protein

MITOSIS

Mitosis is a simple copying process that organizes and redistributes DNA during cell division in all normal growth. It occurs continuously during growth and also as the body replaces old, worn-out cells. During this copying process, one cell produces two daughter cells that are identical to each other and to the parent cell. Cells of the growing embryo multiply by mitosis, as do adult tissues such as skin and intestinal lining.

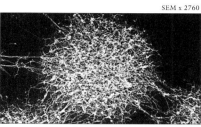

SEM x 2760

Chromatin

The stage that precedes actual cell division is called interphase. During this time, molecules of DNA are loosely organized into a network of extended filaments, which is known as chromatin.

Prophase

DNA strands replicate and coil up, forming spiral filaments called chromatids that join at the centromere. These filaments then condense and form 46 X-shaped pairs of chromosomes.

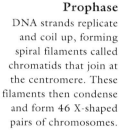

Cytoplasm

Nucleus

Chromatin

Paired chromosomes

Centromere

Threads of the spindle

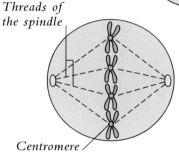

Metaphase

Chromosome pairs line up in the centre of the cell. Thread-like fibres create the spindle that connects the centromere of each chromosome pair to opposite poles of the dividing cell.

Centromere

Anaphase

Each centromere splits, dividing the paired chromosomes so that there are 92 single chromosomes. One-half, that is 46, of these daughter chromosomes move toward each side of the cell.

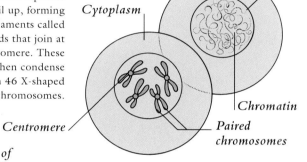

Daughter chromosomes

Telophase

Spindle fibres disappear, and a nuclear membrane forms around each group of 46 daughter chromosomes. The cell becomes pinched in the middle, and the chromosomes start to uncoil.

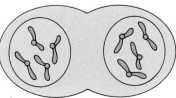

Late telophase

The cytoplasm begins to divide, a cell plate forms between the two groups of chromosomes, and the cell splits into two. Each cell has a set of 46 chromosomes; these revert to chromatin filaments.

Chromatin

Nucleus

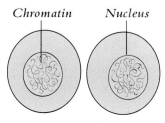

SKIN STRUCTURE *and* EPITHELIAL TISSUES

SKIN IS THE BODY'S PROTECTIVE OUTER BOUNDARY. It is one of the largest organs of the body, is self-repairing, and contains a variety of sensory receptors so that many parts are sensitive to the lightest touch. Skin plays an essential role in regulating body temperature. The appearance of the skin alters with emotional state and general health, and can reveal many signs of a wide range of disorders.

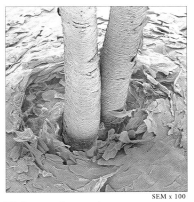

SEM x 100

Hair on the scalp
Hair grows from follicles located in the dermis. The scaly cells covering each hair are lubricated by oil glands.

THE STRUCTURE OF SKIN

The skin is composed of two main layers. The outer layer is stratified squamous epithelial tissue, and consists of sheets of cells that are flatter and more scaly near the surface. The inner dermis comprises fibrous and elastic tissue pierced by blood vessels, nerve fibres, hair follicles, and sweat glands; its deepest layer anchors the skin to underlying tissues.

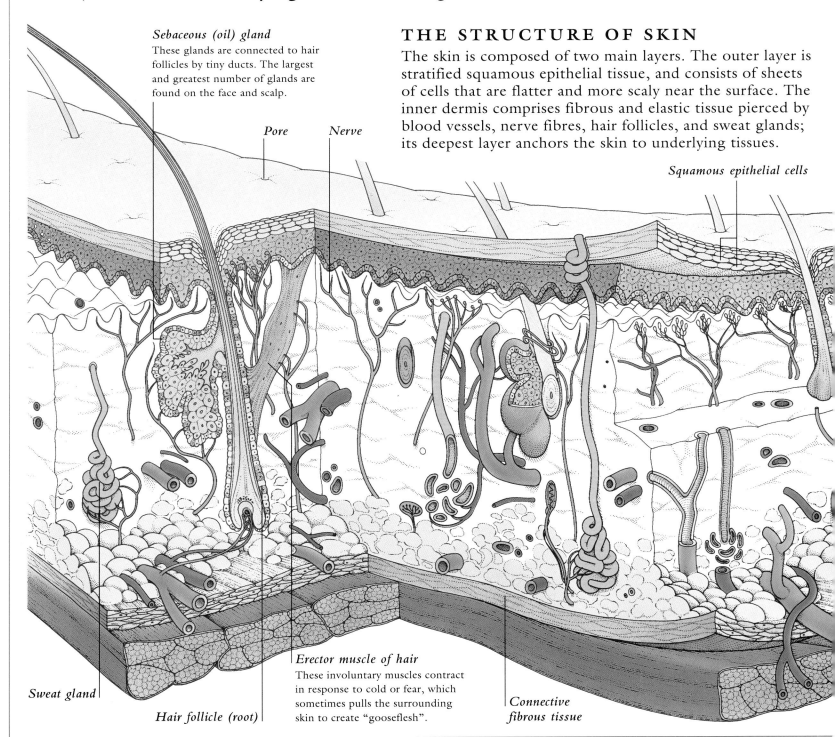

Sebaceous (oil) gland
These glands are connected to hair follicles by tiny ducts. The largest and greatest number of glands are found on the face and scalp.

Pore

Nerve

Squamous epithelial cells

Sweat gland

Hair follicle (root)

Erector muscle of hair
These involuntary muscles contract in response to cold or fear, which sometimes pulls the surrounding skin to create "gooseflesh".

Connective fibrous tissue

Nail Structure

Nails are made of keratin, a hard, fibrous protein, which is also the main constituent of hair. The nails rest on a bed served by blood vessels, which creates the pink colour; they grow from a matrix of active cells under skin folds at their base and sides.

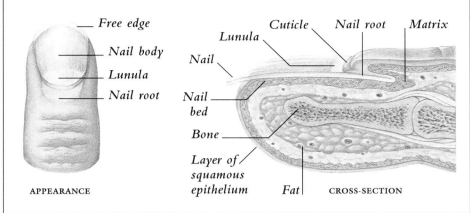

APPEARANCE

Free edge
Nail body
Lunula
Nail root

CROSS-SECTION

Cuticle   _Nail root_   _Matrix_
Lunula
Nail
Nail bed
Bone
Layer of squamous epithelium   _Fat_

Pseudostratified Epithelium

This type of columnar epithelial tissue appears to be stratified, but actually consists of a single layer of cells of different heights. Sometimes the taller cells are specialized; they are either goblet cells, which secrete mucus, or ciliated cells, which have tiny surface hairs to trap or move foreign particles.

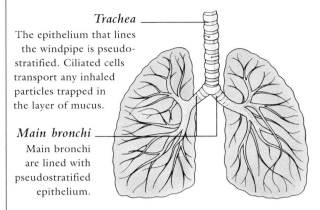

Trachea
The epithelium that lines the windpipe is pseudo-stratified. Ciliated cells transport any inhaled particles trapped in the layer of mucus.

Main bronchi
Main bronchi are lined with pseudostratified epithelium.

Basal cell layer
In this layer, cells constantly divide. The new cells push toward the upper surface, replacing dead or worn-out cells of the outermost layer.

Epidermis

Prickle cell layer
To strengthen the skin, epithelial cells in this layer are bound together by tiny cells with filaments.

Dermis

Arteriole

Venule

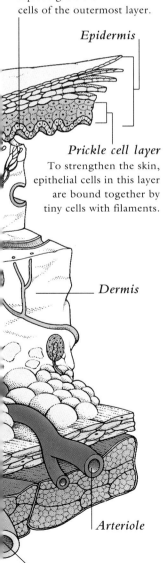

EPITHELIAL TISSUES

Epithelial tissue, also called epithelium, is an important structural element that acts as a lining or covering for other body tissues. Epithelium can be classified according to cell type and arrangement of cells into one or more layers. These tissues are specialized for protection, absorption, or secretion.

Simple and Stratified Epithelium

Simple epithelium is composed of a single layer of cells, which are called squamous (plate-like or flattened), cuboidal (cube-shaped), or columnar (tall and thin). Simple epithelium is often found in areas where substances need to pass through easily. Stratified epithelium has more than one layer, and is thus well adapted for protection.

The eye

There are two types of epithelium in the eye. Simple cuboidal epithelium occurs in the pigmented layer of the retina, whereas stratified squamous epithelium is found in the outer cornea.

Retina
Cornea

The cornea

The cornea is covered by about five layers of stratified squamous epithelial cells, which form a transparent coating that permits light rays to enter the eye. Tiny ridges, called microplicae (seen on the surface of the cell at lower centre), hold fluid, which helps to refract the incoming rays of light.

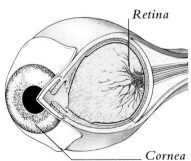

SEM x 1170

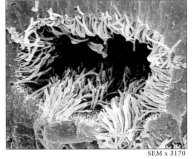

SEM x 3170

Tracheal epithelium
Cilia that project from tracheal epithelial cells are seen here in green. Mucus-secreting goblet cells between the cilia possess tiny microvilli (seen here in yellow).

Transitional Epithelium

This kind of epithelial tissue is similar to stratified squamous epithelium, but has the ability to stretch without tearing. It is particularly well suited to the urinary system. Covering the columnar cells at the base are progressively rounder surface cells that flatten, or become more squamous, as they stretch.

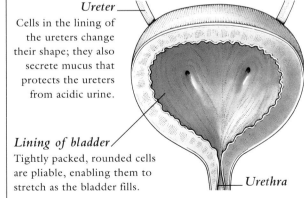

Ureter
Cells in the lining of the ureters change their shape; they also secrete mucus that protects the ureters from acidic urine.

Lining of bladder
Tightly packed, rounded cells are pliable, enabling them to stretch as the bladder fills.

Urethra

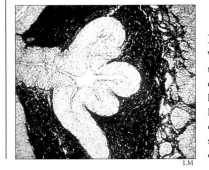

LM

Inside a ureter
When the muscles of the ureters are relaxed, epithelial cells in the lining appear folded; here they are seen to curve around the star-shaped white interior of the relaxed ureter.

23

SKIN DISORDERS

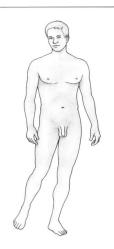

SKIN MAY BE AFFECTED BY A WIDE RANGE OF DISORDERS – from physical injury to chemical damage. It is susceptible to infection by viruses, bacteria, fungi, and protozoa, and to infestation by mites and other parasites. Skin may also develop tumours and may be affected by an inadequate blood supply. Its own glands, blood vessels, and nerves may become disordered, and skin may show various allergic reactions. Rashes and skin discoloration may reflect general body disorders.

COMMON SWELLINGS

Skin swellings may be small,. inflamed, pus-filled spots known as pustules, or larger ones called boils. A cluster of boils may link, forming a larger lump called a carbuncle. Other swellings may be caused by a local increase in cell numbers, as in warts, moles, or malignant tumours. Swellings may also result from acne, cysts, allergies, and chilblains.

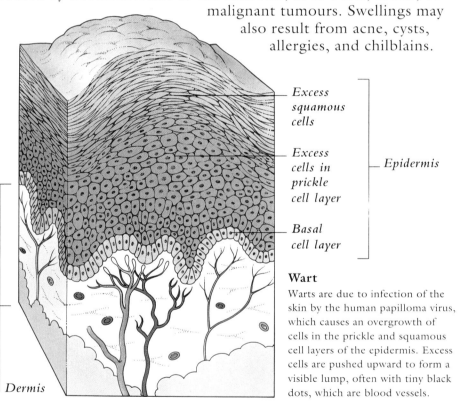

Excess squamous cells

Excess cells in prickle cell layer

Basal cell layer

Epidermis

Dermis

Mole

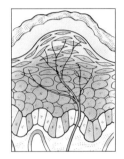

A mole, also called a naevus, is an aggregate of pigment cells (melanocytes) or of tiny blood vessels. Moles rarely become malignant, but any change in size, shape, or colour should be discussed with a doctor.

Boil

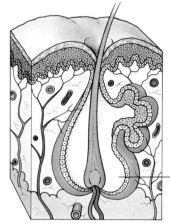

This collection of pus inside a hair follicle or a sebaceous gland is most often due to infection by staphyloccocal bacteria, which results in acute inflammation of the area.

Pus-filled follicle

Wart

Warts are due to infection of the skin by the human papilloma virus, which causes an overgrowth of cells in the prickle and squamous cell layers of the epidermis. Excess cells are pushed upward to form a visible lump, often with tiny black dots, which are blood vessels.

Cyst

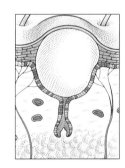

Cysts are sac-like structures containing fluid or semi-solid material. Most have a strong capsule. The commonest cyst of the skin is a "wen", which is full of sebaceous secretions.

ACNE VULGARIS

In acne vulgaris, the sebaceous (oil-secreting) glands of the skin produce excessive amounts of their secretion, known as sebum. The sebum oxidizes and forms a blackened plug in the skin pore. Trapped sebum, dead cells, and infection by bacteria inflame the area and can cause a pustule to form. Acne can be treated with skin medications, for example tretinoin, or drugs that can be taken orally, such as tetracycline.

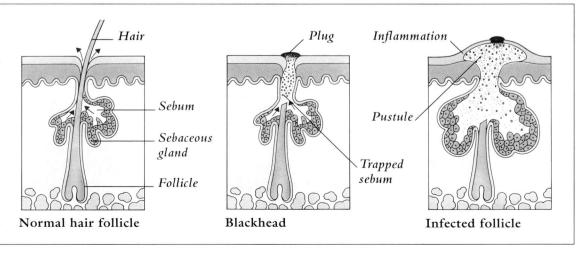

Hair

Plug

Inflammation

Sebum

Sebaceous gland

Follicle

Pustule

Trapped sebum

Normal hair follicle

Blackhead

Infected follicle

WOUNDS

Damage to or removal of part of the skin surface to variable depths is called a wound, and may occur by accident or as a result of an operation. How well a wound heals depends upon the alignment of the edges and the prevention of infection. Well-closed, clean wounds usually heal in a few weeks, while open wounds heal more slowly and usually result in a puckered scar.

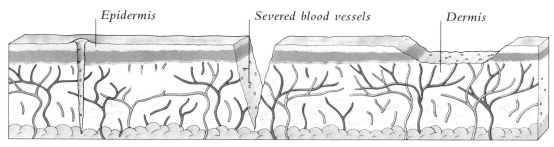

Epidermis   *Severed blood vessels*   *Dermis*

Puncture wounds
Punctures usually heal quickly but infection is a risk. Because tetanus sometimes follows puncture wounds, immunization may be necessary.

Cuts
Deep cuts often need stitching if scarring is to be avoided. Clean cuts will heal with only minimal scarring if they are well closed.

Abrasions
Abrasions involving only the epidermis usually heal without a scar. Any deeper abrasion is likely to leave a scar.

RASHES

Rashes are areas of skin inflammation or groups of spots. They may occur in small patches, or cover a large part of the body. Among the main causes of rashes are skin conditions, including eczema and psoriasis, infectious diseases, and allergic reactions. Some types are accompanied by fever or itching.

Eczema

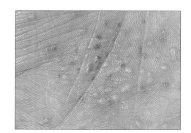

The term eczema refers to various skin inflammations with common features; these include itching, red patches, and small blisters that burst so that the skin becomes moist and crusty. The commonest type, atopic eczema, is an allergic reaction and often appears in the first year of life.

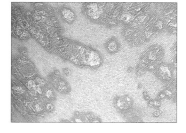

Psoriasis

This common, non-infectious skin disease of unknown cause features sharply outlined, bright red or pink, dry, non-itchy plaques with silvery, scaly surfaces. These inflamed areas occur mainly on the elbows, knees, shins, scalp, and lower back.

INFECTIOUS RASHES

Common infectious diseases such as measles, rubella (German measles), and chickenpox – as well as other less common diseases, including typhoid and scarlet fever – have a toxic effect on the skin that produces a characteristic, temporary rash. The rashes are due to organisms in the skin or their circulating toxins.

Chickenpox rash

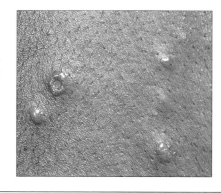

The photograph seen at right is a close-up view of a typical chickenpox rash. The spots are itchy, fluid-filled blisters that dry out and form scabs after a few days. The rash, which is most dense on the trunk, is accompanied by a low fever.

SKIN CANCER

Skin cancers are related to excessive exposure to sunlight. Ultraviolet light can damage DNA, and change the cell's genetic material. The type that occurs most frequently is basal cell carcinoma, which spreads only locally and not to other parts of the body. Squamous cell carcinoma and the rarer malignant melanoma are more dangerous. Skin cancers may be treated by excising (cutting away), radiation, or cryocautery (freezing).

Cancer cells   *Surface of epidermis*

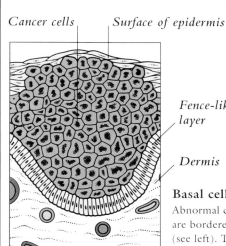

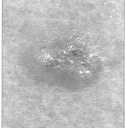

Fence-like layer

Dermis

TYPICAL APPEARANCE

Basal cell carcinoma

Abnormal cells grow in the epidermis and are bordered by a fence-like layer of cells (see left). The tumour, also called a rodent ucler, is typically firm and pearly-looking, and occurs most frequently on the face.

Cancer cells in epidermis

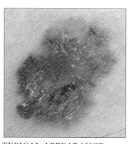

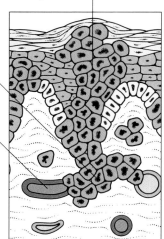

Cancer cells spreading into dermis

Blood vessel

TYPICAL APPEARANCE

Malignant melanoma

This skin cancer develops in pigment cells (melanocytes). Tumour cells break through the layers of skin (see right). A malignant melanoma is often very dark in colour and asymmetrical, with an indistinct border. It can grow rapidly and spread to distant sites.

CHAPTER TWO

The SKELETAL SYSTEM

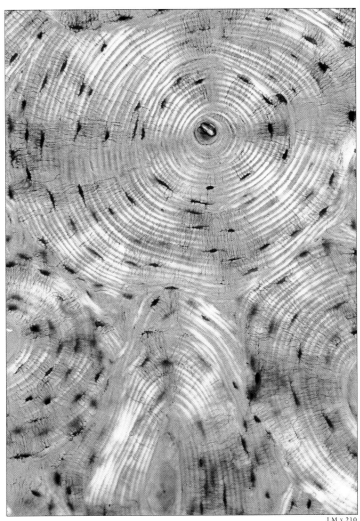

The structure of hard bone

LM x 210

INTRODUCTION

There is more life in a bone than most people think. The living skeleton, though tough, is a flexible structure with blood flowing through every part, and it is in a state of constant growth and renewal. Even the bones of skeletons discovered by archaeologists tell a story: they often reveal a great deal about the dead person's age, sex, height and weight, activities, and whether he or she was a meat-eater or a vegetarian. Fossil bones also provide clear evidence that such bone disorders as rickets and arthritis have a long history. Diseases of the bones and joints have always been among the most common causes of poor health and disability, especially in older people. However, many are preventable: the bulk and strength of bones in later life depends critically on a person's health in earlier adult life. Being overweight, for example, increases the risk of developing osteoarthritis, while a calcium-rich diet combined with moderate, regular exercise reduces the risk of a variety of bone diseases. An important recent advance in treating arthritis and some other bone disorders has been the development of artificial replacements for many joints in the body. Scientists are also exploring the complex interactions between human genes and environmental factors to find out why some bone disorders affect only a small fraction of the population.

A lumbar vertebra

X-RAY

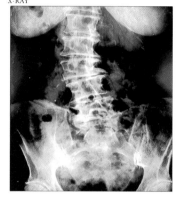

Osteoarthritis of the lumbar spine

THE SKELETAL SYSTEM

BONES of the BODY I

BOTH STRONG ENOUGH to support weight and light enough to facilitate movement, bones also offer protection to internal organs and store most of the calcium, phosphorus, and some other minerals, such as magnesium salts, that the body needs. While the bones seen in a museum appear dry and rigid, living bones are actually a moist hive of activity. The marrow in bones is the site where red blood cells and some white cells are produced.

THE SKELETON

The precise number of bones in the adult human skeleton varies from one person to another, but on average there are 206 bones of varying shapes and sizes. The skeleton is divided into two main parts. The central bones of the skull, ribs, vertebral column, and sternum form the axial skeleton. The bones of the arms and legs, along with the scapula, clavicle, and pelvis, make up the appendicular skeleton.

SPINAL LINK

The cylindrical, linked vertebrae of the spinal column offer strong, bony protection for the spinal cord. Aided by muscles and ligaments, they support the skull, hold the body upright, and permit twisting and bending of the trunk.

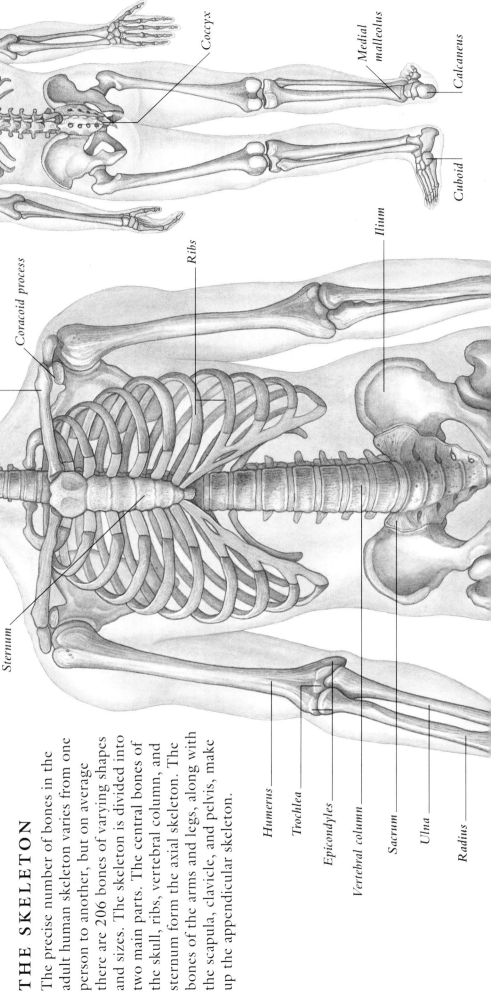

Parietal bones

Occipital bone

Coccyx

Medial malleolus

Calcaneus

Cuboid

Acromion

Scapula

Clavicle

Coracoid process

Ribs

Ilium

Sternum

Humerus

Trochlea

Epicondyles

Vertebral column

Sacrum

Ulna

Radius

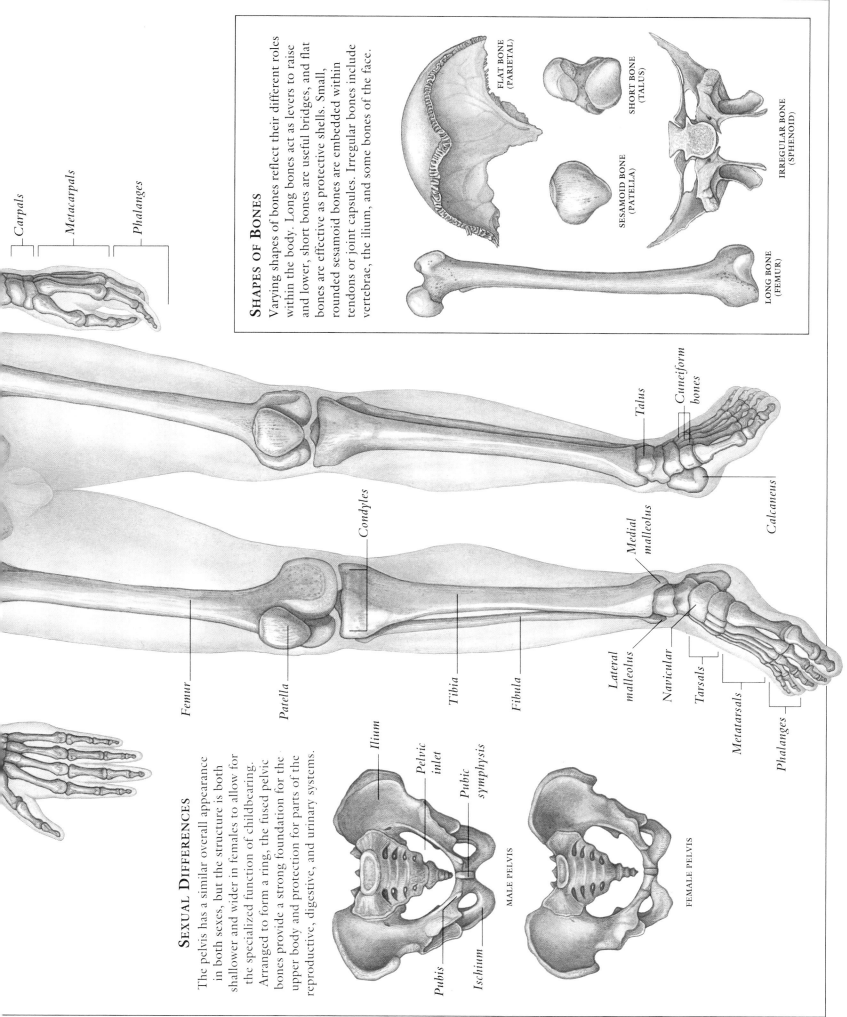

Carpals

Metacarpals

Phalanges

SHAPES OF BONES

Varying shapes of bones reflect their different roles within the body. Long bones act as levers to raise and lower, short bones are useful bridges, and flat bones are effective as protective shells. Small, rounded sesamoid bones are embedded within tendons or joint capsules. Irregular bones include vertebrae, the ilium, and some bones of the face.

FLAT BONE
(PARIETAL)

SHORT BONE
(TALUS)

IRREGULAR BONE
(SPHENOID)

SESAMOID BONE
(PATELLA)

LONG BONE
(FEMUR)

Talus

Cuneiform bones

Condyles

Medial malleolus

Lateral malleolus

Navicular

Tarsals

Metatarsals

Phalanges

Calcaneus

Femur

Patella

Tibia

Fibula

SEXUAL DIFFERENCES

The pelvis has a similar overall appearance in both sexes, but the structure is both shallower and wider in females to allow for the specialized function of childbearing. Arranged to form a ring, the fused pelvic bones provide a strong foundation for the upper body and protection for parts of the reproductive, digestive, and urinary systems.

Ilium

Pelvic inlet

Pubic symphysis

MALE PELVIS

FEMALE PELVIS

Pubis

Ischium

BONES *of the* BODY II

A CAGE OF BONES within the thorax, or chest, demonstrates both the supportive and protective functions of the skeleton. The ribcage and its muscles form the chest wall while shielding vital internal organs such as the heart, lungs, and liver. Most people have 12 pairs of ribs, but about 5 per cent are born with one or more extra ribs. Some people, such as Down's syndrome sufferers, have one pair of ribs less than is usual.

THE RIBCAGE

All 12 pairs of ribs attach to the spine. The upper seven pairs, known as "true ribs", link directly to the sternum by costal cartilage. The next two to three pairs of "false ribs" connect indirectly to the sternum by means of cartilage to the ribs above; the remaining "floating ribs" do not have any link to the sternum. (The lower two pairs of ribs are hidden by the liver and the stomach in this illustration.)

HOW RIBS ATTACH

Each rib links to its corresponding thoracic vertebra at two points. Flexible costal cartilage attaches some of the ribs to the sternum, allowing the ribcage to move during breathing.

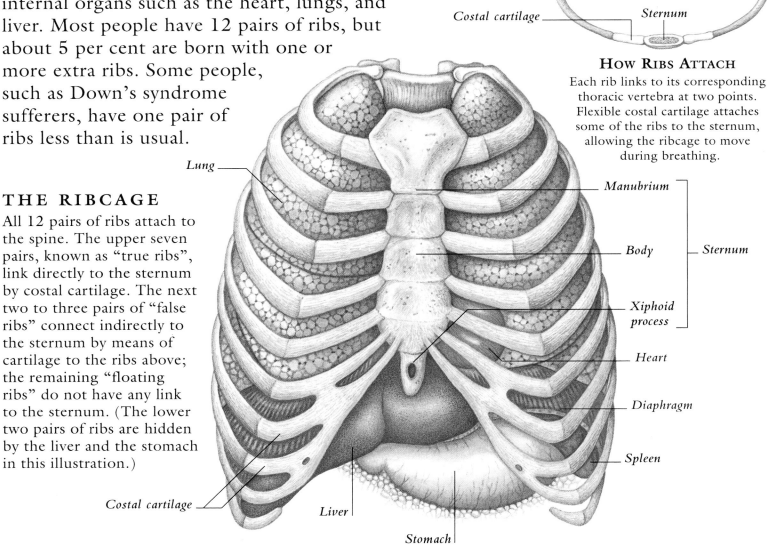

Thoracic vertebra
Rib
Costal cartilage
Points of attachment
Sternum

Lung
Manubrium
Body — Sternum
Xiphoid process
Heart
Diaphragm
Spleen
Costal cartilage
Liver
Stomach

BONES OF THE HAND AND FOOT

A similar arrangement of bones is repeated in the hand and foot, but with some key differences. For example, the phalanges in toes are generally shorter than those in fingers.

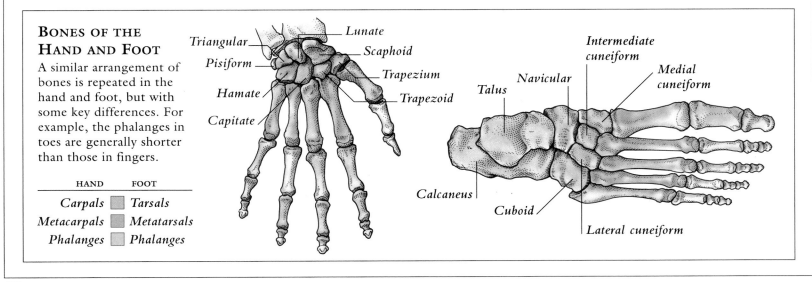

Triangular
Pisiform
Hamate
Capitate
Lunate
Scaphoid
Trapezium
Trapezoid

Talus
Navicular
Intermediate cuneiform
Medial cuneiform
Calcaneus
Cuboid
Lateral cuneiform

HAND	FOOT
Carpals	Tarsals
Metacarpals	Metatarsals
Phalanges	Phalanges

THE BONES OF THE SKULL

Two separate sets of bones form the intricate structure of the skull. The eight bones enclosing and protecting the brain are called the cranial vault, while the other 14 bones comprise the skeleton of the face.

Wiggly lines that appear on the surface of the skull are actually joints known as sutures. While flexible in very young children to allow for growth, these sutures become virtually fixed with age. The mandible bone of the lower jaw is the only skull bone secured by a more movable joint. The ossicles (tiny bones) of the middle ear are not technically part of the skull. They conduct sound waves from the eardrum to the inner ear.

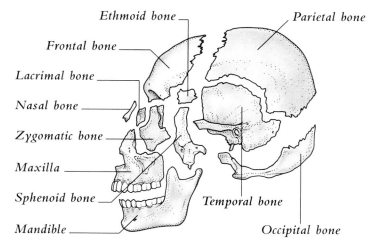

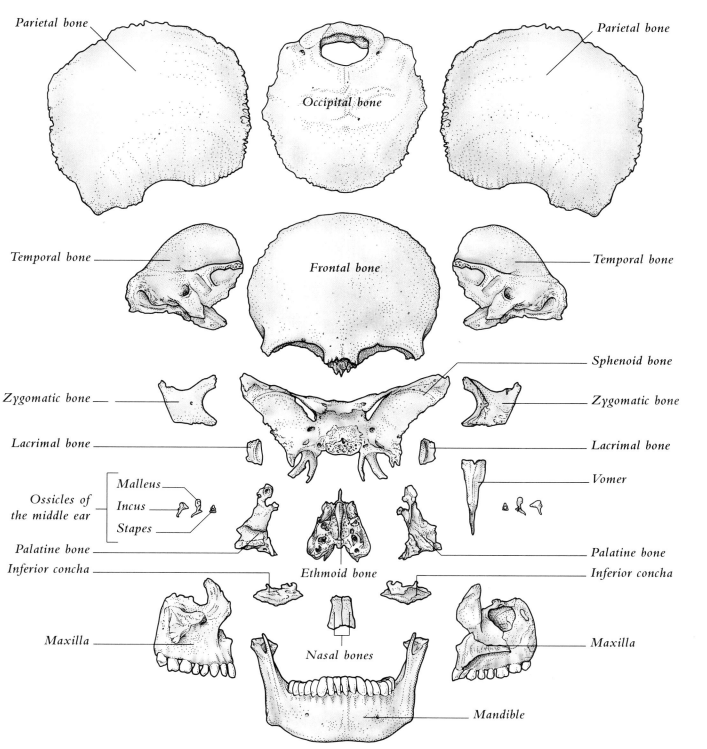

31

BONE STRUCTURE *and* GROWTH

BONE IS A TYPE OF CONNECTIVE TISSUE that is as strong as steel but as light as aluminium. It is made of specialized cells and protein fibres interwoven in a gel-like matrix composed of water, mineral salts, and carbohydrates. Bone tissue is not completely rigid. It continually breaks down and rebuilds, renewing its shape and proportion during the growing process and after an injury.

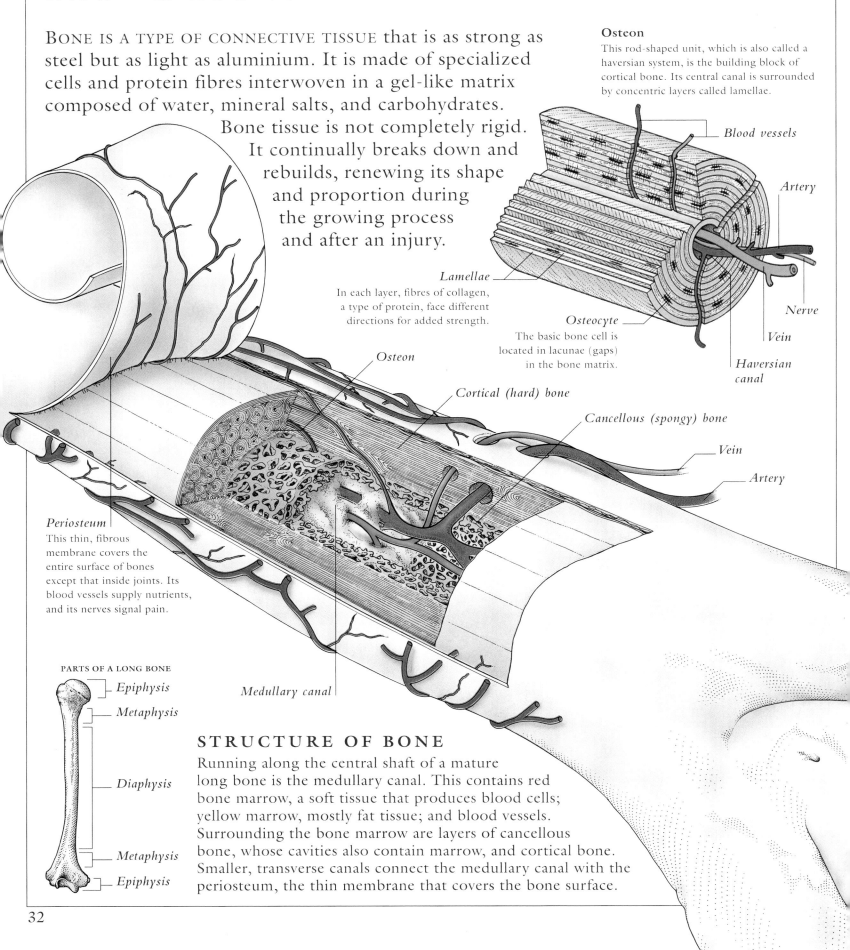

Osteon
This rod-shaped unit, which is also called a haversian system, is the building block of cortical bone. Its central canal is surrounded by concentric layers called lamellae.

Blood vessels

Artery

Nerve

Vein

Haversian canal

Lamellae
In each layer, fibres of collagen, a type of protein, face different directions for added strength.

Osteocyte
The basic bone cell is located in lacunae (gaps) in the bone matrix.

Osteon

Cortical (hard) bone

Cancellous (spongy) bone

Vein

Artery

Periosteum
This thin, fibrous membrane covers the entire surface of bones except that inside joints. Its blood vessels supply nutrients, and its nerves signal pain.

PARTS OF A LONG BONE
Epiphysis
Metaphysis
Diaphysis
Metaphysis
Epiphysis

Medullary canal

STRUCTURE OF BONE

Running along the central shaft of a mature long bone is the medullary canal. This contains red bone marrow, a soft tissue that produces blood cells; yellow marrow, mostly fat tissue; and blood vessels. Surrounding the bone marrow are layers of cancellous bone, whose cavities also contain marrow, and cortical bone. Smaller, transverse canals connect the medullary canal with the periosteum, the thin membrane that covers the bone surface.

Bone marrow

The microscopic image at right shows red bone marrow dotted with red blood cells, which are (with white blood cells) produced here. At birth, red marrow is present in all bones, but in the long bones it gradually becomes yellow marrow and loses its capacity to produce blood cells.

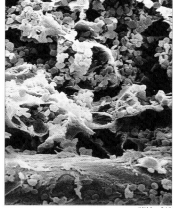

SEM x 340

Cortical bone

Cortical bone consists of many closely packed osteons. The central canals (black) in each osteon contain blood vessels and nerves. The tiny black dots located between the concentric lamellae are lacunae (gaps) which contain osteocytes (bone cells).

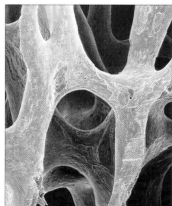

LM x 100

Cancellous bone

Shown at right is the latticework structure of cancellous bone, which consists of bony spikes called trabeculae ("little beams"). The trabeculae are arranged along the lines of greatest pressure or stress, making bones both strong and light.

SEM x 40

BONE LENGTHENING

Near the ends of the long bones, which are covered with cartilage instead of periosteum, is an area known as the epiphyseal plate. Cartilage cells (chondrocytes) proliferate here and form columns that push older cells toward the middle of the bone shaft. As the chondrocytes enlarge and die, the space they occupied is filled by new bone cells.

Articular cartilage

The process of bone growth

Bone growth continues until about the age of 17. If the epiphyseal plate is injured during adolescence, a shortened bone and impaired movement may result.

GROWTH

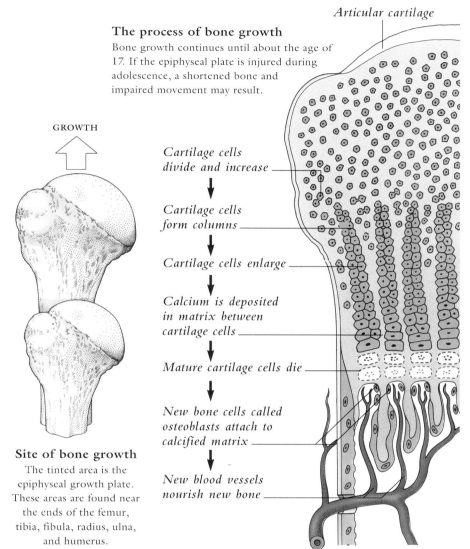

Cartilage cells divide and increase

Cartilage cells form columns

Cartilage cells enlarge

Calcium is deposited in matrix between cartilage cells

Mature cartilage cells die

New bone cells called osteoblasts attach to calcified matrix

New blood vessels nourish new bone

Site of bone growth

The tinted area is the epiphyseal growth plate. These areas are found near the ends of the femur, tibia, fibula, radius, ulna, and humerus.

Epiphysis

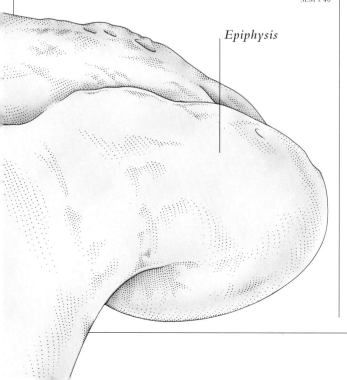

THE GROWTH OF BONES

Most bones develop from cartilage precursors. Ossification is the process by which cartilage is converted into bone as a result of the deposition of mineral salts, mainly calcium. Bones do not become completely ossified until early into adult life when bone growth has come to an end.

Fetal skeleton

In this 12-week-old fetus, the lighter areas in the hands, feet, and knees are pieces of bone-shaped cartilage that will not harden until after the baby is born. Suture joints between the skull bones will also not harden until much later.

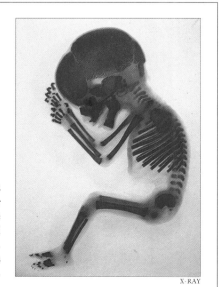

X-RAY

FRACTURES

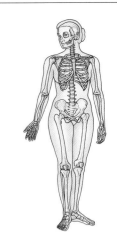

BROKEN BONES – FRACTURES – ARE A COMMON INJURY and can occur at any age. Injuries may range from minor cracks in the surface, known as fissures, to complete breaks through the entire bone. Fractures may be caused by a sudden, unusual impact, or by compression. So-called "stress" fractures are caused by prolonged or repeated force straining the bone, and are known to occur during long-distance walks. Nutritional deficiencies or certain chronic diseases, which can weaken bone, may increase the likelihood of fractures.

HOW BONES BREAK

If a broken bone remains beneath the skin, the fracture is described as closed (simple); if the ends of the fractured bones project outside the skin, the injury is described as open (also called compound). A displaced fracture occurs when the bones are forced from their normal anatomical position.

TYPES OF FRACTURE

Bones break in different ways depending on the angle and degree of force to which they are subjected, and on the part affected. From these patterns, a surgeon can usually gauge the probable stability of the bone fragments, and the easiest way in which to reposition the injury.

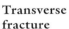

Transverse fracture
A powerful direct or angular force may cause a break straight across the width of a bone. Such fractures are usually stable.

Comminuted fracture
A powerful direct impact can shatter a bone into several fragments. This type of fracture can easily occur during a road traffic accident.

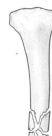

Spiral fracture
A sharp sudden twist may break a bone diagonally across the shaft, and sometimes leave jagged ends.

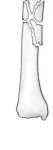

Greenstick fracture
Strong force may cause long bones to bend and crack obliquely on only one side. This fracture is most common in young children but heals well.

BONES COMMONLY INJURED

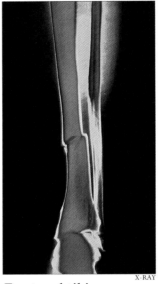

Fractured tibia
A younger person is especially likely to injure a lower leg bone during active movement, such as playing sports. The image above shows a displaced tibial fracture. This type of injury is frequently accompanied by a fracture of the fibula.

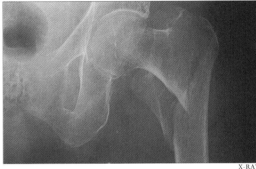
X-RAY

Fractured neck of femur
Bones naturally become thinner and more brittle with age, and are more likely to fracture from only minimal force. The hip joint is especially vulnerable.

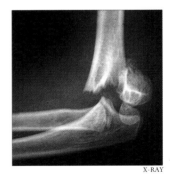
X-RAY

Elbow fracture
An injury that often occurs in childhood, a supracondylar fracture of the humerus (upper arm bone) just above the elbow may damage the brachial artery and affect circulation of the forearm and hand.

Colles' fracture
Flexing a hand to cushion a fall sometimes breaks the end of the radius and occasionally the tip of the ulna. This injury can occur at any age, but it is especially likely to occur in older people with thin bones and whose balance may be unsteady.

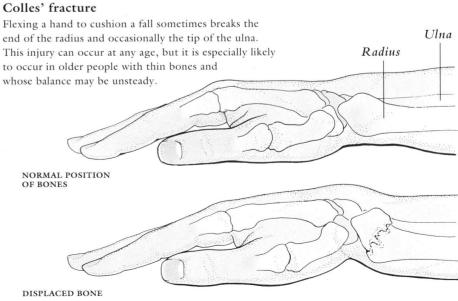

Ulna

Radius

NORMAL POSITION
OF BONES

DISPLACED BONE

REPAIRING FRACTURES

How fractures are treated depends upon the nature of the injury, the particular bone(s) affected, and the extent of tissue damage. If the bones are displaced, manipulation to restore their normal position may be performed under general anaesthesia. Physiotherapy often encourages healing and prevents deformity.

METHODS OF IMMOBILIZATION

Some fractures need to be immobilized in order to ensure that bones unite soundly in a good position. In most cases this is achieved with a splint or a cast made from plaster of Paris or plastic. Certain fractures, particularly those with many bone fragments, require an operation to reposition and fix bones securely so that surrounding tissues heal.

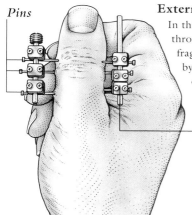

Pins

External fixation

In this form of fixation, pins are inserted through the skin into repositioned bone fragments. These are held firmly in place by an external metal frame positioned outside the skin. Pins and frame are removed when the bone has healed.

External metal frame

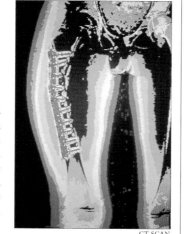

Internal fixation

This type of fixation may be used if a bone is severely fractured in several places. An incision is made in the skin to expose the injured bone, and some combination of plates, wires, screws, rods, and nails is inserted. The image at right shows a fractured femur held in place by a metal plate and screws.

CT SCAN

TRACTION

Pulling on the ends of a broken bone in order to realign them is like straightening a string of beads by tugging at each end. Traction is the force generated by a mechanical system of weights and pulleys to perform this necessary realignment. If rapid repositioning of a fracture is needed, traction may be applied while a patient is anaesthetized.

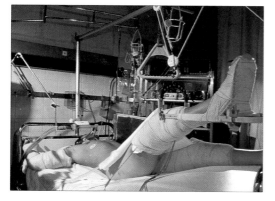

Gradual traction

A fractured femur is often treated by the application of gradual traction, as shown left. This helps to prevent the large muscles from going into spasm and pulling the correctly repositioned bones out of alignment.

INTERNAL FIXATION: FRACTURED SHAFT OF FEMUR

The strong, weight-bearing femur (thighbone) is the largest bone in the body. If the femoral shaft is severely fractured, it may be necessary to insert a rod into the central medullary canal to hold the repositioned bone in place while it heals. The rod may be left permanently in place or removed at a later date. In patients who are fit, full use of the leg usually follows within 3 months.

Traction pin

1 With the patient anaesthetized, a temporary traction pin is attached to the lower end of the fractured femur just above the knee. The ends of the fractured bone are then repositioned gradually to restore normal alignment.

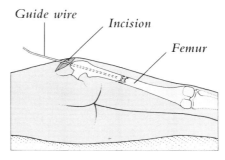

Guide wire   *Incision*   *Femur*

2 After an incision is made, a hole is drilled in the top of the exposed femur. A wire is guided down into the medullary canal at the centre of the bone, passing the fracture and stopping just above the knee.

3 Using an instrument known as a reamer, the surgeon enlarges the medullary canal and then passes a hollow metal rod of the correct length down over the guide wire. Once this rod is in place, the guide wire is removed.

Screws

Rod

4 The bones are held in position by screws that pass through each end of the femur and the intramedullary rod.

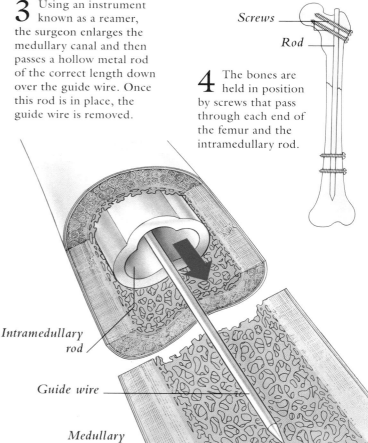

Intramedullary rod

Guide wire

Medullary canal

BONE DISORDERS

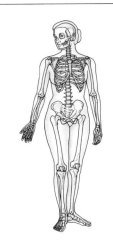

BONE STRENGTH AND STRUCTURE may be affected by nutritional, hormonal, and other disorders that can occur throughout life. These include rickets, osteomalacia, osteoporosis, and cancers. Some people are born with a bone deformity such as a shortened or partially absent limb. While birth defects of this kind affect only a small minority of people, the bone-weakening disorder called osteoporosis occurs gradually with advancing age in virtually everyone. Exercise and calcium supplements may slow the effects of this condition.

OSTEOPOROSIS

After middle age, bones become notably thinner and more porous, causing loss of bone mass in both sexes. Oestrogen levels fall rapidly in women after the menopause, often leading to severe osteoporosis. The decline in testosterone in men is gradual and they suffer less osteoporosis.

EFFECTS OF OSTEOPOROSIS

Because of their decreased density, bones affected by osteoporosis are much more prone to fractures. Crush fractures in the spine may lead to spinal curvature; hip or wrist fractures may occur after falls.

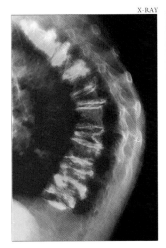

X-RAY

Osteoporotic spine
Osteoporosis may cause some vertebrae suddenly to collapse, even after coughing, sneezing, or some other minor activity.

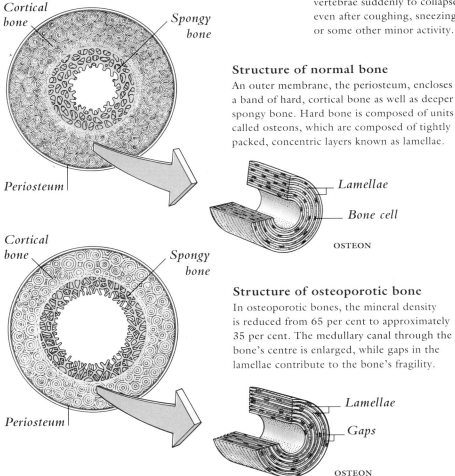

Structure of normal bone
An outer membrane, the periosteum, encloses a band of hard, cortical bone as well as deeper spongy bone. Hard bone is composed of units called osteons, which are composed of tightly packed, concentric layers known as lamellae.

Structure of osteoporotic bone
In osteoporotic bones, the mineral density is reduced from 65 per cent to approximately 35 per cent. The medullary canal through the bone's centre is enlarged, while gaps in the lamellae contribute to the bone's fragility.

WHY OSTEOPOROSIS OCCURS

Bones are continually being broken down and then rebuilt in order to facilitate growth and repair. In young people, the rate of bone formation exceeds the rate at which cells are reabsorbed. This process begins to change in early adulthood, with the rate of reabsorption becoming greater than formation. Bones gradually become weaker and lighter.

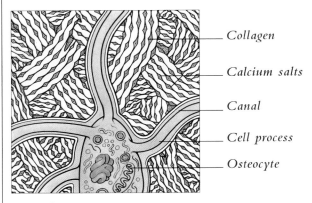

Bone formation
Bone is built up by the deposition of minerals (mainly calcium salts) on an organic matrix of collagen fibres. Osteocytes, or bone cells, form the collagen and also aid in the laying down of calcium. Canals in the bone permit calcium to move in or out of the blood in response to hormones that regulate the body's needs.

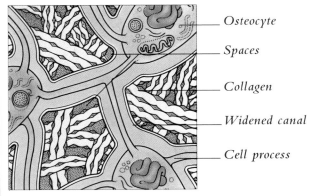

Bone reabsorption
As osteoporosis develops with age, both the collagen framework and deposited minerals are broken down much faster than they are formed. The canals that connect the osteocytes become wider and new spaces appear in the collagen matrix. These changes weaken the bone.

OSTEOMALACIA

In osteomalacia, bones are weakened by the loss of calcium and phosphorus. The condition differs from osteoporosis in that there is not any loss of the bone's protein matrix. In children, this is called rickets. A primary cause is a shortage of vitamin D, essential to enable the body to deal with calcium and phosphorus. Inadequate sunlight may be a factor.

Pelvic deformity
When the pelvic bones are softened as a result of osteomalacia, they may become weakened and severely deformed. Someone with such an abnormal pelvis would probably find walking difficult and painful.

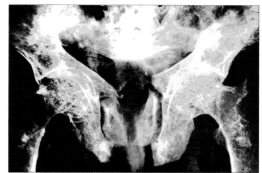
X-RAY

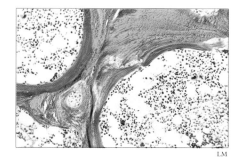
LM

Bone biopsy
This stained sample of bone tissue reveals distinctive signs of osteomalacia. The areas that have reduced deposits of calcium are shown as brown, while normal areas are green. This irregular structure may result in tiny fractures on the surface of affected bones.

PAGET'S DISEASE

The normal formation of bone is disturbed in Paget's disease, also called osteitis deformans. Bone is broken down at an increased rate and is replaced rapidly by abnormal bone. This condition occurs less frequently in younger people, but it affects up to 3 per cent of those over the age of 40. Paget's disease occurs most commonly in the skull, spine, pelvis, and leg bones.

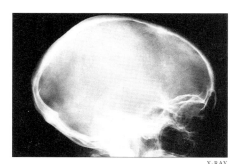
X-RAY

X-RAY

Bone enlargement and thickening
One effect of Paget's disease may be the enlargement and thickening of certain bones. Contrast the normal skull (top) with an affected skull (below), in which areas of increased bone density are seen as white patches. Bone enlargement has various effects, such as hearing loss as the cranial nerves become compressed. Affected parts may also feel hot due to an increased blood supply.

BONE CANCER

Cancer may originate in a bone, when it is described as primary. More frequently, a malignant tumour in bone is the result of cancer cells that have spread from a primary tumour elsewhere in the body; this type of bone cancer is known as secondary or metastatic.

PRIMARY BONE CANCER

Cancers that start in bone are most likely to occur in younger people. Osteosarcoma is the most common type, and affects long bones such as the femur. Another primary bone cancer, chondrosarcoma, occurs mainly in the pelvis, ribs, and breastbone. Treatment for primary bone cancer may include replacement by a bone graft.

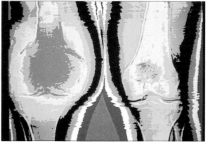
CT SCAN

Osteosarcoma
The most common site of osteosarcoma is just above the knee at the lower end of the femur. The first sign of the tumour is usually a painful, visible swelling (shown as the blue area at left centre).

SECONDARY BONE CANCER

Secondary bone cancer is more likely to occur in older people. Commonly affected areas are the skull, sternum, pelvis, vertebrae, ribs, and, less often, the upper ends of the femur and humerus. Treatment for secondary bone cancer may include anticancer drugs and radiotherapy in order to reduce tumour size, and painkillers.

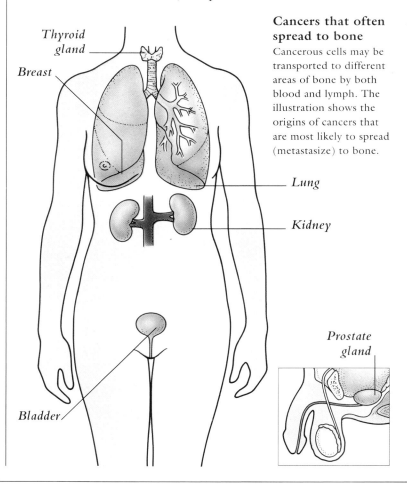

Cancers that often spread to bone
Cancerous cells may be transported to different areas of bone by both blood and lymph. The illustration shows the origins of cancers that are most likely to spread (metastasize) to bone.

Thyroid gland
Breast
Lung
Kidney
Bladder
Prostate gland

The SPINE

THE SPINE IS A STRONG but flexible support that holds the head and body upright, and allows the upper body to bend and twist. Thirty-three ring-like bones called vertebrae are linked by a series of mobile joints. Sandwiched between the vertebrae are springy discs of tough, fibrous cartilage that squash down under pressure to absorb shocks. These discs are subjected to enormous forces: as much as several hundred kilograms per square centimetre during strenuous movements. Strong ligaments and muscles around the spine stabilize the vertebrae and help to control movement.

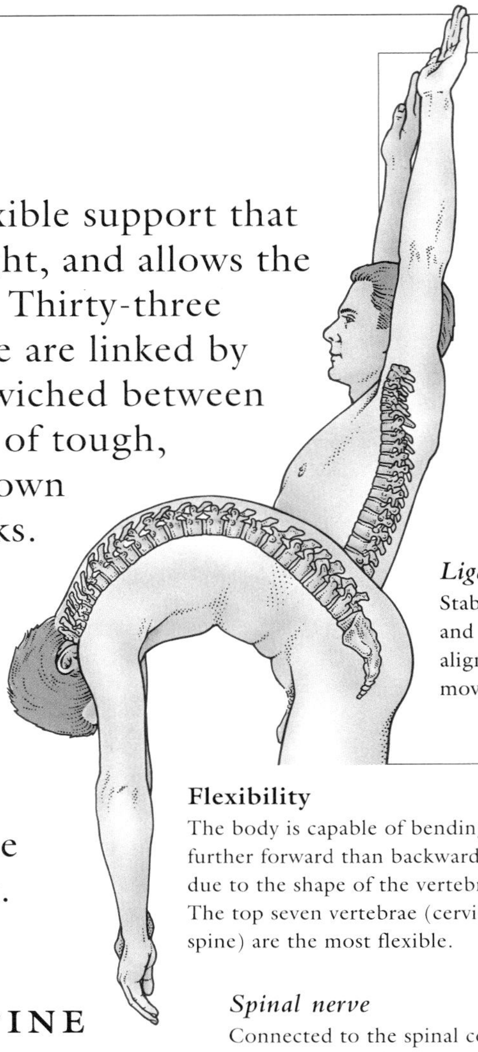

STRUCTURE OF THE SPINE

Three main types of individual vertebrae, each a different shape, make up the spine: cervical in the neck, thoracic in the upper back, and lumbar in the lower back. Both the wedge-shaped sacrum and the tail-like coccyx at the base of the spine consist of several fused vertebrae. Cartilage discs separate these bony components of the spine and cushion them from pressure during twisting, weight-bearing, or jumping.

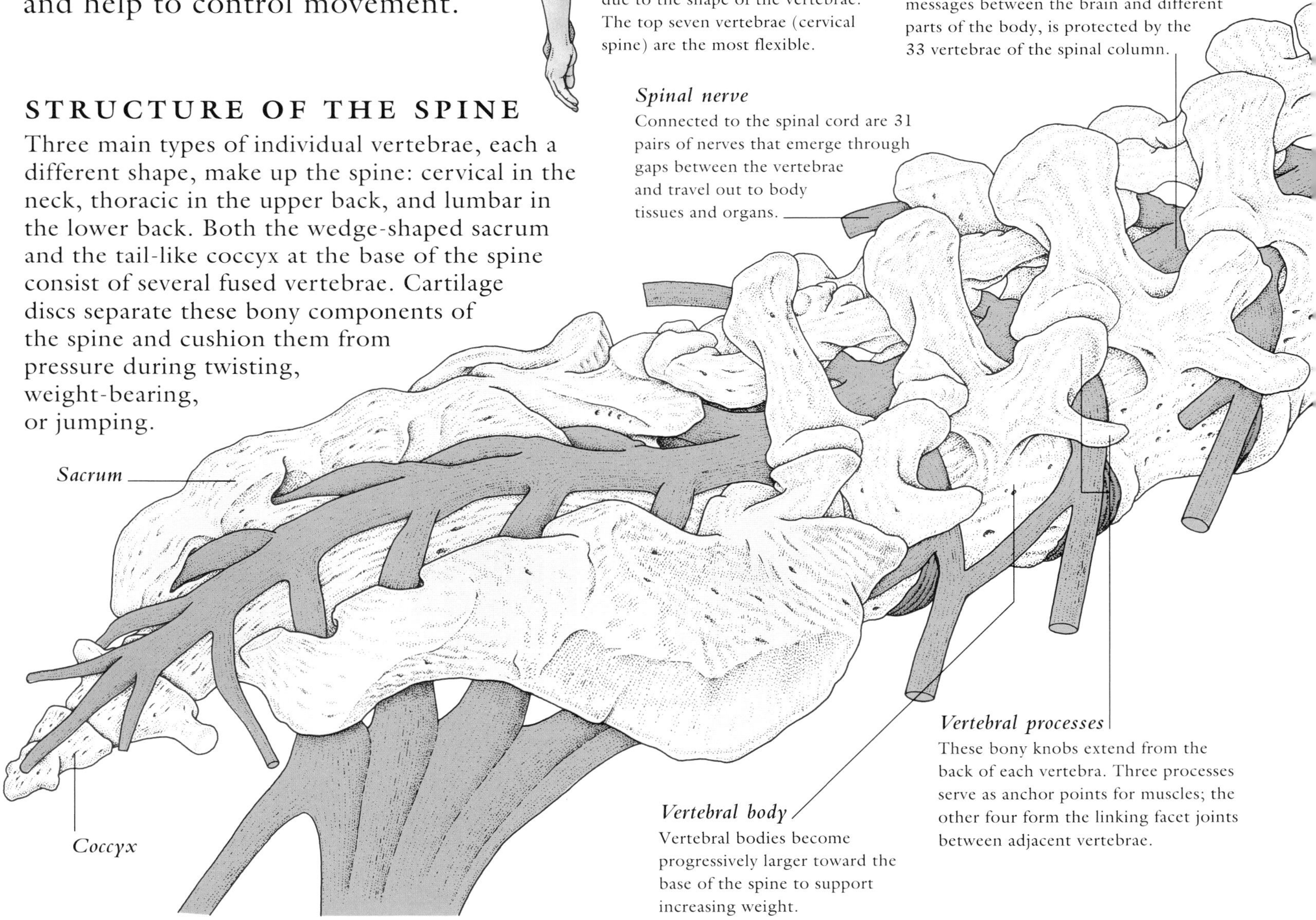

MOVEMENT OF SPINAL JOINTS

Individual spinal joints do not have a wide range of movement, but working together they give the spine great flexibility, letting it arch backward, twist around, or curve forward for toe-touching.

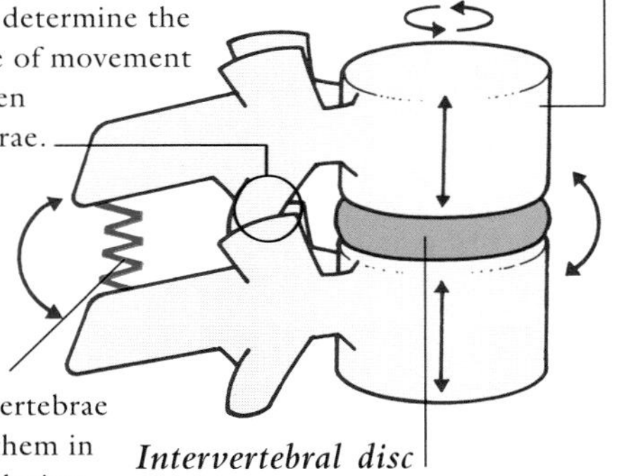

Facet joint
Helps determine the degree of movement between vertebrae.

Vertebral body

Ligament
Stabilizes vertebrae and holds them in alignment during movement.

Intervertebral disc
Absorbs forces directed through its axis and acts like a ball-bearing during bending or twisting.

Flexibility
The body is capable of bending further forward than backward, due to the shape of the vertebrae. The top seven vertebrae (cervical spine) are the most flexible.

Spinal cord
This vital cable of nerve tissue, which relays messages between the brain and different parts of the body, is protected by the 33 vertebrae of the spinal column.

Spinal nerve
Connected to the spinal cord are 31 pairs of nerves that emerge through gaps between the vertebrae and travel out to body tissues and organs.

Sacrum

Coccyx

Vertebral body
Vertebral bodies become progressively larger toward the base of the spine to support increasing weight.

Vertebral processes
These bony knobs extend from the back of each vertebra. Three processes serve as anchor points for muscles; the other four form the linking facet joints between adjacent vertebrae.

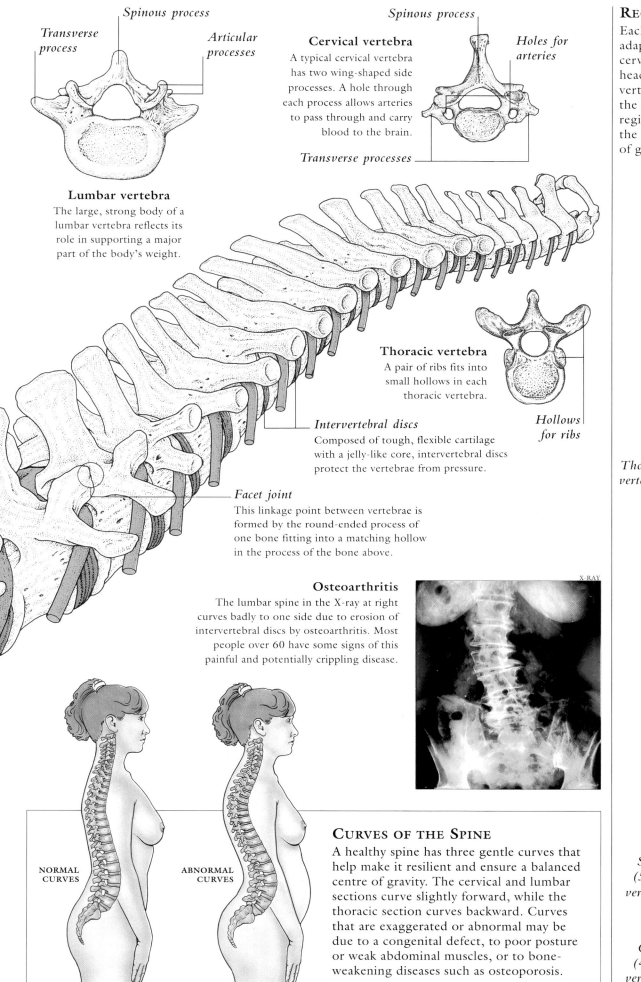

Transverse process

Spinous process

Articular processes

Lumbar vertebra
The large, strong body of a lumbar vertebra reflects its role in supporting a major part of the body's weight.

Spinous process

Cervical vertebra
A typical cervical vertebra has two wing-shaped side processes. A hole through each process allows arteries to pass through and carry blood to the brain.

Holes for arteries

Transverse processes

Thoracic vertebra
A pair of ribs fits into small hollows in each thoracic vertebra.

Hollows for ribs

Intervertebral discs
Composed of tough, flexible cartilage with a jelly-like core, intervertebral discs protect the vertebrae from pressure.

Facet joint
This linkage point between vertebrae is formed by the round-ended process of one bone fitting into a matching hollow in the process of the bone above.

Osteoarthritis
The lumbar spine in the X-ray at right curves badly to one side due to erosion of intervertebral discs by osteoarthritis. Most people over 60 have some signs of this painful and potentially crippling disease.

X-RAY

NORMAL CURVES

ABNORMAL CURVES

CURVES OF THE SPINE
A healthy spine has three gentle curves that help make it resilient and ensure a balanced centre of gravity. The cervical and lumbar sections curve slightly forward, while the thoracic section curves backward. Curves that are exaggerated or abnormal may be due to a congenital defect, to poor posture or weak abdominal muscles, or to bone-weakening diseases such as osteoporosis.

REGIONS OF THE SPINE
Each section of the spine is adapted to its function. The cervical vertebrae support the head and neck, the thoracic vertebrae anchor the ribs, and the strong, weight-bearing regions toward the bottom of the spine provide a stable centre of gravity during movement.

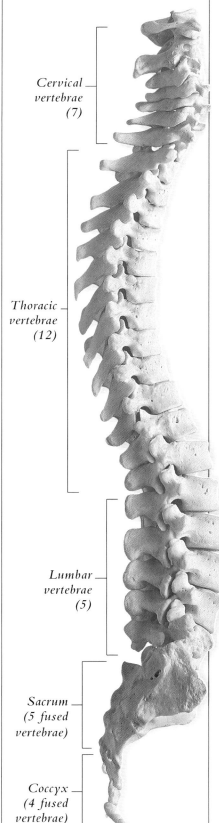

Cervical vertebrae (7)

Thoracic vertebrae (12)

Lumbar vertebrae (5)

Sacrum (5 fused vertebrae)

Coccyx (4 fused vertebrae)

SPINAL INJURIES *and* DISORDERS

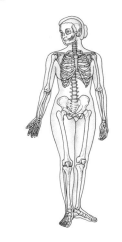

MANY INJURIES TO THE SPINE ARE MINOR and cause only slight bruising, but a severe fall or an accident may dislocate or fracture vertebrae. If the spinal cord or specific nerves are damaged, a loss of bodily sensation or function, or even paralysis, may result. Bone diseases, for example osteoporosis, and deformities can affect the spine and may increase the likelihood of fractures.

SPINAL FRACTURES

Most major spinal injuries occur as a result of severe forces of compression or of rotation or bending beyond the spine's normal range of movement. The most important consideration in assessing a spinal injury is whether a fracture is stable (unlikely to shift) or unstable, in which case damage to the spinal cord or nerves is more likely.

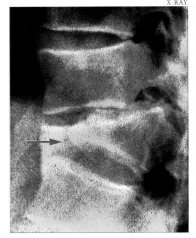

X-RAY

Compression fracture
A compression force through the longitudinal axis of the spine may cause the front part of a vertebral body to collapse (arrow).

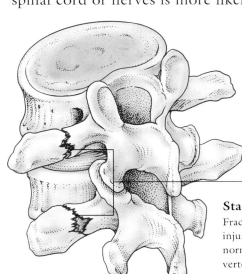

Fractures of transverse processes

Stable fracture
Fracture of a transverse process is usually a minor injury because the vertebra does not shift from its normal position. Most commonly affecting lumbar vertebrae, these injuries are often the result of a direct blow. They rarely cause nerve damage.

SPINAL FUSION

An operation to fuse vertebrae may be needed to treat unstable fractures or to correct spinal distortions or deformity. Bone taken from the back of the pelvis is placed on either side of the spine so that it bridges the two vertebrae to be fused. The bone is held in its new position by muscles in the back, and a metal plate and wire may also be used if greater stability is needed.

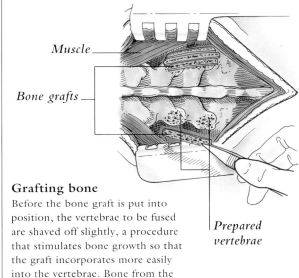

Muscle

Bone grafts

Prepared vertebrae

Grafting bone
Before the bone graft is put into position, the vertebrae to be fused are shaved off slightly, a procedure that stimulates bone growth so that the graft incorporates more easily into the vertebrae. Bone from the individual's own body is readily compatible with the new location.

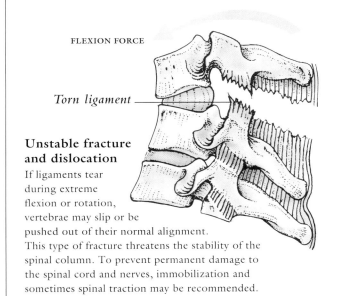

FLEXION FORCE

Torn ligament

Unstable fracture and dislocation
If ligaments tear during extreme flexion or rotation, vertebrae may slip or be pushed out of their normal alignment. This type of fracture threatens the stability of the spinal column. To prevent permanent damage to the spinal cord and nerves, immobilization and sometimes spinal traction may be recommended.

WHIPLASH INJURY

Suddenly forcing the neck forward and then backward often sprains the ligaments and/or partially dislocates a cervical joint. Following a whiplash injury, often the result of a car accident, an orthopaedic neck collar may be worn for several weeks until the neck moves freely and there is no pain. Usually, physiotherapy and analgesics are prescribed, and may be supplemented by muscle-relaxants.

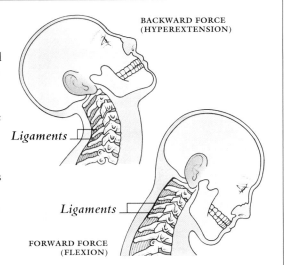

BACKWARD FORCE (HYPEREXTENSION)

Ligaments

Ligaments

FORWARD FORCE (FLEXION)

DISC PROLAPSE

The cartilage discs that separate adjacent vertebrae have a hard outer covering and a jelly-like centre. Wear and tear or pressure may rupture the outer layer, forcing the centre through and causing pressure on a spinal nerve root. If the symptoms are not relieved by rest, the protruding disc can be removed by opening the vertebral canal or by a less invasive procedure (see right).

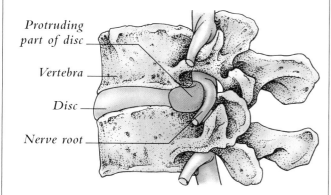

Protruding part of disc

Vertebra

Disc

Nerve root

Pressure on a nerve root

A so-called "slipped disc" may cause severe back pain if it presses on a nerve root. The pain may be aggravated by even simple activities such as coughing, bending, or sitting for a long time.

SCIATICA

Pain that affects the buttock and back of the thigh can be caused by pressure on the spinal roots of the sciatic nerve. The source of this pressure is usually a prolapsed intervertebral disc, but it may be due to a tumour, a blood clot, a muscle spasm, or just sitting in an awkward position.

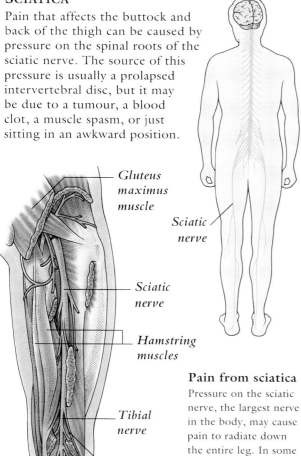

Gluteus maximus muscle

Sciatic nerve

Sciatic nerve

Hamstring muscles

Tibial nerve

Peroneal nerve

Pain from sciatica

Pressure on the sciatic nerve, the largest nerve in the body, may cause pain to radiate down the entire leg. In some severe cases, numbness and weakness of the muscles also occur.

OPERATION

MICRODISCECTOMY

In this operation for relieving symptoms caused by a disc prolapse, the surgeon makes a tiny incision in the patient's back. He or she uses an operating microscope and special small instruments to remove the protruding intervertebral disc tissue.

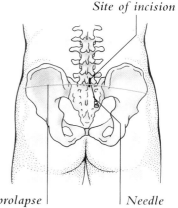

Site of incision

Level of prolapse

Needle

1 The anaesthetized patient is placed face down. A needle is inserted into the spine at the level of the prolapse, and an X-ray taken to confirm the level. The confirmed disc level and incision site are marked on the skin.

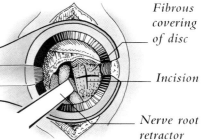

Guide

2 After making an incision at the site marked, the surgeon inserts a guiding instrument into the space between the vertebrae adjacent to the disc. The procedure is viewed through an operating microscope.

Vertebra

Prolapsed disc

Nerve root

3 The compressed nerve root is pulled aside using a retractor to reveal the underlying prolapsed intervertebral disc. A tiny, cross-like incision is then made in the fibrous covering of the disc.

Fibrous covering of disc

Incision

Nerve root retractor

Rongeur

4 A rongeur – a scissor-like cutting instrument – is passed through the guide into the incision in order to reach the protruding disc tissue that needs to be removed.

Instrument to protect nerve root

5 The disc tissue is trimmed away using the rongeur and is removed through the guide. The instruments are withdrawn, and the incision is closed. The patient is usually able to get out of bed the next day.

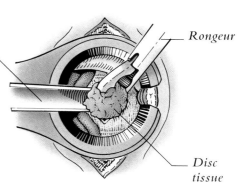

Rongeur

Disc tissue

JOINTS *of the* BODY

THE PLACE WHERE TWO BONES MEET is called a joint, also known as an articulation. Joints are classified by their structure or by the way they move. In the freely movable synovial joints, the surfaces in contact slide over each other easily. Less mobile joints, such as those in the spine, are more firmly linked by fibrous tissue or cartilage to permit growth or provide stability.

OTHER JOINTS
Not all joints have a wide range of movement. Some types allow for growth or for limited flexibility where greater stability is needed.

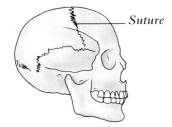

— *Suture*

Fixed joints
After growth is complete, all the separate bone plates of the skull are securely connected by interlocking fibrous tissue, forming so-called suture joints.

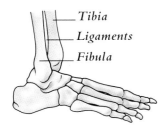

— *Tibia*
— *Ligaments*
— *Fibula*

Slightly movable joints
Bones with limited movement may be stabilized by pads of cartilage, as between spinal vertebrae, or by slightly flexible ligaments, as in the lower leg.

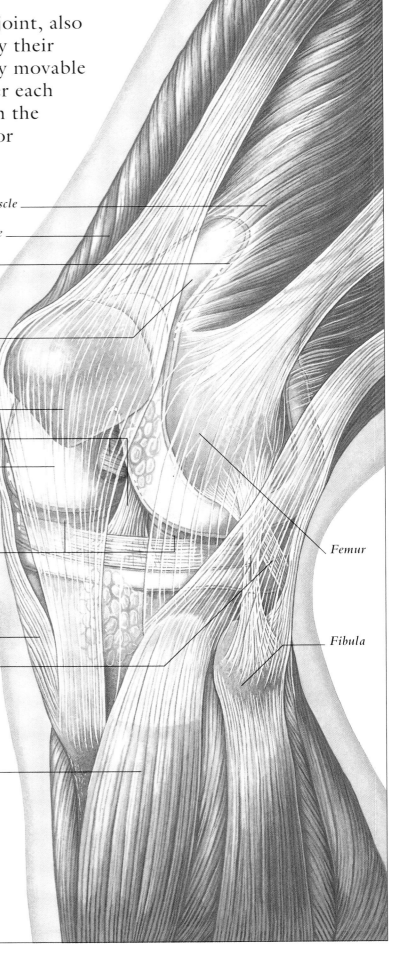

Vastus lateralis muscle ——————

Vastus medialis muscle ——————

Synovial membrane ——————
Tissue that lines the non-contact surfaces within the joint capsule secretes lubricating synovial fluid.

Synovial fluid ——————
This clear fluid lubricates and nourishes all the tissues inside the joint capsule.

Patella ——————

Internal ligaments ——————

Articular cartilage ——————
Where the bone ends are in contact, connective tissue provides a smooth, protective surface for ease of movement.

Menisci (articular discs) ——————
Unique to the knee and wrist are pads of fibrous cartilage. Called menisci, they help the weight-bearing bones to absorb shock.

Joint capsule (cut away) ——————

External ligaments ——————
Thickenings of the capsule form these fibrous cords. They stabilize the joint, especially during movement. Some joints, such as the knee, have internal ligaments for added stability.

Tibialis anterior muscle ——————

Femur

Fibula

SYNOVIAL JOINT STRUCTURE
Most of the joints in the body are synovial joints. These are movable, highly versatile, lubricated joints. Articular cartilage covers and protects the bone ends, ligaments help provide stability, and a fibrous capsule encloses the structure. Muscles around the joint contract to produce movement. The knee, shown here, is the largest joint.

TYPES OF SYNOVIAL JOINT

The shape of articular cartilage surfaces in a synovial joint and the way they fit together determine the range and the direction of the joint's movement. Hinge and pivot joints move in only one plane (from side to side, for example, or up and down), while ellipsoidal joints are able to move in two planes at right angles to each other. Most joints in the body can move in more than two planes, which allows for a wide range of motion.

RANGE OF MOVEMENT

The shoulder is one of the most mobile and most complex joints of the body: it moves up and down, forward and backward, and can rotate in a complete circle at the side of the body. Joints like this that move in more than two planes are called multiaxial.

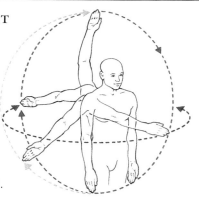

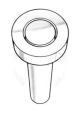 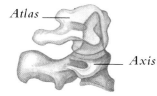

Atlas

Axis

Pivot joint

A projection from one bone turns within a ring-shaped socket of another bone, or the ring turns around the bony projection. A pivot joint formed by the top two cervical vertebrae allows the head to turn from side to side, as when shaking the head "no".

Scapula

Humerus

Ball-and-socket joint

The rounded head of one bone fits into the cup-like cavity of another bone. Of all joint structures, a ball-and-socket type allows for the greatest range of movement. The shoulder and the hip are both ball-and-socket joints.

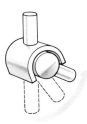

Humerus

Ulna

Radius

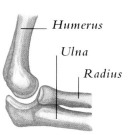

Hinge joint

In this simplest of joints, the convex surface of one bone fits into the concave surface of another bone. This allows for movement like a hinged door in only one plane. Both the elbow and the knee are modified hinge joints: they bend up and down in one plane quite easily, but are also capable of very limited rotation.

Trapezium of wrist

First metacarpal bone of thumb

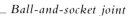

Saddle joint

The joint surface of each bone has both concave and convex areas so that the bones can rock back and forth and from side to side, but they have limited rotation. The only saddle joints in the body are at the base of the thumbs.

Radius

Scaphoid

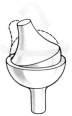 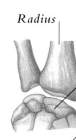

Ellipsoidal joint

An ovoid, or egg-shaped, bone end is held within an elliptical cavity. The radius bone of the forearm and the scaphoid bone of the hand meet in an ellipsoidal joint. This type of joint can be flexed or extended and moved from side to side, but rotation is limited.

Tarsals

Metatarsals

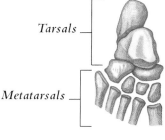 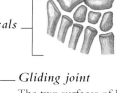

Gliding joint

The two surfaces of bones that meet in a gliding joint are almost flat, and slide over one another. Movement is limited, however, by strong encasing ligaments. Some joints in the foot and wrist move in this way.

JOINT INJURIES
and DISORDERS

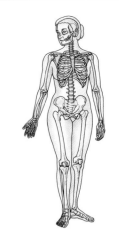

JOINTS ARE MADE TO WORK IN SPECIFIC WAYS, and any movement beyond the normal range, or in an unnatural direction, often causes an injury. Certain injuries may result from a direct blow or fall, or, occasionally, from overuse. Arthritis is a general term used to describe several different disorders that cause painful, swollen joints. The most common disorder is osteoarthritis.

LIGAMENT INJURIES

Ligaments, which are strong bands of fibrous tissue, link bone ends together. If the bones within a joint are pulled too far apart, often as a result of a sudden or unexpected movement, or one that is too forceful, fibres may be overstretched or torn. This commonly results in swelling, pain, or muscle spasm, and, if the injury is severe, joint instability or even dislocation.

Ankle sprain

A sprain is a partial tearing of a ligament. The ankle may be sprained as a result of a fall or stumble that forces the full weight of the body onto the outer edge of the foot. Rest, ice, compression, and elevation are the steps used to treat sprains.

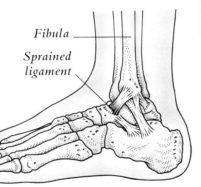

Fibula

Sprained ligament

TREATING PAIN AND INFLAMMATION

Inflamed tissue triggers the release of prostaglandins, which stimulate nerve endings, cause blood vessels to dilate, and attract white blood cells to the area. The result is pain and inflammation. These symptoms are often treated with non-steroidal anti-inflammatory drugs, which act to block the synthesis of prostaglandins. If pain is severe, corticosteroid drugs, which reduce inflammation, may be injected.

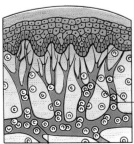

Before medication

Abundant white blood cells flow through dilated blood vessels to the injured area, causing heat, redness, pain, and swelling.

Dilated blood vessels

Increased white blood cells

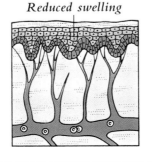

Reduced swelling

After medication

Drugs inhibit the production of white blood cells, and thus help to reduce swelling, by blocking the synthesis of prostaglandins.

TORN CARTILAGE

One type of cartilage found in the body consists of firm, flexible, slightly elastic connective tissue. In the knee, discs called menisci made of this fibrocartilage cushion the bones from excessive force. If a meniscus is torn, which may occur by twisting the knee while playing sports, a meniscectomy to remove part or all of the damaged cartilage may be performed.

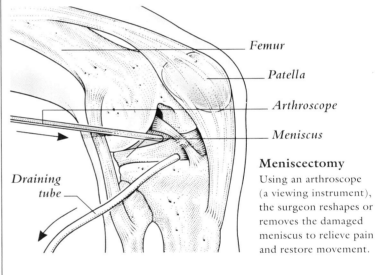

Femur

Patella

Arthroscope

Meniscus

Draining tube

Meniscectomy

Using an arthroscope (a viewing instrument), the surgeon reshapes or removes the damaged meniscus to relieve pain and restore movement.

DISLOCATED JOINTS

A drastic shift of two bone ends out of their normal end-to-end position, particularly of a bone from its complementary socket, is called a dislocation. Often painful, a dislocation frequently can tear ligaments in the joint and fracture of one or both bones. This can damage nerves or adjacent blood vessels. The area around the joint may also appear misshapen.

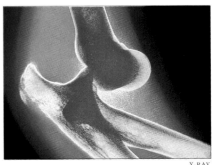

Dislocated elbow

Usually caused by a fall onto an outstretched hand, a dislocated elbow is a common injury that affects both children and adults. It is treated by repositioning the bones and then immobilizing the joint for about 3 to 6 weeks. Exercises are recommended to regain movement and strength.

X-RAY

RHEUMATOID ARTHRITIS

This autoimmune form of arthritis develops when the immune system, usually triggered by an antigen in a genetically predisposed person, begins to attack body tissues. The joints become inflamed, swollen, stiff, and deformed. Early symptoms include fever, pallor, and weakness. If the disease is chronic, tissues of the eyes, skin, heart, nerves, and lungs may be affected.

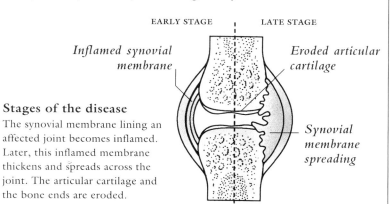

EARLY STAGE   LATE STAGE

Inflamed synovial membrane

Eroded articular cartilage

Synovial membrane spreading

Stages of the disease
The synovial membrane lining an affected joint becomes inflamed. Later, this inflamed membrane thickens and spreads across the joint. The articular cartilage and the bone ends are eroded.

EFFECTS OF RHEUMATOID ARTHRITIS

Characteristically, many of the small joints are affected in a symmetrical pattern; for example, the hands and feet may be inflamed to the same degree on both sides. Stiffness is often worse in the mornings, but eases during the day. A doctor will suspect the disease from these well-recognized features. The diagnosis is confirmed if a blood test detects an antibody associated with rheumatoid arthritis.

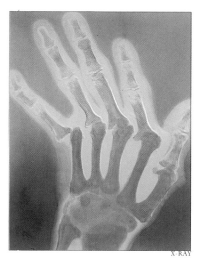

X-RAY

Painful deformity
In severe rheumatoid arthritis, joint spaces disappear and the angle at which bone ends meet changes as a result of ligament laxity. Bone ends are roughened and eroded, and nodules, which are aggregates of inflamed tissue cells, collect around the bone ends. Above the nodules, the skin is thin and fragile. These features all restrict movement.

GOUT

Gout, also called crystal-induced arthritis, may cause sudden and severe pain, swelling, and redness in one joint, usually at the base of the big toe. More common in men than in women, it is caused by excess uric acid in the body. Normally, uric acid is dissolved and excreted in urine. In gout, however, this substance collects in the synovial fluid of a joint, forming needle-like crystals.

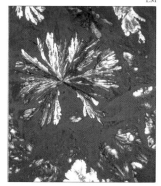

LM

Crystals of uric acid

TREATMENT

Although there is no cure yet, it is currently believed that if powerful immunosuppressant drugs are given at an early stage, the disease may go into prolonged remission. Rest and drugs to relieve inflammation and pain are often prescribed during an acute attack, while gentle exercise during remission helps to keep affected joints mobile.

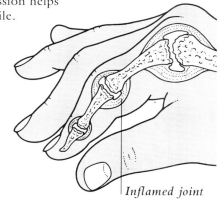

Types of drugs
Certain drugs aim to reduce the swelling that is caused by inflammation of the synovial membrane and the production of excess synovial fluid. Other drugs are used to slow down cartilage and bone destruction.

Inflamed joint

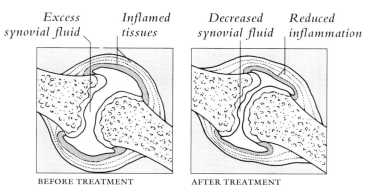

Excess synovial fluid   *Inflamed tissues*   *Decreased synovial fluid*   *Reduced inflammation*

BEFORE TREATMENT   AFTER TREATMENT

SURGERY

When inflammation of the synovial membrane cannot be controlled by drugs, surgery may be carried out to alleviate symptoms and to slow down further joint deterioration. Contracted tendons can be released to permit greater movement, or the inflamed synovial membrane may be removed in a procedure called a synovectomy. Joint replacement surgery is very occasionally carried out for severely deformed, immobile, and painful joints.

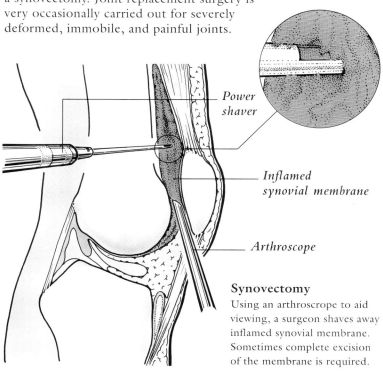

Power shaver

Inflamed synovial membrane

Arthroscope

Synovectomy
Using an arthroscope to aid viewing, a surgeon shaves away inflamed synovial membrane. Sometimes complete excision of the membrane is required.

OSTEOARTHRITIS

Unlike rheumatoid arthritis, which affects several body systems at once, osteoarthritis may affect only a single joint, and can be triggered by localized "wear and tear". The joint degeneration may be hastened by a congenital defect, injury or infection, or obesity. Because cartilage normally wears away as the body ages, a mild form of osteoarthritis affects most people by about age 60.

STAGES IN OSTEOARTHRITIS

The process by which articular cartilage begins to break down is not yet fully understood, but it gradually becomes thinner and roughened. The bone underneath the cartilage eventually erodes so that bone surfaces rub against one another, causing severe discomfort. Joints may become painfully inflamed only from time to time. Minor degrees of this condition are quite common, and can usually be treated; only a few people have progressive joint damage.

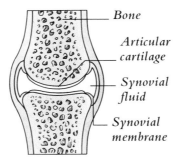

Bone
Articular cartilage
Synovial fluid
Synovial membrane

Normal joint structure
Healthy articular cartilage is lubricated by synovial fluid for ease of movement.

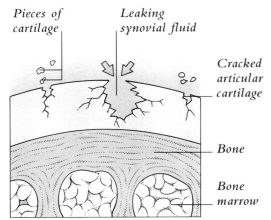

Pieces of cartilage
Leaking synovial fluid
Cracked articular cartilage
Bone
Bone marrow

1 When articular chondrocytes (cartilage cells) die, surface cracks appear; this allows synovial fluid to leak in, causing greater cartilage degeneration. Pieces of this weakened cartilage break off, inflaming the synovial membrane.

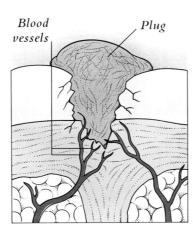

Blood vessels
Plug

2 Eventually, a gap developing in the cartilage reaches the underlying bone. Blood vessels begin to grow, and a plug made of fibrocartilage fills the gap.

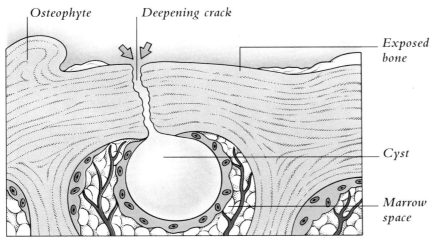

Osteophyte
Deepening crack
Exposed bone
Cyst
Marrow space

3 The fibrocartilage plug wears away, thus exposing the bone surface. If surface cracks deepen, synovial fluid can leak into the marrow space, and may form a cyst surrounded by weakened bone. Small outgrowths called osteophytes may further deform the bone surface.

OSTEOARTHRITIS OF THE HIP

In weight-bearing or frequently used joints, the articular cartilage is more likely to erode with age. The hip is particularly vulnerable to osteoarthritic changes, which may severely inhibit movement; obesity may also accelerate this process in the hip.

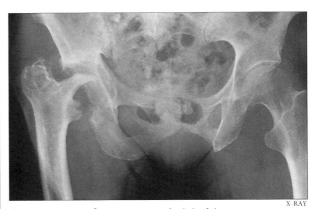

X-RAY

Appearance of an osteoarthritic hip
Here osteoarthritis has eroded the hip socket and almost completely flattened the normally convex curve of the femoral head.

DRUGS FOR OSTEOARTHRITIS

Although drugs cannot repair damaged bone and cartilage, they reduce any inflammation and control pain to help maintain joint mobility and minimize deformity. Non-steroidal anti-inflammatory drugs (NSAIDs), for example ibuprofen, are prescribed first; these may then be followed by injections of corticosteroid drugs into severely inflamed joints.

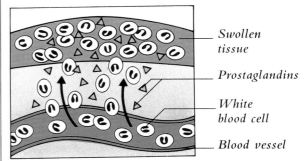

Swollen tissue
Prostaglandins
White blood cell
Blood vessel

Before corticosteroids
Prostaglandins are released from damaged tissues, attracting numerous white blood cells to repair the injury. The prostaglandins cause swelling, an increase in blood flow, and pain.

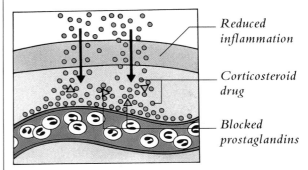

Reduced inflammation
Corticosteroid drug
Blocked prostaglandins

After corticosteroids
Injected corticosteroids inhibit the production of prostaglandins; this reduces the number and activity of the white blood cells. Inflammation and pain are relieved, and mobility increases.

OPERATION

HIP JOINT REPLACEMENT

In older people, a stiff, painful hip that does not respond well to treatment with drugs may be replaced by an artificial joint, or prosthesis. Joint replacement may also be used to treat hip fractures. Made up of a metallic femoral shaft and a cup-like pelvic socket, a prosthesis is frequently cemented in place; newer prostheses stimulate bone growth and can be fitted without cement.

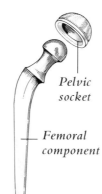

Pelvic socket

Femoral component

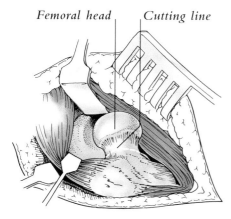

Femoral head *Cutting line*

1 The surgeon makes an incision over the affected hip. Ligaments and muscles are pushed aside or cut through so that the entire hip joint may be seen. The head of the femur, which is often eroded or broken, is subsequently removed.

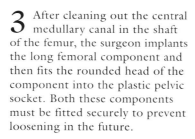

Pelvic bone *Reamer*

2 The surgeon employs an instrument called a reamer to shave and shape the cavity in the pelvic bone that normally holds the femoral head in place. The plastic pelvic socket is fitted and may be cemented in place.

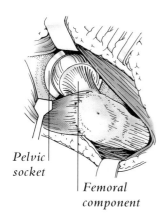

3 After cleaning out the central medullary canal in the shaft of the femur, the surgeon implants the long femoral component and then fits the rounded head of the component into the plastic pelvic socket. Both these components must be fitted securely to prevent loosening in the future.

Pelvic socket

Femoral component

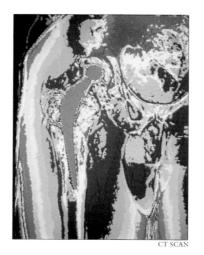

CT SCAN

4 A postoperative X-ray or CT scan is taken after the incision is closed in order to confirm that components are well positioned. Exercises to strengthen muscles in the hip area are often suggested. The operation usually relieves pain; after muscle strength has been regained, it helps to restore ease of movement.

HIP PROBLEMS IN CHILDREN

Although most of the bone and joint abnormalities occurring in children are caused by injuries, a painful or misshapen hip may also be due to some congenital defect, a bone infection, or an acquired disorder such as juvenile rheumatoid arthritis, also known as Still's disease. In a child who walks, the most obvious sign of hip malformation is a limp, which may be due to pain or to shortening of the affected leg.

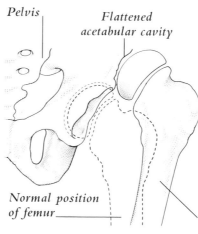

Pelvis *Flattened acetabular cavity*

Normal position of femur *Displaced femur*

CONGENITAL HIP DISLOCATION

This condition is the result of a flattened or misplaced acetabular cavity that fails to enclose the head of the femur. Although normally detected and treated with splints soon after birth, hip dislocation is occasionally missed and is detected only when a child begins to walk with a limp.

Appearance of a dislocated hip
A flattened acetabular cavity and an upwardly displaced hip (left side of image) were the result of an untreated congenital hip dislocation. If severe, misalignment of the hips causes obvious limping.

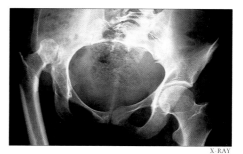

X-RAY

PERTHES' DISEASE

This disorder, which is more common in boys, is thought to be due to abnormal blood circulation in the epiphyseal growth plate. The head of the femur softens and becomes deformed, causing pain in the thigh and groin and a limp. The disease often affects only one hip, and must be treated as soon as possible by rest, splinting, and possibly surgery to prevent osteoarthritis later.

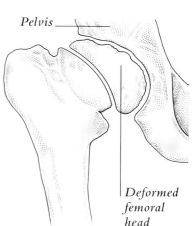

Pelvis

Deformed femoral head

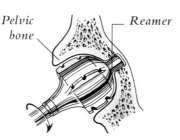

NORMAL POSITION OF EPIPHYSIS **SLIPPED EPIPHYSIS**

SLIPPED EPIPHYSIS

The upper growing end of the femur, the epiphysis, may slip out of position as a result of a fall or injury. More often, the displacement occurs gradually, possibly due to tissue-softening caused by the growth hormones produced during adolescence. Operative repair repositions the displaced bone, which is then secured with metal pins.

CHAPTER THREE

C H A P T E R   3

The MUSCULAR SYSTEM

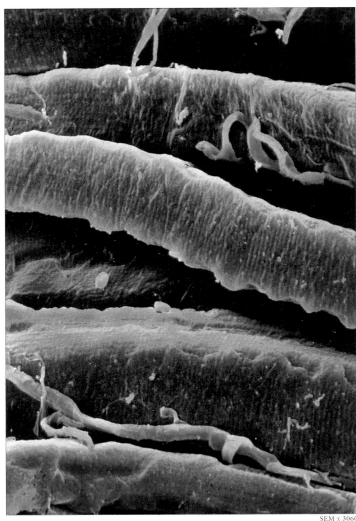

Skeletal muscle fibres
(with accompanying
capillaries seen in blue)

SEM x 3060

INTRODUCTION

Muscles make up the bulk of the body and account for about half its weight. They are divided into three distinct types: skeletal muscle, involuntary (or smooth) muscle, and cardiac muscle. Muscles of all three kinds have in common the ability to be stretched, to contract, to be excited by a stimulus, and to return to their original size and shape. Involuntary muscles are those that handle the unconscious routine of the body: they constantly perform tasks such as propelling food down the alimentary canal into the stomach, keeping the eyes in focus, or controlling the calibre of the arteries. Cardiac muscle is found only in the heart and is unique for its branched interconnections. Skeletal muscle, the subject of this section of the book, is also called voluntary muscle because we can usually choose to contract or relax it. All muscles in the trunk and limbs are kept in a partly contracted state, known as muscle tone, by a steady flow of nerve impulses from the spinal cord. If a muscle loses its nerve supply, it will shrink to around two-thirds of its bulk within a few months. Many of the diseases affecting muscles, such as poliomyelitis and myasthenia gravis, are really diseases of the nervous system rather than the muscles. Muscles are more often injured than diseased, and they are capable of self-repair: if one is partly destroyed, the remaining part will grow larger and stronger in order to compensate.

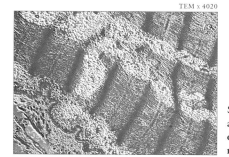

TEM x 4020

Striated appearance of skeletal muscle

Muscles of the hand and lower arm

THE MUSCULAR SYSTEM

MUSCLES *of the* BODY I

OVER 600 SKELETAL MUSCLES make up nearly half the weight of the human body. By working with skeletal bones, these muscles provide the vital forces that enable the body to move. A skeletal muscle usually attaches onto one end of a bone, stretches across a joint, and then tapers to attach to another bone. As a muscle contracts, it moves one bone while the other bone remains reasonably stable. The muscle's point of attachment on the more stable bone is called its origin; the point where it attaches to the more movable bone is its insertion. Many muscles have more than one point of origin and insertion.

SUPERFICIAL AND DEEP

Layers of skeletal muscles overlap each other in intricate patterns. Those just below the skin and its underlying fat are described as superficial (on right side of illustration); beneath these are the deep muscles (on left side of illustration). The muscles of the abdominal wall form three layers; the fibres of each run in a different direction. These provide a strong barrier that is flexible enough to accommodate changes of volume in the intestines, bladder, and uterus.

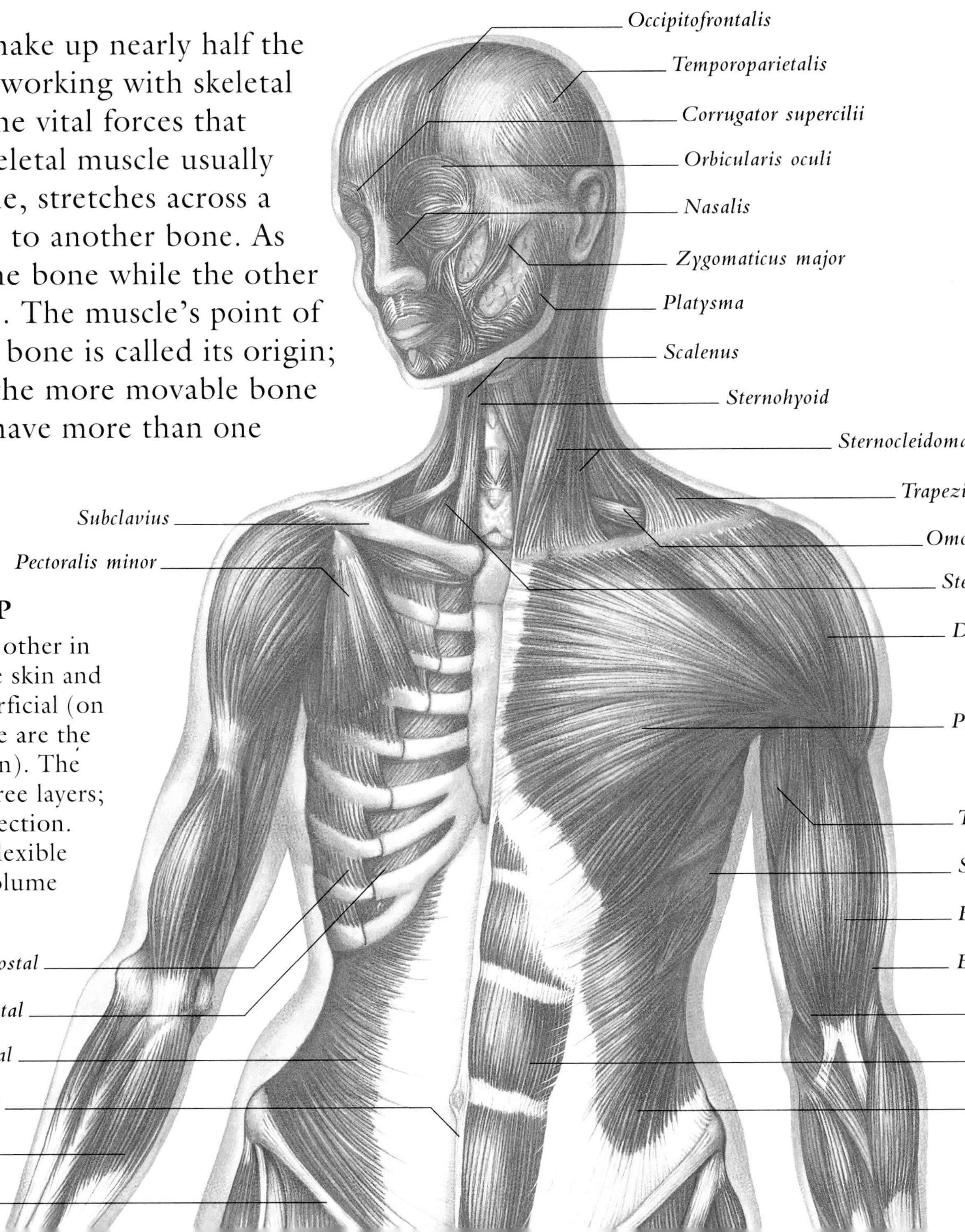

Occipitofrontalis

Temporoparietalis

Corrugator supercilii

Orbicularis oculi

Nasalis

Zygomaticus major

Platysma

Scalenus

Sternohyoid

Sternocleidomastoid

Trapezius

Omohyoid

Sternothyroid

Deltoid

Pectoralis major

Triceps (long head)

Serratus anterior

Biceps brachii

Brachialis

Triceps (medial head)

Rectus abdominis

External oblique abdominal

Subclavius

Pectoralis minor

External intercostal

Internal intercostal

Internal oblique abdominal

Linea alba

Flexor digitorum profundus

Inguinal ligament

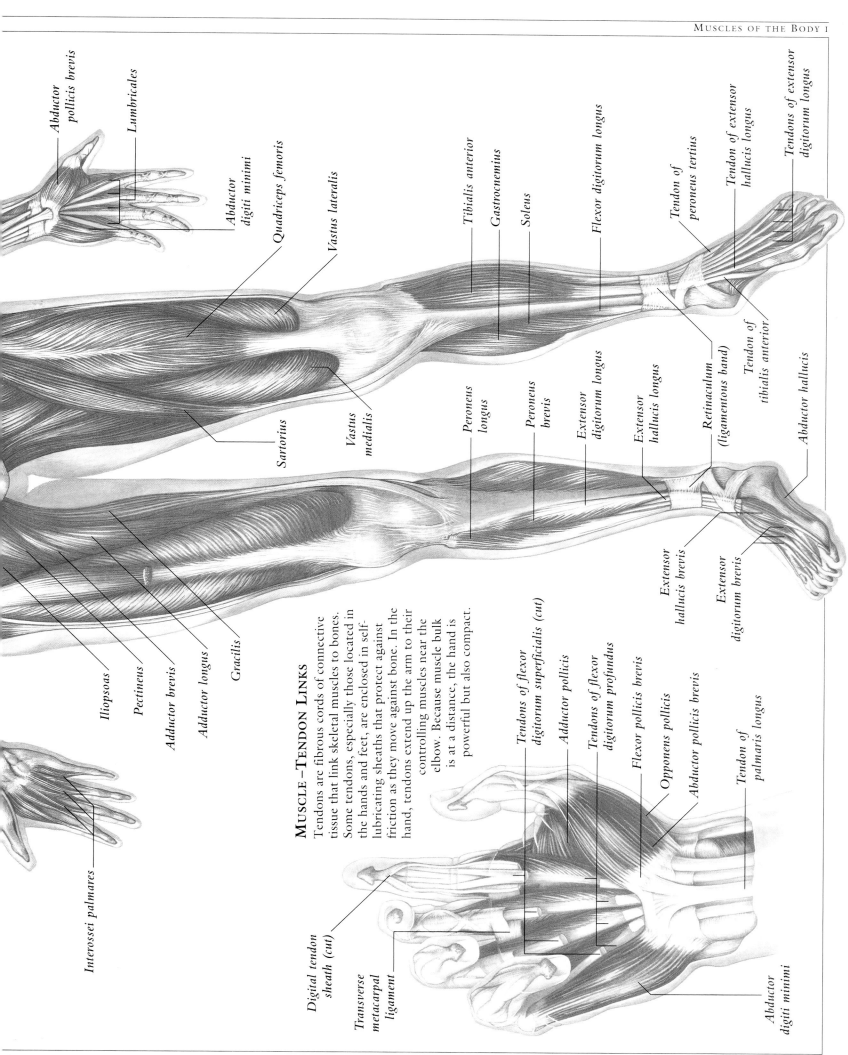

Abductor pollicis brevis

Lumbricales

Abductor digiti minimi

Quadriceps femoris

Vastus lateralis

Tibialis anterior

Gastrocnemius

Soleus

Flexor digitorum longus

Tendon of peroneus tertius

Tendon of extensor hallucis longus

Tendons of extensor digitorum longus

Sartorius

Vastus medialis

Peroneus longus

Peroneus brevis

Extensor digitorum longus

Extensor hallucis longus

Retinaculum (ligamentous band)

Tendon of tibialis anterior

Abductor hallucis

Iliopsoas

Pectineus

Adductor brevis

Adductor longus

Gracilis

Extensor hallucis brevis

Extensor digitorum brevis

MUSCLE–TENDON LINKS

Tendons are fibrous cords of connective tissue that link skeletal muscles to bones. Some tendons, especially those located in the hands and feet, are enclosed in self-lubricating sheaths that protect against friction as they move against bone. In the hand, tendons extend up the arm to their controlling muscles near the elbow. Because muscle bulk is at a distance, the hand is powerful but also compact.

Tendons of flexor digitorum superficialis (cut)

Adductor pollicis

Tendons of flexor digitorum profundus

Flexor pollicis brevis

Opponens pollicis

Abductor pollicis brevis

Tendon of palmaris longus

Interossei palmares

Digital tendon sheath (cut)

Transverse metacarpal ligament

Abductor digiti minimi

51

MUSCLES *of the* BODY II

MUSCLE APPEARANCE VARIES GREATLY, from the massive triangles of the upper back to the slender cables of the small, dexterous hand. The shape of a muscle determines the strength with which it contracts, and thus influences its specific function. The most powerful muscles are those that run along the spine; they maintain posture and provide the strength for lifting and pushing. The smallest is the stapedius inside the ear.

STRONG, STABILIZING MUSCLES

Muscles in the neck and upper back provide strength and permit complex movement. Those in the neck support the head and keep it upright. Upper-back muscles that attach to the wing-like scapula help stabilize the shoulder, the body's most mobile joint.

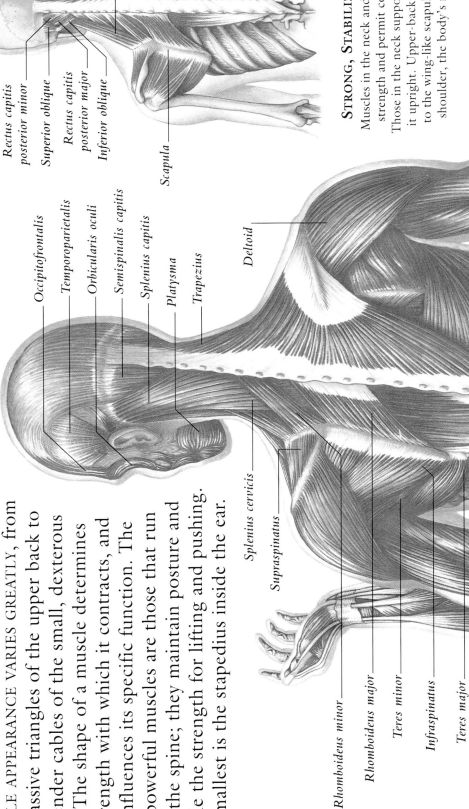

Semispinalis capitis

Splenius capitis

Levator scapulae

Rectus capitis posterior minor

Superior oblique

Rectus capitis posterior major

Inferior oblique

Scapula

Occipitofrontalis

Temporoparietalis

Orbicularis oculi

Semispinalis capitis

Splenius capitis

Platysma

Trapezius

Deltoid

Latissimus dorsi

Triceps

External oblique abdominal

Anconeus

Extensor digitorum

Flexor carpi ulnaris

Extensor carpi ulnaris

Splenius cervicis

Supraspinatus

Rhomboideus minor

Rhomboideus major

Teres minor

Infraspinatus

Teres major

External intercostal

Spinalis thoracis

Longissimus thoracis

Erector spinae

Internal oblique abdominal

Gluteus minimus

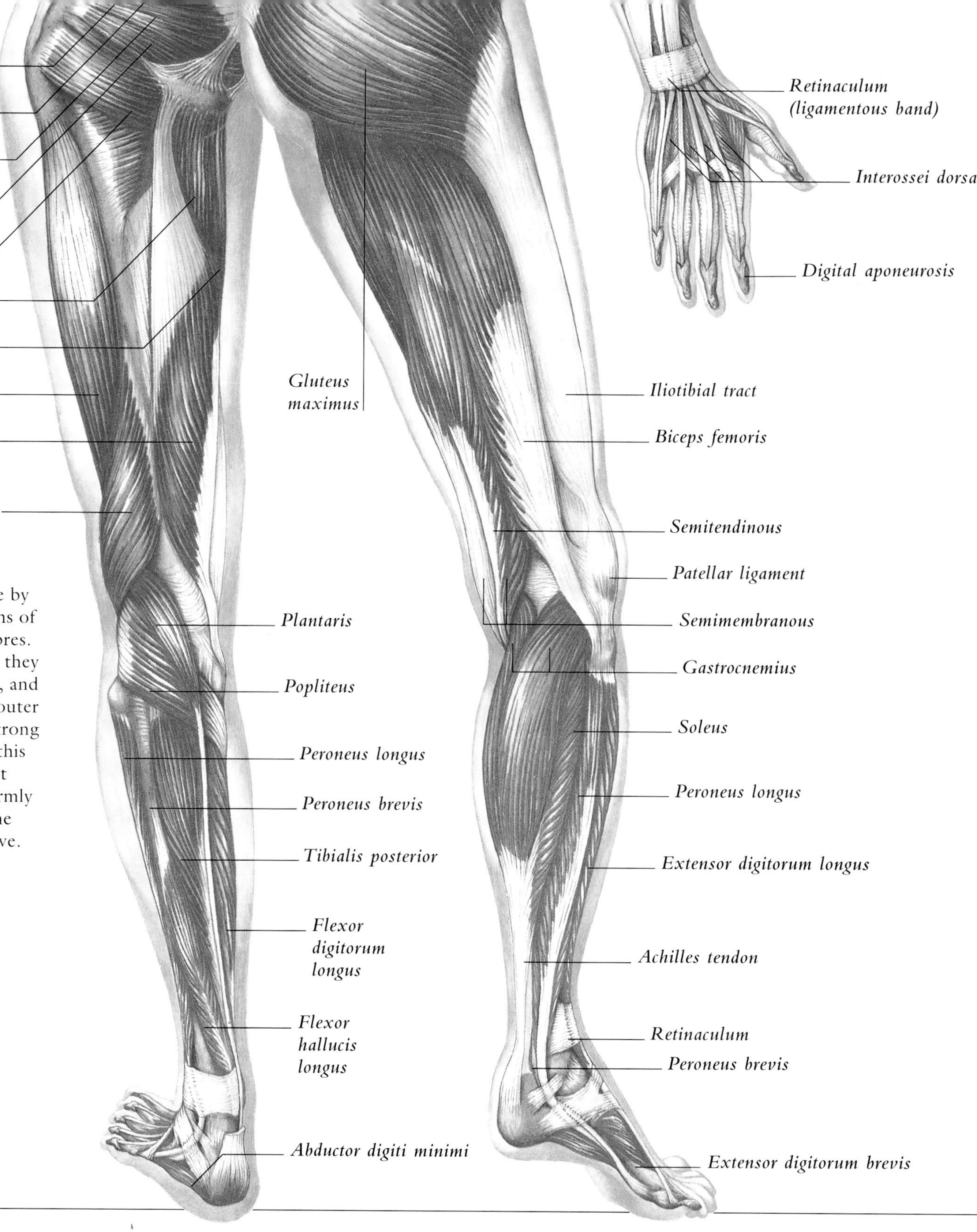

Retinaculum
(ligamentous band)

Interossei dorsales

Digital aponeurosis

Iliotibial tract

Biceps femoris

Semitendinous

Patellar ligament

Semimembranous

Gastrocnemius

Soleus

Peroneus longus

Extensor digitorum longus

Achilles tendon

Retinaculum

Peroneus brevis

Extensor digitorum brevis

Gluteus maximus

Plantaris

Popliteus

Peroneus longus

Peroneus brevis

Tibialis posterior

Flexor digitorum longus

Flexor hallucis longus

Abductor digiti minimi

Piriformis

Gemellus superior

Internal obturator

Gemellus inferior

Quadratus femoris

Adductor magnus

Gracilis

Vastus lateralis

Semimembranous

Biceps femoris
(short head)

TENDON–BONE LINKS

Tendons are linked strongly to bone by Sharpey's fibres, which are extensions of the tendon's collagen (a protein) fibres. Also known as perforating fibres, they pass through the periosteum, and are embedded within the outer parts of the bone. The strong anchorage provided by this arrangement means that tendons remain very firmly attached even when the underlying bones move.

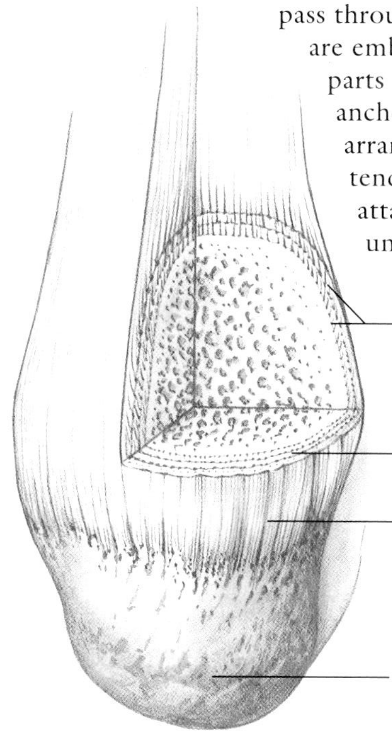

Sharpey's fibres

Periosteum

Tendon

Bone

MUSCLE STRUCTURE *and* CONTRACTION

THE STRUCTURE OF SKELETAL MUSCLES enables them to contract when stimulated by nerve impulses, pulling some part of the skeleton in the same direction as the contraction. Because muscles can only pull, not push, they are arranged in opposition to each other. This means that the movement produced by a group of muscles can always be reversed by its opposing group.

MUSCLE STRUCTURE

Skeletal muscles consist of densely packed groups of elongated cells known as muscle fibres held together by fibrous connective tissue. Numerous capillaries penetrate this connective tissue to keep muscles supplied with the abundant quantities of oxygen and glucose needed to fuel muscle contraction.

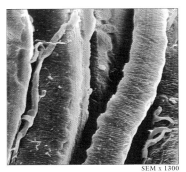

SEM x 1300

Striated muscle
The alternation of thick and thin myofilaments gives skeletal muscle fibres their striated (striped) appearance, as shown at left. The thin, blue tubular structures are capillaries.

HOW MUSCLES CONTRACT
In a relaxed muscle, the thick and thin myofilaments overlap a little. When a muscle contracts, the thick filaments slide farther in between the thin filaments, rather like interlacing fingers, and move closer to the Z bands. This action shortens the myofibril and the entire muscle fibre. The more shortened muscle fibres there are, the greater the contraction in the muscle as a whole.

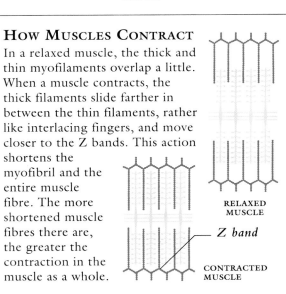

RELAXED MUSCLE

Z band

CONTRACTED MUSCLE

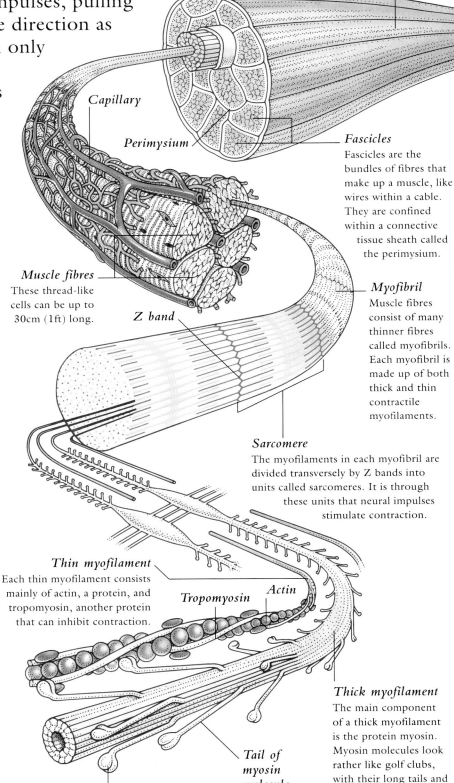

Muscle

Capillary

Perimysium

Muscle fibres
These thread-like cells can be up to 30cm (1ft) long.

Z band

Fascicles
Fascicles are the bundles of fibres that make up a muscle, like wires within a cable. They are confined within a connective tissue sheath called the perimysium.

Myofibril
Muscle fibres consist of many thinner fibres called myofibrils. Each myofibril is made up of both thick and thin contractile myofilaments.

Sarcomere
The myofilaments in each myofibril are divided transversely by Z bands into units called sarcomeres. It is through these units that neural impulses stimulate contraction.

Thin myofilament
Each thin myofilament consists mainly of actin, a protein, and tropomyosin, another protein that can inhibit contraction.

Tropomyosin

Actin

Thick myofilament
The main component of a thick myofilament is the protein myosin. Myosin molecules look rather like golf clubs, with their long tails and oval-shaped heads.

Tail of myosin molecule

Head of myosin molecule

LEVER SYSTEMS

Most bodily movements employ the mechanical principles by which a force applied to one part of a rigid lever arm is transferred via a pivot point, or fulcrum, to a weight elsewhere on the lever. In the body, muscles apply force, bones serve as levers, and joints function as fulcrums in order to move a body part. Lever systems in the body sacrifice mechanical advantage for range of movement.

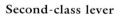

First-class lever

A first-class lever works like a see-saw, with the fulcrum lying between the force and the weight. One rare example in the body is the action of the posterior neck muscles tilting back the head. The lever at the base of the skull pivots on the fulcrum of the atlanto-occipital joint.

Second-class lever

In a second-class lever, the weight lies between the force and the fulcrum. The action of raising the heel from the ground is an example of this type of system in the body. The calf muscles are the force to lift the body weight, the heel and most of the foot form the lever, and the metatarsal-phalangeal joints provide the fulcrum.

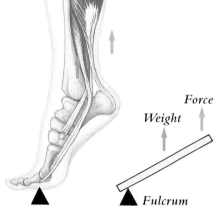

Third-class lever

In a third-class lever, which is the most common type in the body, the force is applied to the lever between the weight and the fulcrum. A typical example is flexing the elbow joint (the fulcrum) by contracting the biceps brachii muscle in order to lift the forearm and hand.

MUSCLES WORK TOGETHER

In order to lift the upper arm away from the trunk, the anterior and posterior sectors of the deltoid muscle balance each other, while the middle sector carries out the work. When a muscle contracts to produce movement it is called the agonist and its opposite, relaxing muscle is known as the antagonist. Sometimes stabilizing muscles also play an important role in creating this coordinated muscle action.

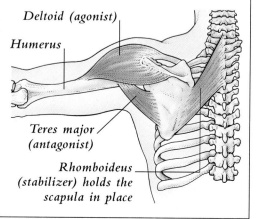

Deltoid (agonist)
Humerus
Teres major (antagonist)
Rhomboideus (stabilizer) holds the scapula in place

FACIAL EXPRESSIONS

For humans and other primates, varying facial expressions are a significant means of communication. The musculature involved is highly complex, allowing for many subtle nuances of expression. Facial muscles have their insertions (attachments to moving parts) within the skin, which means that even a slight degree of muscle contraction can produce movement of facial skin.

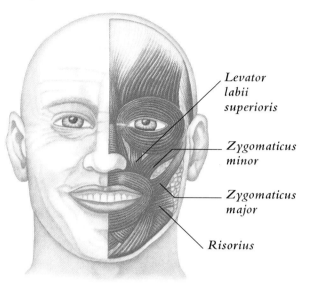

Levator labii superioris
Zygomaticus minor
Zygomaticus major
Risorius

Smiling

The smile is a very ambiguous and versatile expression, which can convey a wide range of emotions apart from just pleasure. The levator labii superioris elevates the upper lip, while the zygomaticus major, the zygomaticus minor, and the risorius muscles pull the angle of the mouth and the corners of the lips upward and sideways.

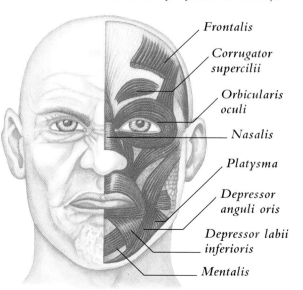

Frontalis
Corrugator supercilii
Orbicularis oculi
Nasalis
Platysma
Depressor anguli oris
Depressor labii inferioris
Mentalis

Frowning

A frown can express various feelings, including disapproval and confusion. The frontalis and corrugator supercilii furrow the brow, the nasalis widens the nostrils, while the orbicularis oculi narrows the eye. The platysma and depressors pull the mouth and corners of the lips downward and sideways, and the mentalis puckers the chin.

MUSCLE INJURIES *and* DISORDERS

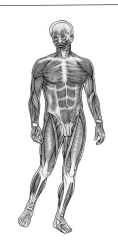

INJURIES TO MUSCLES and their tendon attachments are usually the result of overexertion during daily activities or from sudden pulling or twisting movements, such as those occurring during sports. Various work actions can also damage muscles and tendons. A number of rare muscle disorders may be responsible for muscle weakness and progressive degeneration.

MUSCLE STRAINS AND TEARS

Muscle strain is the term used for a moderate amount of damage to muscle fibres. Limited bleeding inside the muscle causes tenderness and swelling, which may be accompanied by painful spasms. Visible bruising may follow. More severe damage that involves a larger number of torn fibres is called a muscle tear.

Muscle tear

A torn muscle causes severe pain and swelling. Extensive bleeding may result in the formation of a blood clot, which a doctor may need to remove through a hollow needle (aspiration). Vigorous shoulder movements may cause tearing of a deltoid or pectoral muscle where it attaches to the humerus.

Deltoid muscle

Tear

Pectoral muscle

Humerus

TENDON INFLAMMATION

Inflammation involving tendons may affect the tendon itself (tendinitis) or inner lining of the fibrous sheaths that enclose some tendons (tenosynovitis). Tendinitis may occur when strong or repeated movement creates excessive friction between the tendon's outer surface and an adjacent bone. Tenosynovitis may be the result of overstretching or repeated movements.

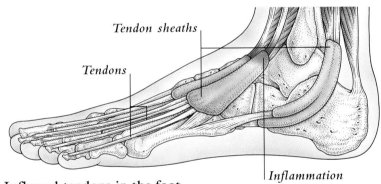

Tendon sheaths

Tendons

Inflammation

Inflamed tendons in the foot

The complexity of the foot makes it susceptible to tendon damage. Activities that involve running or kicking, and any awkward or complex movements (such as dancing) may cause tendon inflammation as can friction from ill-fitting shoes. Symptoms include pain, swelling, and restricted movement.

REPETITIVE STRAIN INJURY

Repetitive strain injury (RSI) describes a range of conditions caused by the constant repetition of particular movements. Irritation of the flexor and extensor tendons is a common injury that often affects keyboard operators and some musicians. Pain occurs when the fingers are moved. Another type of RSI may be due to pressure on the median nerve as it passes through a gap under a ligament at the front of the wrist, a condition known as carpal tunnel syndrome.

Ulnar extensor muscle of wrist

Tendon of flexor muscles

Tendons of extensor muscles

Extensor muscle of fingers

Ulnar flexor muscle of wrist

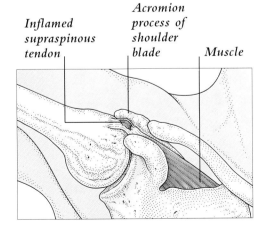

Inflamed supraspinous tendon

Acromion process of shoulder blade

Muscle

Inflamed supraspinous tendon

Anyone who plays much tennis or squash risks tendinitis of the shoulder. Repeated arm lifting causes the supraspinous tendon in the shoulder to rub against the shoulder blade's acromion process, creating friction.

TENDON TEARS

A sudden, powerful muscle contraction can severely damage a tendon, and can even tear it away from the bone. For example, the strain of lifting a heavy weight may result in tearing of the tendons attached to the biceps or of the main tendon at the front of the thigh (the quadriceps tendon) that stretches across the knee.

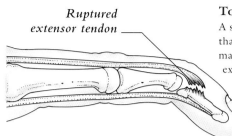

Ruptured extensor tendon

Torn finger tendon
A solid object, such as a hard ball, that strikes the end of a fingertip may bend it forward so that the extensor tendon is torn from its attachment. With this kind of tear, it may be necessary to immobilize the finger for several months.

OPERATION

TORN ACHILLES TENDON

A minor tear of the Achilles tendon may heal with rest and physiotherapy, but a serious injury often requires surgery and months of convalescence. A torn Achilles tendon is a familiar injury to tennis players when rising abruptly onto their toes in order to serve. It is also a constant threat to sprinters, who frequently subject the calf muscles to explosive bursts of muscle contraction.

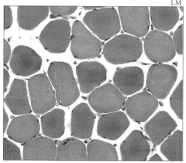

Location of tendon
The Achilles tendon runs from the base of the gastrocnemius muscle of the calf down to the calcaneus bone of the heel. If the tendon is torn, it becomes impossible to raise the heel.

- *Gastrocnemius muscle*
- *Achilles tendon*
- *Calcaneus (heel bone)*

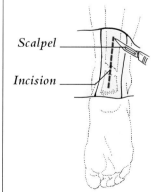

Scalpel

Incision

1 To reattach the torn ends of the tendon, the surgeon first applies a tourniquet around the thigh, to keep the injured area free of blood. An incision over the area of the tear exposes the separated tendon ends.

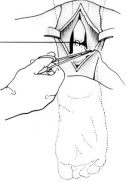

Stitches

2 After removing any blood clots and damaged tissue, the surgeon stitches together the separated ends of the tendon. Sometimes tendon tissue from elsewhere in the body may be used to reinforce the repair.

MUSCULAR DYSTROPHY

Muscular dystrophy is a term that describes a group of inherited disorders in which there is progressive degeneration of skeletal muscles. Common symptoms are increasing wasting of muscles and loss of muscle function. There is no effective treatment. However, stretching exercises and surgery to release shortened muscles and tendons can benefit some sufferers.

DIAGNOSIS

The patient's symptoms and history help in diagnosing muscular dystrophy. Tests include genetic screening for any abnormalities and blood tests to identify an enzyme released by damaged muscle. A muscle biopsy involves the removal of a small piece of tissue, while an electrical recording is used to demonstrate muscle activity.

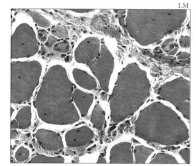

NORMAL MUSCLE FIBRES   ABNORMAL MUSCLE FIBRES

Muscle biopsy
A small tissue sample is removed, using either a biopsy needle or scalpel incision, and is then examined under a microscope. The muscle fibres above right show the degeneration characteristic of muscular dystrophy.

MYASTHENIA GRAVIS

This autoimmune disorder is marked by severe muscle weakness and fatigue. This is caused by antibodies that gradually reduce the number of receptors in the fibres that stimulate muscle contractions. A thymus disorder may trigger the disease; the gland may be removed and immunosuppressant drugs given as part of the treatment.

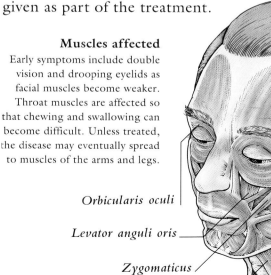

Muscles affected
Early symptoms include double vision and drooping eyelids as facial muscles become weaker. Throat muscles are affected so that chewing and swallowing can become difficult. Unless treated, the disease may eventually spread to muscles of the arms and legs.

Orbicularis oculi

Levator anguli oris

Zygomaticus

Sternohyoid

CHAPTER FOUR

C H A P T E R   4

The NERVOUS SYSTEM

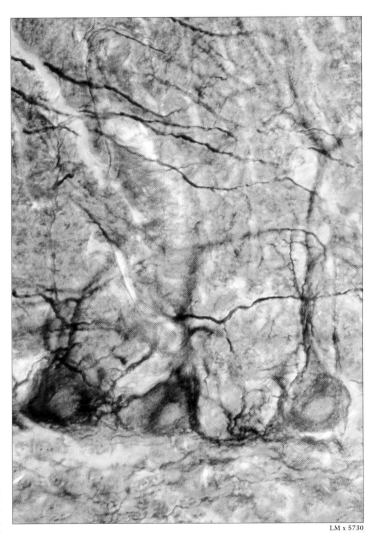

Two large nerve cells
from the cerebellum,
a part of the brain

LM x 5730

INTRODUCTION

Our brains – not our hearts – are where we feel emotions such as love and anger. They are also where we think, decide, and initiate and control our actions. Nerve impulses are constantly flashing into the brain, around it, and away from it via the spinal cord and a network of cable-like nerves that are distributed throughout the body. The brain, which monitors and regulates these impulses, is sometimes thought of as a computer, but the comparison is rather misleading. Communication between the billions of nerve cells in the brain is by means of chemical signals as well as electrical ones, which is why alcohol and drugs affect us. More significantly, the complex connections between nerve cells are capable of growth and development, and so are able to react to events for which the brain has not been programmed. The brain is capable of creativity in a way that no computer has yet achieved. But it is delicate: nerve tracts damaged by injury or disease cannot repair themselves. Although the brain has long been slow to give up its secrets, recent advances in biochemistry and modern imaging techniques have helped to reveal its workings; and they have helped clarify our understanding of various conditions such as stroke, tumours, and Alzheimer's disease.

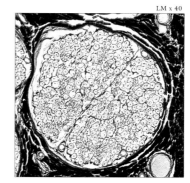

LM x 40

Cross-section of the sciatic nerve

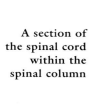

A section of the spinal cord within the spinal column

THE NERVOUS SYSTEM

ORGANIZATION
of the NERVOUS SYSTEM

THE BODY AND BRAIN ARE CONSTANTLY ALIVE with billions of electrical and chemical signals. This incessant signalling is the result of activity from neurons, or nerve cells, and their filamentous but far-reaching fibres. Along with support cells called neuroglia, neurons make up the brain and spinal cord, also called the central nervous system or CNS. Neurons also make up the peripheral nerves that connect the CNS with the rest of the body. Most nerve signalling occurs unconsciously and is responsible for keeping the human body safe and functioning properly.

NERVE NETWORKS

The long, slender nerve fibres of individual neurons band together in groups outside the CNS to form the cable-like peripheral nerves. This body-wide network reports to the CNS on the state of events outside and inside the body. Most of the peripheral nerves divide and branch in order that nerve fibres make contact with as many parts and tissues as possible. Some form groups, called plexuses, so that important areas, such as the hand and fingers, are under finely tuned control.

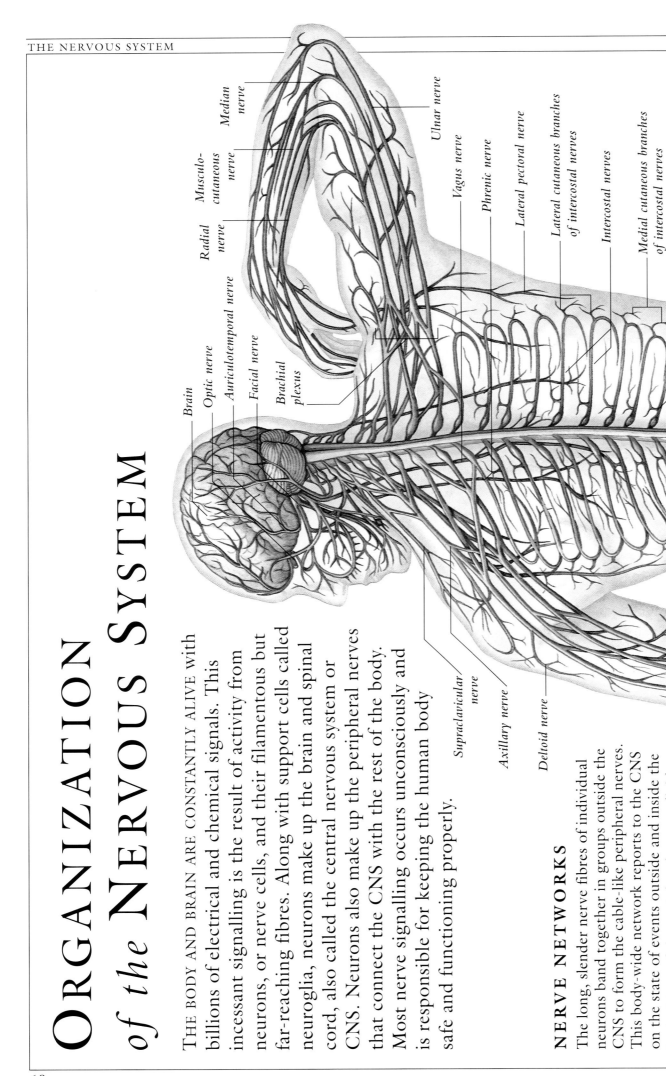

Median nerve

Ulnar nerve

Radial nerve

Musculo-cutaneous nerve

Auriculotemporal nerve

Facial nerve

Optic nerve

Brain

Brachial plexus

Vagus nerve

Phrenic nerve

Lateral pectoral nerve

Lateral cutaneous branches of intercostal nerves

Intercostal nerves

Medial cutaneous branches of intercostal nerves

Dorsal branches of intercostal nerves

Subcostal nerve

Iliohypogastric nerve

Ilioinguinal nerve

Spinal ganglion

Spinal cord

Supraclavicular nerve

Axillary nerve

Deltoid nerve

Radial nerve

Muscular branches of median nerve

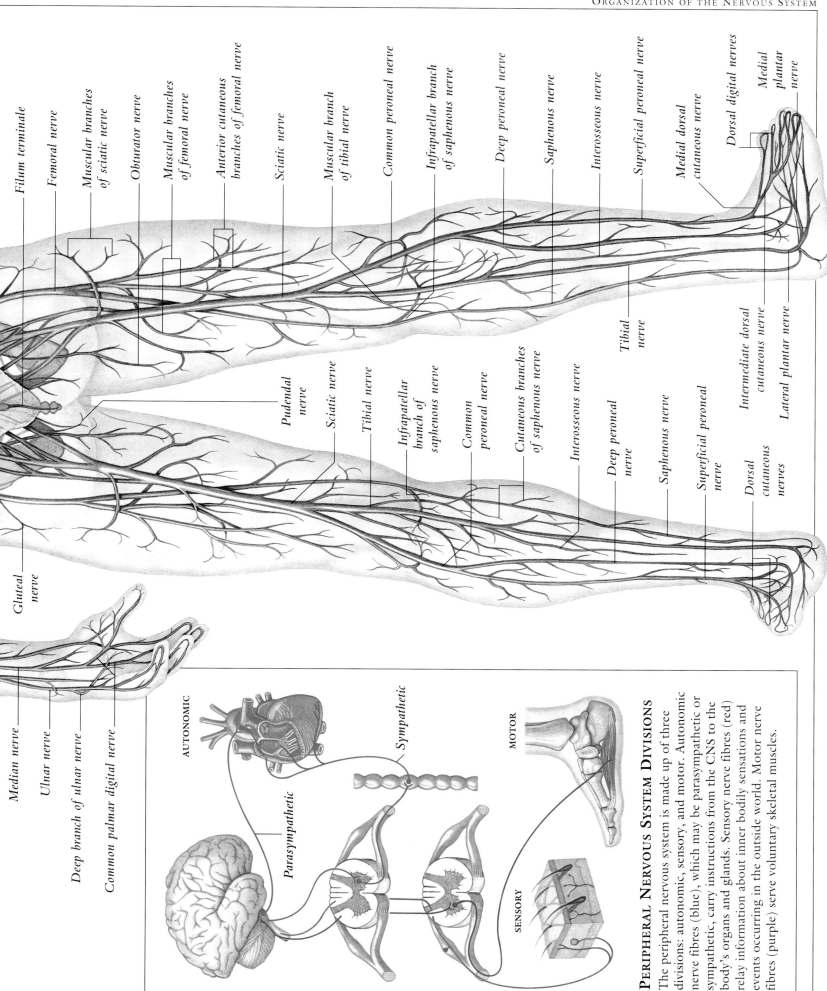

Filum terminale

Femoral nerve

Muscular branches of sciatic nerve

Obturator nerve

Muscular branches of femoral nerve

Anterior cutaneous branches of femoral nerve

Sciatic nerve

Muscular branch of tibial nerve

Common peroneal nerve

Infrapatellar branch of saphenous nerve

Deep peroneal nerve

Saphenous nerve

Interosseous nerve

Superficial peroneal nerve

Medial dorsal cutaneous nerve

Dorsal digital nerves

Medial plantar nerve

Tibial nerve

Intermediate dorsal cutaneous nerve

Lateral plantar nerve

Pudendal nerve

Sciatic nerve

Tibial nerve

Infrapatellar branch of saphenous nerve

Common peroneal nerve

Cutaneous branches of saphenous nerve

Interosseous nerve

Deep peroneal nerve

Saphenous nerve

Superficial peroneal nerve

Dorsal cutaneous nerves

Gluteal nerve

Median nerve

Ulnar nerve

Deep branch of ulnar nerve

Common palmar digital nerve

AUTONOMIC

Sympathetic

Parasympathetic

MOTOR

SENSORY

PERIPHERAL NERVOUS SYSTEM DIVISIONS

The peripheral nervous system is made up of three divisions: autonomic, sensory, and motor. Autonomic nerve fibres (blue), which may be parasympathetic or sympathetic, carry instructions from the CNS to the body's organs and glands. Sensory nerve fibres (red) relay information about inner bodily sensations and events occurring in the outside world. Motor nerve fibres (purple) serve voluntary skeletal muscles.

NERVE CELLS *and* NERVES

THE BASIC UNIT OF THE NERVOUS SYSTEM is the neuron. The body of this specialized nerve cell has projections that either receive electrical messages from or transmit messages to other neurons, muscles, or glands. The billions of interconnecting neurons that make up the nervous system are protected by other supporting nerve cells known as glial cells. These non-excitable cells, located between and around neurons, account for over half of all nerve cells in the nervous system.

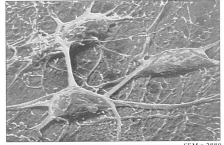
SEM x 2880

Three neurons in the cerebral cortex

NEURON STRUCTURE

Like other body cells, neurons have a cell body with a central nucleus and a number of other structures that are important for the maintenance of cell life. Extending from the cell body are a variable number of projections, called processes or neurites. Neurites that carry impulses away from the cell body are called axons, while processes that receive impulses are called dendrites.

TYPES OF NEURON

The shape and size of neuron cell bodies vary greatly as do the type, number, and length of their processes. Some general types of neuron are shown in the illustrations below.

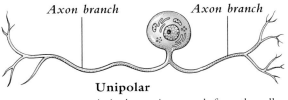

Axon branch   *Axon branch*

Unipolar
A single neurite extends from the cell body and subsequently divides into two distinct branches of a single axon.

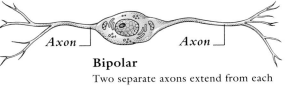

Axon   *Axon*

Bipolar
Two separate axons extend from each end of a slightly elongated cell body.

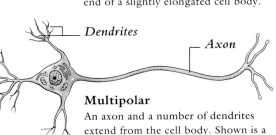

Dendrites

Axon

Multipolar
An axon and a number of dendrites extend from the cell body. Shown is a neuron of this type, called a pyramidal cell, found in the cerebral cortex.

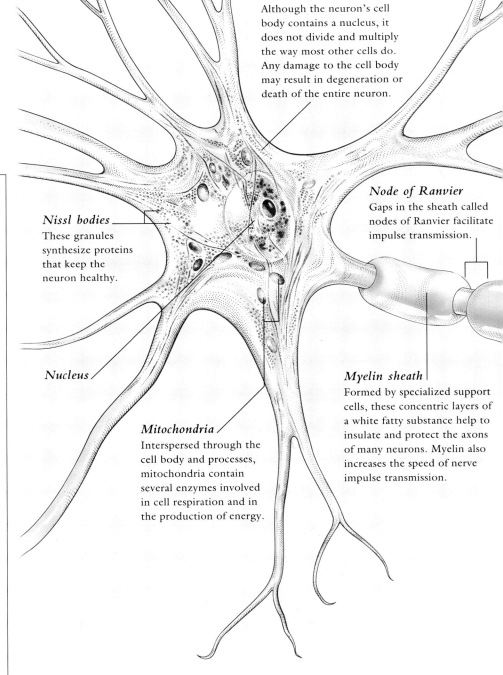

Cell body
Although the neuron's cell body contains a nucleus, it does not divide and multiply the way most other cells do. Any damage to the cell body may result in degeneration or death of the entire neuron.

Node of Ranvier
Gaps in the sheath called nodes of Ranvier facilitate impulse transmission.

Nissl bodies
These granules synthesize proteins that keep the neuron healthy.

Nucleus

Mitochondria
Interspersed through the cell body and processes, mitochondria contain several enzymes involved in cell respiration and in the production of energy.

Myelin sheath
Formed by specialized support cells, these concentric layers of a white fatty substance help to insulate and protect the axons of many neurons. Myelin also increases the speed of nerve impulse transmission.

SUPPORT CELLS

Unlike neurons, supporting nerve cells, known as glial cells, are not involved with the transmission of nerve impulses. Instead, they act to protect and nourish the neurons. Several types of these specialized cells exist. The smallest cells are called microglia: they engulf and destroy microorganisms. Other cells help to insulate axons or to regulate the flow of cerebrospinal fluid.

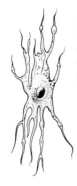

Oligodendrocytes

These cells wrap their plasma membranes around neurons of the brain and spinal cord to form myelin sheaths.

Astrocytes

Delicate projections of cytoplasm give these star-shaped cells their name ("astro" means star). Some cell processes connect with capillaries and help regulate the flow of substances from the blood to the brain and spinal cord.

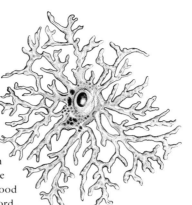

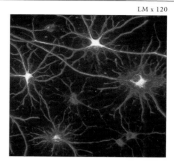

LM x 120

"Star-cell" constellation

Astrocytes, which are the most numerous type of glial cell, form complex networks in the grey matter of the brain.

Dendrite

Branching from the cell body are tapering filaments called dendrites, which receive electrical signals from other neurons.

Synaptic knobs

These bulges at the ends of the axon's terminal fibres contain vesicles, or sacs, of chemicals known as neurotransmitters that help transmit information from one cell to another.

Axon terminal fibre

Axon

The longest process extending from a cell body is the axon, also known as a nerve fibre. Axons conduct impulses in one direction only. Some grow to reach a length of over 1m (3ft), and those with a large diameter can conduct impulses very quickly.

NERVE STRUCTURE

Cordlike nerves are formed from bundles, called fascicles, of axons that project from several neurons. Most nerves travel to a particular site in the body and carry two types of fibre: sensory (afferent) fibres, which convey impulses from receptors in the skin, sense organs, and internal organs back to the brain and spinal cord; and motor (efferent) fibres, which transmit signals from the brain and spinal cord to a muscle or gland.

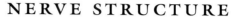

Epineurium

Ganglion

A cluster of neuron cell bodies creates a ganglion. Axons that run in parallel to one another extend from the cell bodies.

Myelin sheath

Axon

Fascicle

The word "fascicle" means bundle; a nerve fascicle is composed of a bundle of neuronal axons.

Perineurium

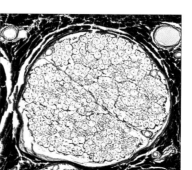

LM x 40

A major nerve

This cross-section shows the sciatic nerve with its numerous fascicles. The thickest nerve in the body, it measures 2cm (less than 1in) in diameter when it emerges from the spinal cord. The branches of the sciatic nerve innervate the muscles and skin of the leg.

NEURON BEHAVIOUR

IN ORDER TO PRODUCE ELECTRICAL NERVE IMPULSES
neurons must be triggered by a stimulus, which is
anything inside or outside the body that evokes a
physical or a psychological response. A neuron's
capacity to respond to a stimulus is known as
excitability. Electrical nerve impulses may
also be blocked, or inhibited, by some
neurotransmitters or by drugs.

TEM x 14,000

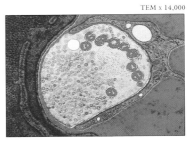

The synaptic cleft
Tiny sacs, called vesicles, containing
chemicals cluster near the canal-like
synaptic cleft between an axon (seen
in yellow) and a muscle fibre (red).

THE SYNAPSE

To "fire" a neuron, a stimulus must convert
the electrical charge on the inside of the cell
membrane from negative to positive. The
nerve impulse travels down the axon to a
synaptic knob, and triggers the release
of chemicals that may stimulate a
response in the target cell.

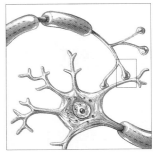

The synapse
This communication point
between neurons (above and
enlarged at left) comprises the
synaptic knob, the synaptic
cleft, and the target site.

*Axon
terminal fibre*

Neurofilaments
These act as scaffolding to help
give the nerve cell its shape.

Cell membrane
This conveys electrical impulses
away from the cell body.

Microtubules
These structures are thought to help
in the transport of neurotransmitter
molecules to the synaptic membrane.

Synaptic vesicles
These sacs contain molecules of
the neurotransmitter and are
drawn toward the synaptic
cleft by calcium ions.

Receptor sites
The neurotransmitter
combines with protein
receptors on the target
cell membrane, which
then becomes permeable
to specific ions.

Synaptic knob
Each knob at the end of an axon
terminal fibre lies close to the
neuron cell body, its axons
or dendrites, another
synaptic knob, or a
muscle fibre.

Mitochondrion

*Neurotransmitter
molecules*
These chemical molecules
are released from the
vesicles into the synaptic
cleft, where they influence
impulse transmission.

Synaptic cleft

Membrane channels
Excitation occurs when enough positive
sodium ions (Na⁺) have passed through
channels in the membrane to change the
charge on the inside of the cell membrane
from negative to positive.

Na⁺

Na⁺

Na⁺

Target cell membrane

SENDING A NERVE IMPULSE

The level at which a stimulus begins to transmit an electrical impulse is called a threshold. If a stimulus is too weak, or below the threshold, there is only a very brief local response in the membrane. If, however, the threshold is reached, the impulse travels along the entire length of the fibre. The speed of transmission can vary: fibres that are cold (as when ice is applied in order to dull pain), those with small diameters, and those without myelin sheaths conduct impulses more slowly.

REGENERATION

Peripheral nerve fibres that are crushed or only partially cut may slowly regenerate if the cell body and the hollow segments of the myelin sheath remain undamaged. Regeneration does not occur in nerves in the brain or spinal cord; instead, injured nerve fibres are wrapped in scar tissue.

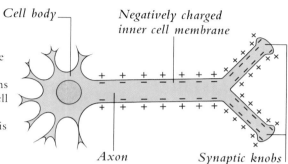

Cell body — *Negatively charged inner cell membrane* — *Axon* — *Synaptic knobs*

1 In a neuron's "resting" state when no impulse is being transmitted, positive sodium ions diffuse from the inside of the cell membrane at a continuous rate; the inner membrane of the cell is thus negatively charged.

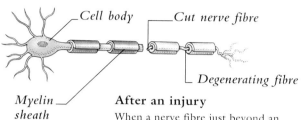

Cell body — *Cut nerve fibre* — *Myelin sheath* — *Degenerating fibre*

After an injury
When a nerve fibre just beyond an injury and farthest from the cell body no longer receives vital proteins and enzymes, it begins to degenerate and the myelin sheath becomes hollow.

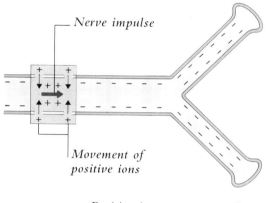

Nerve impulse — *Movement of positive ions*

2 When stimulated by a nerve impulse, positively charged ions in the fluid outside the membrane cross the cell membrane. At these local sites the electrical charge on the inside of the cell membrane changes from negative to positive.

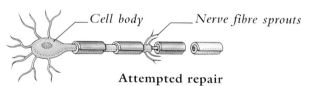

Cell body — *Nerve fibre sprouts*

Attempted repair
The undamaged neuron cell body stimulates the growth of several nerve sprouts in the remaining portion of the fibre. One of these sprouts may eventually find its way through the empty but intact myelin sheath.

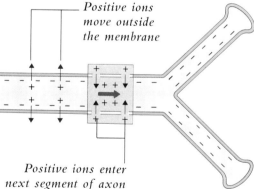

Positive ions move outside the membrane — *Positive ions enter next segment of axon*

3 This localized reversal of charge across the membrane stimulates similar changes in the next segment of the membrane. The electrical impulse continues down the axon; as it passes along, previous segments of the membrane revert back to the original "inside-negative" state.

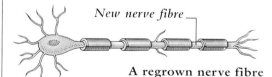

New nerve fibre

A regrown nerve fibre
Growing at a rate of about 1.5mm a day, the new nerve fibre reaches its previous connection. Function and sensation are slowly restored, and unused nerve sprouts degenerate.

4 The impulse reaches the synaptic cleft. At right is a microscopic image of the branching terminal fibres of a motor neuron axon (pink); these fibres end in synaptic knobs that lie very close to skeletal muscle fibres (red). When a neurotransmitter is released from vesicles in the synaptic knob, it crosses the synaptic cleft and stimulates the muscle fibres to contract.

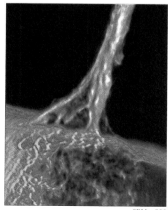

SEM x 900

INHIBITION

During inhibition, or blockage of electrical impulses, channels that are sensitive to chloride or potassium ions may open rather than channels that are sensitive to sodium. Positive potassium ions (shown as K^+) escape from the target cell, or else negative chloride ions (shown as Cl^-) permeate the cell membrane. In both instances, the electrical charge inside the target cell membrane stays negative, the neuron cannot be "fired", and the nerve impulse is inhibited.

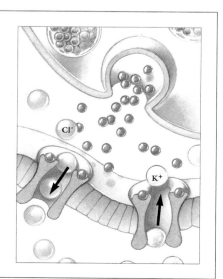

Cl^- — K^+

The BRAIN I

LOCATED IN THE SKULL, THE BRAIN contains over 12 billion neurons and 50 billion supporting glial cells, but weighs less than 1.4kg (3lb). With the spinal cord, the brain monitors and regulates many unconscious bodily processes, such as heart rate, and coordinates most voluntary movement. Most importantly, it is the site of consciousness and all the different intellectual functions that allow human beings to think, learn, and create.

Halves of the brain
A longitudinal fissure, seen from above, divides the brain into two halves, called hemispheres, that communicate with each other.

OUTER BRAIN STRUCTURE

The most obvious feature about the cerebrum – the largest part of the brain – is its heavily folded surface, the pattern of which is different in each human being. The grooves are called sulci when shallow and fissures when deep. Fissures and some of the large sulci outline specific functional areas called lobes. A ridge on the surface of the brain is called a gyrus.

Central sulcus

Cerebral cortex
The entire cerebrum is covered by a layer of grey matter about 2 to 6mm thick. Underneath is the brain's white matter as well as islands of grey matter.

Parietal lobe
Bodily sensations such as touch, temperature, pressure, and pain are perceived and interpreted in this area.

Gyrus

Occipital lobe
This area detects and interprets visual images.

Frontal lobe
Speech production, the elaboration of thought and emotion, and skilled movements are controlled by neurons found in this part of the brain.

Temporal lobe
The recognition of sounds, and their tones and loudness, takes place here. This lobe also plays a role in the storage of memory.

Sylvian or lateral fissure

Cerebellum
This is the second largest part of the brain. Its neurons link up with other regions of the brain and the spinal cord to facilitate smooth, precise movement, and to control balance and posture.

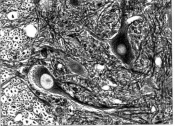

Cells of the cerebral cortex
Higher intellectual functions such as memory and the interpretation of sensory impulses are assisted by the complex network of neurons that make up the cerebral cortex.

LM x 360

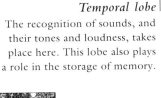

The tree of life
This image shows a section through the cerebellum, which is made up of many myelinated nerve fibres. The distinctive pattern resembles the veins of a leaf and is described as the arbor vitae ("tree of life").

INNER BRAIN STRUCTURES

The thalamus, which lies in the centre of the brain, acts as the brain's information relay station. Surrounding this is a group of structures, the limbic system, which is involved in survival behaviour and emotions, such as rage and fright. Closely linked with the limbic system is the hypothalamus, which has overall control of automatic body processes.

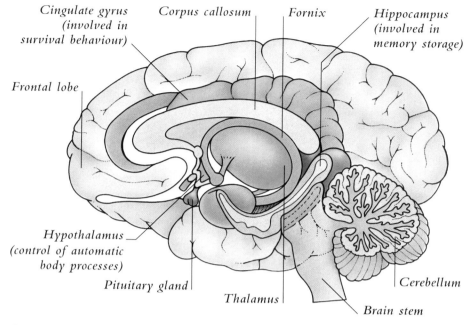

Cingulate gyrus (involved in survival behaviour)
Corpus callosum
Fornix
Hippocampus (involved in memory storage)
Frontal lobe
Hypothalamus (control of automatic body processes)
Pituitary gland
Thalamus
Brain stem
Cerebellum

GREY AND WHITE MATTER

The brain's grey matter is made up of groups of neuron cell bodies. White matter, by contrast, is composed mainly of the myelin-covered axons, or nerve fibres, that extend from the neuron cell bodies. The fatty, insulating myelin sheaths act to increase the speed of the transmission of nerve impulses.

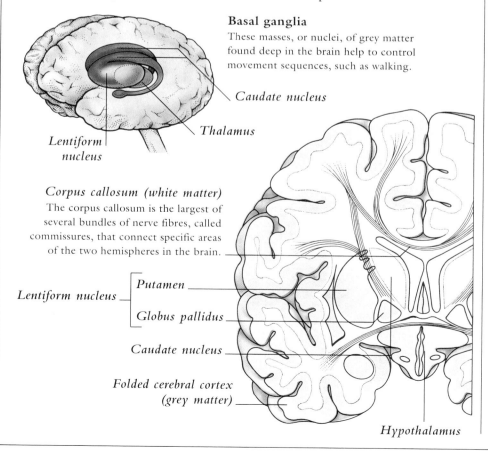

Basal ganglia

These masses, or nuclei, of grey matter found deep in the brain help to control movement sequences, such as walking.

Caudate nucleus
Thalamus
Lentiform nucleus

Corpus callosum (white matter)

The corpus callosum is the largest of several bundles of nerve fibres, called commissures, that connect specific areas of the two hemispheres in the brain.

Lentiform nucleus
Putamen
Globus pallidus
Caudate nucleus
Folded cerebral cortex (grey matter)
Hypothalamus

VERTICAL LINKS

Myelinated fibres organized into so-called projection tracts transmit impulses to and from the spinal cord and lower brain areas to the cerebral cortex. These nerve tracts pass through a communication link called the internal capsule, a compact band of fibres, and intersect the corpus callosum.

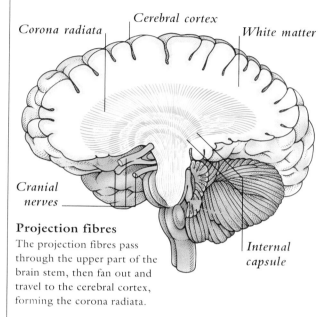

Corona radiata
Cerebral cortex
White matter
Cranial nerves
Internal capsule

Projection fibres

The projection fibres pass through the upper part of the brain stem, then fan out and travel to the cerebral cortex, forming the corona radiata.

THE THALAMUS AND BRAIN STEM

The thalamus is a relay station that sorts, interprets, and directs sensory nerve signals to and from the midbrain and the spinal cord to the cerebral cortex and appropriate regions of the cerebrum. The brain stem contains centres that regulate several functions that are vital for survival: these include heartbeat, respiration, blood pressure, digestion, and certain reflex actions such as swallowing and vomiting.

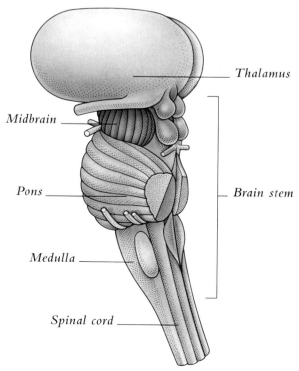

Thalamus
Midbrain
Pons
Brain stem
Medulla
Spinal cord

The BRAIN II

THE SOFT TISSUE OF THE BRAIN FLOATS within the bony casing of the skull in a watery medium. Known as cerebrospinal fluid, this clear liquid, which is renewed four to five times a day, is produced inside the ventricles (chambers) of the brain. It contains proteins and glucose that provide energy for brain cell function as well as lymphocytes that guard against infection. This fluid protects and nourishes both the brain and spinal cord as it flows around them.

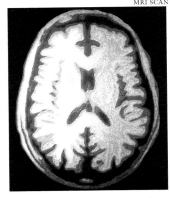

MRI SCAN

View of lateral ventricles
Each of the two lateral ventricles, one in each hemisphere, has a front and a longer back horn, which extend from the centre of the brain. When seen from above, these ventricles have the appearance of a large X.

Site of fluid production (choroid plexuses)
Cerebrospinal fluid is produced in clusters of thin-walled capillaries, called choroid plexuses, that line the walls of the ventricles.

Direction of flow
Fluid moves from the lateral ventricles into the third and fourth ventricles. It then flows up the back of the brain, down around the spinal cord, and up the front of the brain (arrows).

Site of reabsorption (arachnoid granulations)
After circulating, cerebrospinal fluid is reabsorbed into blood through arachnoid granulations, projections from the arachnoid layer of the meninges that connect with veins via the venous sinus.

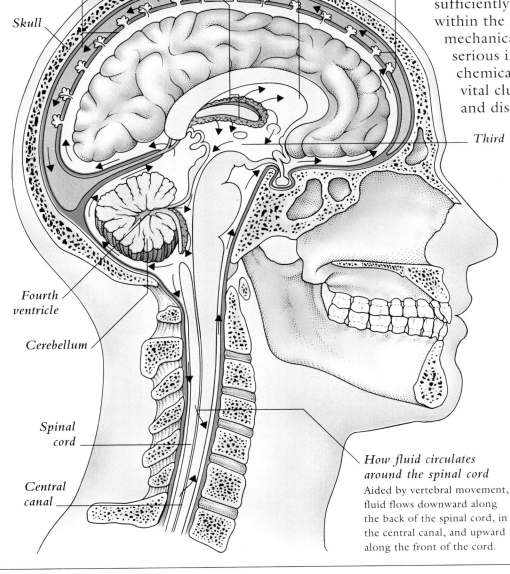

Venous sinus

Dura mater

Skull

Lateral ventricle

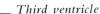

Third ventricle

Fourth ventricle

Cerebellum

Spinal cord

Central canal

How fluid circulates around the spinal cord
Aided by vertebral movement, fluid flows downward along the back of the spinal cord, in the central canal, and upward along the front of the cord.

PROTECTION FOR THE BRAIN

The solid bones of the skull may fracture if struck sufficiently hard. However, the cerebrospinal fluid within the skull absorbs and disperses excessive mechanical forces that might otherwise cause serious injury to the brain. An analysis of its chemical constituents and flow pressure offers vital clues in the diagnosis of many diseases and disorders of the brain, such as meningitis.

FLUID-FILLED CHAMBERS

Fluid produced in the lateral ventricles drains via the interventricular foramen into the third ventricle close to the thalamus. It then flows through the cerebral aqueduct and into the fourth ventricle, which is located in front of the cerebellum. Circulation is aided by the pulsations of the cerebral arteries.

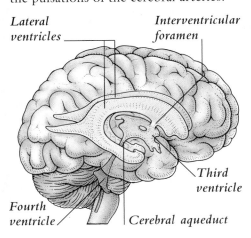

Lateral ventricles

Interventricular foramen

Fourth ventricle

Third ventricle

Cerebral aqueduct

THE MENINGES

Three membranes known as the meninges cover the brain. Lining the inside of the skull is the outermost membrane, the dura mater, which contains veins and arteries that nourish the cranial bones. The middle layer is known as the arachnoid ("spiderlike"); this consists of a type of webbed and elastic connective tissue. Next to the surface of the cerebral cortex is the pia mater; between this delicate, innermost layer and the arachnoid is the subarachnoid space, which contains cerebrospinal fluid as well as blood vessels.

Area shown enlarged

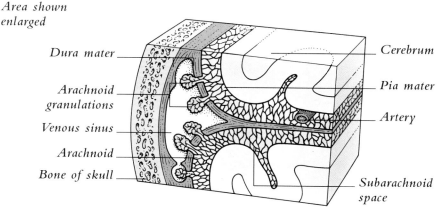

Dura mater — Cerebrum

Arachnoid granulations — Pia mater

Venous sinus — Artery

Arachnoid

Bone of skull — Subarachnoid space

BLOOD SUPPLY TO THE BRAIN

Although the brain accounts for only about 2 per cent of the total weight of the body, it requires 20 per cent of the body's blood. Both oxygen and glucose are transported by blood; without these essential elements, brain function quickly deteriorates, and dizziness, confusion, and loss of consciousness may occur. Within only 4 to 8 minutes of oxygen deprivation, brain damage or death results.

Arteries supplying blood to the brain

Two front and two back arteries join up at the base of the brain to form an arterial ring called the circle of Willis. From this point, branching blood vessels provide the brain with oxygenated blood.

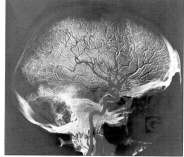

ANGIOGRAM

Blood-brain barrier

For stable brain function, the controlled flow of molecules is necessary. Endothelial cells in the capillary walls impede the flow of substances, creating an almost impermeable barrier. Capillaries are also wrapped in fibres from protective neurons (astrocytes). Oxygen, glucose, and water, which are relatively small molecules, pass through this two-layered barrier easily, but many drugs and chemicals cannot pass through at all.

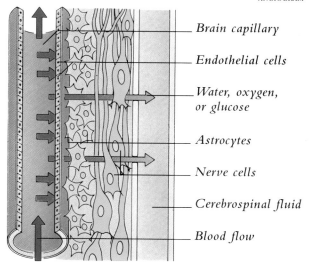

Brain capillary

Endothelial cells

Water, oxygen, or glucose

Astrocytes

Nerve cells

Cerebrospinal fluid

Blood flow

BRAIN DEVELOPMENT

Brain growth, the most important part of embryonic life, occurs much more quickly than the development and growth of the limbs or the internal organs. From small clusters of tissue, highly specialized areas of brain function emerge.

At 3 weeks
A tube of neural tissue develops along the back of the embryo. Three bulges, called the primary vesicles, develop into the main divisions of the brain.

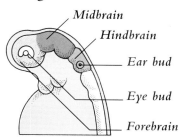

Midbrain
Hindbrain
Ear bud
Eye bud
Forebrain

At 7 weeks
The neural tube flexes, and cranial nerves sprout from the hind-brain. Bulges form on the forebrain, one of which will develop into the cerebrum.

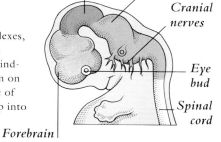

Midbrain
Hindbrain
Cranial nerves
Eye bud
Spinal cord
Forebrain

At 11 weeks
The hindbrain separates into the cerebellum, the pons, and the medulla. The forebrain develops further and the cerebrum starts to grow back over the hindbrain.

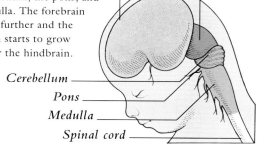

Cerebrum
Midbrain
Cerebellum
Pons
Medulla
Spinal cord

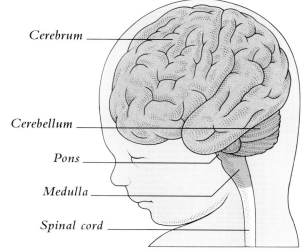

Cerebrum
Cerebellum
Pons
Medulla
Spinal cord

At birth
As the cerebrum enlarges to become the largest part of the brain, folding of the cerebral cortex occurs. Every individual human being has a unique folding pattern.

The SPINAL CORD

THE SPINAL CORD IS A CABLE about 43cm (17in) in length that descends from the brain stem to the lumbosacral part of the back. A slightly flattened cylinder, it is about as wide as a finger for most of its length, tapering to a thread-like tail. Through 31 pairs of spinal nerves, the spinal cord is connected to the rest of the body and relays information received via these nerves about its internal and external environment to and from the brain.

STRUCTURE OF THE SPINAL CORD

The spinal cord consists of two types of tissue. The inner core is grey matter made up of neuron cell bodies, unmyelinated axons, glial cells, and blood vessels. It contains cell bodies of motor neurons that bring about voluntary and reflex movements and control internal functions. Outer white matter is composed of tracts of myelinated axons that relay impulses to and from the spinal cord and specific areas of the brain.

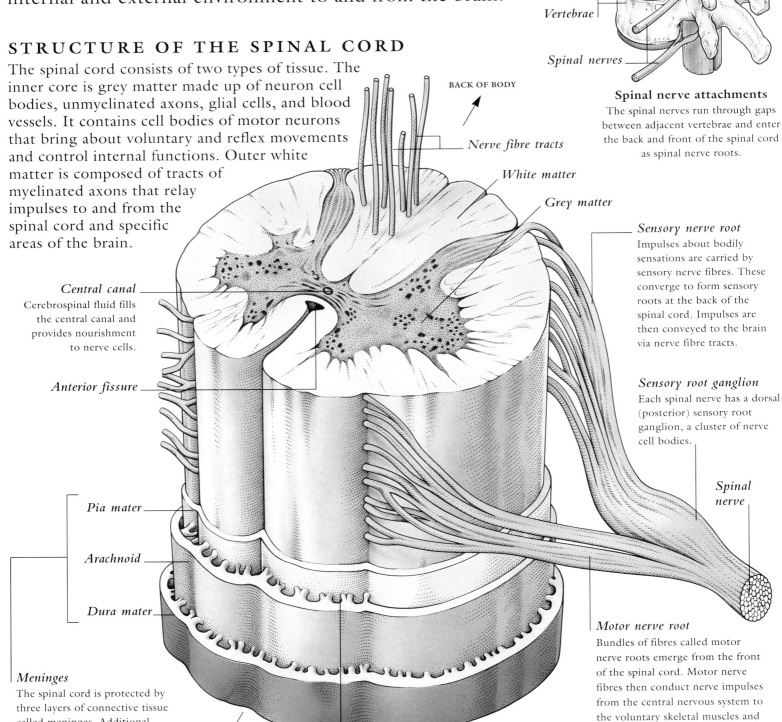

Spinal cord

Vertebrae

Spinal nerves

Spinal nerve attachments
The spinal nerves run through gaps between adjacent vertebrae and enter the back and front of the spinal cord as spinal nerve roots.

BACK OF BODY

Nerve fibre tracts

White matter

Grey matter

Central canal
Cerebrospinal fluid fills the central canal and provides nourishment to nerve cells.

Anterior fissure

Sensory nerve root
Impulses about bodily sensations are carried by sensory nerve fibres. These converge to form sensory roots at the back of the spinal cord. Impulses are then conveyed to the brain via nerve fibre tracts.

Sensory root ganglion
Each spinal nerve has a dorsal (posterior) sensory root ganglion, a cluster of nerve cell bodies.

Spinal nerve

Pia mater

Arachnoid

Dura mater

Meninges
The spinal cord is protected by three layers of connective tissue called meninges. Additional protection is provided by the cerebrospinal fluid circulating in the subarachnoid space.

FRONT OF BODY

Subarachnoid space

Motor nerve root
Bundles of fibres called motor nerve roots emerge from the front of the spinal cord. Motor nerve fibres then conduct nerve impulses from the central nervous system to the voluntary skeletal muscles and to nerves that control involuntary processes such as digestion.

PROTECTION OF THE SPINAL CORD

The spinal cord is protected primarily by the bony segments of the vertebral column and its supporting ligaments. Also protective are the circulating cerebrospinal fluid, which acts as a shock-absorber, and the epidural space, a cushioning layer of fat and connective tissue that lies in between the periosteum (the membrane that covers the vertebral bone) and the dura mater, the outer layer of the meninges.

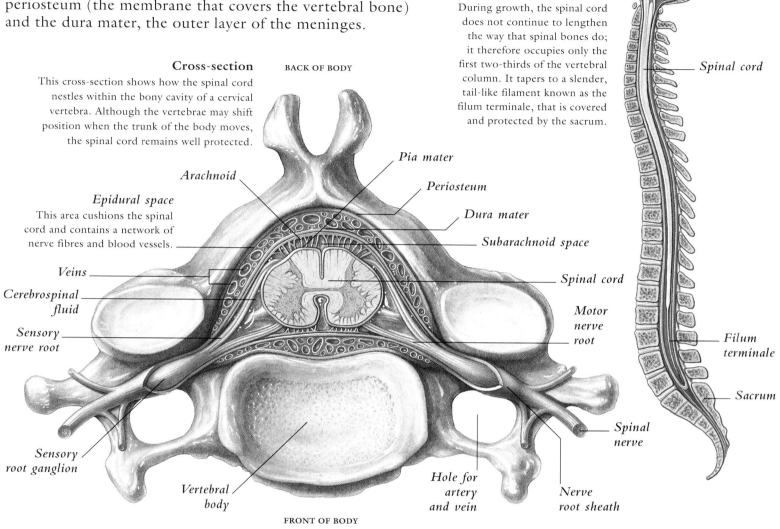

Cross-section
This cross-section shows how the spinal cord nestles within the bony cavity of a cervical vertebra. Although the vertebrae may shift position when the trunk of the body moves, the spinal cord remains well protected.

BACK OF BODY

Epidural space
This area cushions the spinal cord and contains a network of nerve fibres and blood vessels.

Arachnoid

Pia mater

Periosteum

Dura mater

Subarachnoid space

Veins

Cerebrospinal fluid

Sensory nerve root

Spinal cord

Motor nerve root

Sensory root ganglion

Vertebral body

Hole for artery and vein

Nerve root sheath

Spinal nerve

FRONT OF BODY

Extent of spinal cord
During growth, the spinal cord does not continue to lengthen the way that spinal bones do; it therefore occupies only the first two-thirds of the vertebral column. It tapers to a slender, tail-like filament known as the filum terminale, that is covered and protected by the sacrum.

Cerebrum

Skull

Cerebellum

Spinal cord

Filum terminale

Sacrum

ORGANIZATION OF GREY AND WHITE MATTER

Myelinated nerve fibres are grouped together into pathways according to the direction – whether to or from the brain – and the type of impulse they transmit and respond to, such as pain or temperature. Some of these tracts connect and relay impulses between just a few pairs of spinal nerves. Grey matter is organized into horns, also called columns.

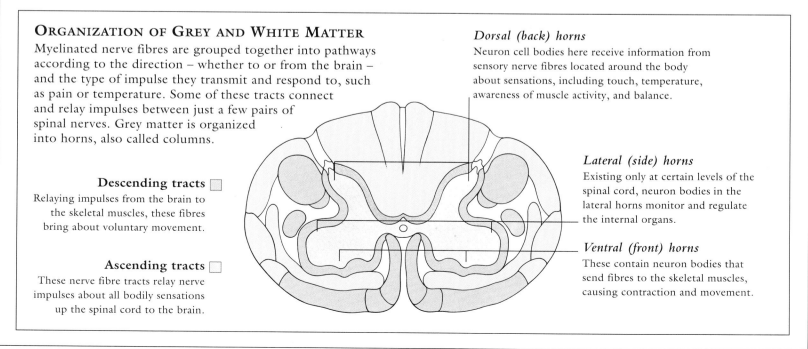

Descending tracts ☐
Relaying impulses from the brain to the skeletal muscles, these fibres bring about voluntary movement.

Ascending tracts ☐
These nerve fibre tracts relay nerve impulses about all bodily sensations up the spinal cord to the brain.

Dorsal (back) horns
Neuron cell bodies here receive information from sensory nerve fibres located around the body about sensations, including touch, temperature, awareness of muscle activity, and balance.

Lateral (side) horns
Existing only at certain levels of the spinal cord, neuron bodies in the lateral horns monitor and regulate the internal organs.

Ventral (front) horns
These contain neuron bodies that send fibres to the skeletal muscles, causing contraction and movement.

The PERIPHERAL NERVES

THE PERIPHERAL NERVES FERRY INFORMATION both to and from the brain and spinal cord. The sensory fibres in the peripheral nerves receive information from the outside world, the skin, and the internal organs, while motor fibres initiate the contraction of skeletal muscle. Autonomic nerve fibres regulate the internal organs and glands, and ensure smooth functioning.

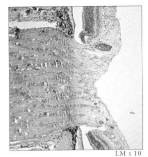

The optic nerve
The image shows the optic nerve as it enters the back of the eyeball. The white area is the vitreous humour, a gel that maintains eye shape; the deep red layer is the choroid, which is filled with blood vessels.

LM x 10

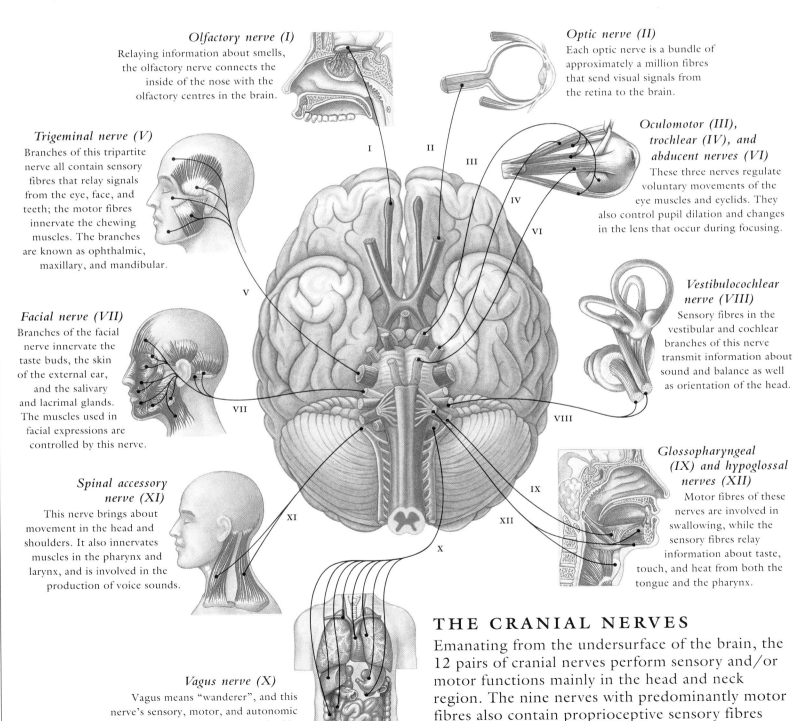

Olfactory nerve (I)
Relaying information about smells, the olfactory nerve connects the inside of the nose with the olfactory centres in the brain.

Optic nerve (II)
Each optic nerve is a bundle of approximately a million fibres that send visual signals from the retina to the brain.

Trigeminal nerve (V)
Branches of this tripartite nerve all contain sensory fibres that relay signals from the eye, face, and teeth; the motor fibres innervate the chewing muscles. The branches are known as ophthalmic, maxillary, and mandibular.

Oculomotor (III), trochlear (IV), and abducent nerves (VI)
These three nerves regulate voluntary movements of the eye muscles and eyelids. They also control pupil dilation and changes in the lens that occur during focusing.

Vestibulocochlear nerve (VIII)
Sensory fibres in the vestibular and cochlear branches of this nerve transmit information about sound and balance as well as orientation of the head.

Facial nerve (VII)
Branches of the facial nerve innervate the taste buds, the skin of the external ear, and the salivary and lacrimal glands. The muscles used in facial expressions are controlled by this nerve.

Glossopharyngeal (IX) and hypoglossal nerves (XII)
Motor fibres of these nerves are involved in swallowing, while the sensory fibres relay information about taste, touch, and heat from both the tongue and the pharynx.

Spinal accessory nerve (XI)
This nerve brings about movement in the head and shoulders. It also innervates muscles in the pharynx and larynx, and is involved in the production of voice sounds.

Vagus nerve (X)
Vagus means "wanderer", and this nerve's sensory, motor, and autonomic fibres are involved in many vital bodily functions, including heartbeat and the formation of stomach acid.

THE CRANIAL NERVES

Emanating from the undersurface of the brain, the 12 pairs of cranial nerves perform sensory and/or motor functions mainly in the head and neck region. The nine nerves with predominantly motor fibres also contain proprioceptive sensory fibres that convey information about the tension of the muscles they serve to the central nervous system.

THE SPINAL NERVES

The 31 pairs of peripheral spinal nerves emerge from the spinal cord and extend through spaces between the vertebrae. Each nerve divides and subdivides into a number of branches; two main subdivisions serve the front and the back of the body in the region innervated by that particular nerve. The branches of one spinal nerve may join up with other nerves to form plexuses ("braids"); these innervate certain areas of complex function or movement, such as the shoulder and neck.

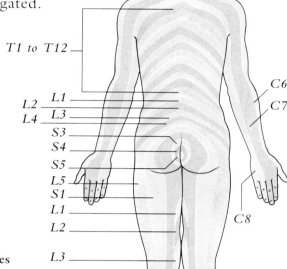

Cervical region (C1 to C8)
The eight pairs of cervical spinal nerves interconnect, forming two networks, the cervical plexus (C1 to C4) and the brachial plexus (C5 to C8 and T1). These innervate the back of the head, the neck, shoulders, arms and hands, as well as the diaphragm.

Thoracic region (T1 to T12)
Apart from T1, which is considered part of the brachial plexus, thoracic spinal nerves are directly connected to the muscles between the ribs, the deep back muscles, and regions of the abdomen.

Lumbar region (L1 to L5)
Four of the five pairs of lumbar spinal nerves (L1 to L4) form the lumbar plexus, which supplies the lower back as well as parts of the thighs and legs. L4 and L5 also interconnect with the first four of the sacral nerves (S1 to S4).

Sacral region (S1 to S5)
Two nerve networks, the sacral plexus (L5 to S3) and the coccygeal plexus (S4, S5, and the coccygeal nerve, Co1), innervate the thighs, the buttocks, the muscles and skin of the legs and feet, and the anal and genital area.

AREAS OF SENSATION

It is possible to create a map that delineates the surface skin into zones, called dermatomes, that are served by specific spinal nerves. Neurologists use pinpricks to identify sites of neural damage; lack of sensation in a particular area may reveal damage far removed from the area being investigated.

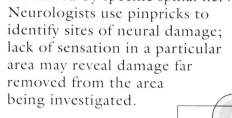

The dermatomes
The dermatomes in the trunk – each served by its own specific pair of spinal nerves – appear roughly horizontal on a schematic "map", while those in the limbs are longitudinal. In real life, the distribution of nerve roots, and thus of sensation, overlaps slightly.

SPINAL REFLEX
A reflex is an involuntary and predictable response to a stimulus. The patellar spinal reflex measures the function of the spine's neural pathways. Tapping the patellar tendon stretches the front thigh muscle, stimulating a sensory neuron that transmits a nerve signal to the spinal cord. Motor nerve fibres then relay the signal to the muscle, which contracts and causes a slight kick.

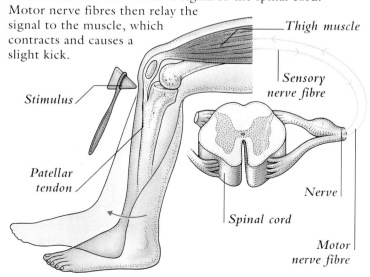

The AUTONOMIC NERVOUS SYSTEM

STRUCTURED TO PROVIDE INVOLUNTARY RESPONSES, both immediate and longer-term, the autonomic nervous system (ANS) regulates body functions to maintain homeostasis (consistency of internal chemistry). Nerve fibres monitor the organs and internal activities, such as heart rate. This information is integrated in the hypothalamus, brain stem, or spinal cord. The two divisions of the ANS – the sympathetic and the parasympathetic – then send commands to involuntary smooth muscles of many organs, blood vessels, and glands, and to heart muscle.

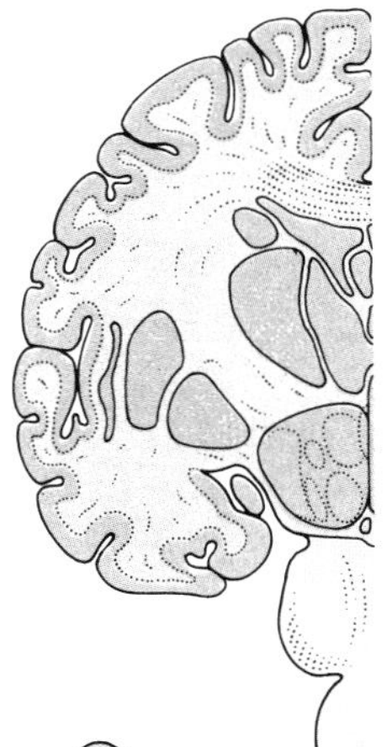

THE TWO DIVISIONS

The sympathetic division is principally an excitatory system that prepares the body for stress. The parasympathetic division maintains or restores energy. Although both divisions innervate many organs and structures, the number and position of ganglia – clusters of nerve cells where axons communicate in a synapse – are different. The activating chemicals, called neurotransmitters, and their effects are also different.

GUIDE TO ILLUSTRATION

The two divisions of the autonomic nervous system connect to both sides of the spinal cord; for clarity, the illustration shows one division on each side. Only skin and blood vessels are innervated at all levels. More details of neural organization are explained in the box, Pathway Structures, on the facing page.

KEY

�	Sympathetic division
☐	Parasympathetic division
——	Preganglionic axon
- - -	Postganglionic axon
•—	Synapse
⊸	Terminal ganglion
⊙	Collateral ganglion

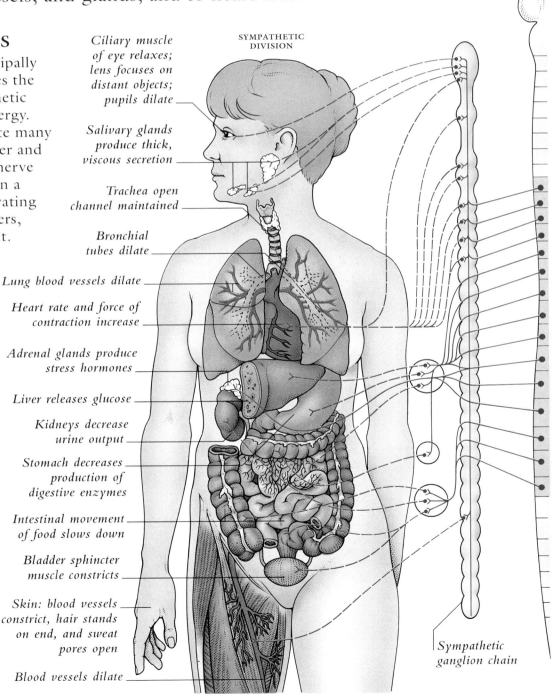

SYMPATHETIC DIVISION

Ciliary muscle of eye relaxes; lens focuses on distant objects; pupils dilate

Salivary glands produce thick, viscous secretion

Trachea open channel maintained

Bronchial tubes dilate

Lung blood vessels dilate

Heart rate and force of contraction increase

Adrenal glands produce stress hormones

Liver releases glucose

Kidneys decrease urine output

Stomach decreases production of digestive enzymes

Intestinal movement of food slows down

Bladder sphincter muscle constricts

Skin: blood vessels constrict, hair stands on end, and sweat pores open

Blood vessels dilate

Sympathetic ganglion chain

PATHWAY STRUCTURES

In the sympathetic division, ganglia are located some distance from their target organs. Many are linked in a chain near the spinal cord. In the parasympathetic division, ganglia lie close to or within the organs.

Preganglionic axon   Postganglionic axon

Sympathetic ganglion chain

Visceral organ (urinary bladder)

SYMPATHETIC

PARASYMPATHETIC

Collateral ganglion

Smooth muscle cell

Terminal ganglion

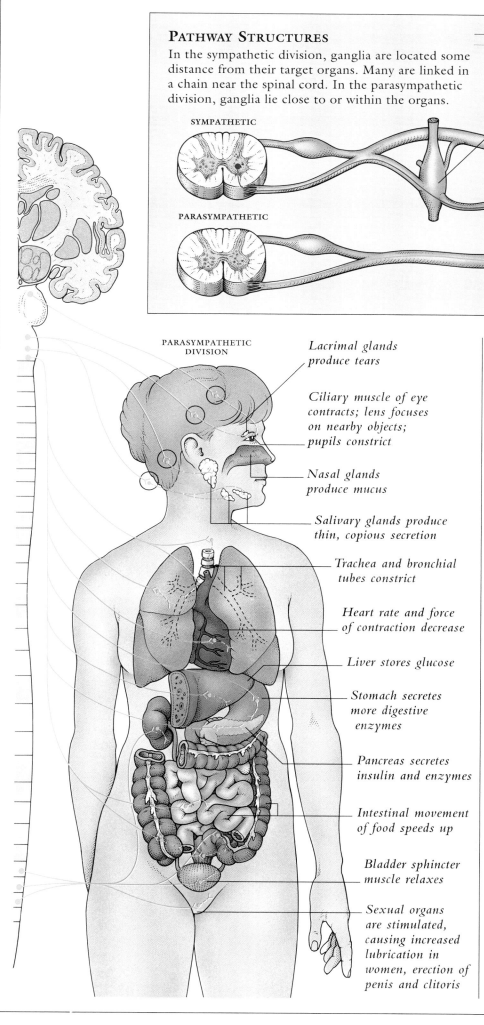

PARASYMPATHETIC DIVISION

Lacrimal glands produce tears

Ciliary muscle of eye contracts; lens focuses on nearby objects; pupils constrict

Nasal glands produce mucus

Salivary glands produce thin, copious secretion

Trachea and bronchial tubes constrict

Heart rate and force of contraction decrease

Liver stores glucose

Stomach secretes more digestive enzymes

Pancreas secretes insulin and enzymes

Intestinal movement of food speeds up

Bladder sphincter muscle relaxes

Sexual organs are stimulated, causing increased lubrication in women, erection of penis and clitoris

COORDINATION OF RESPONSE

In the eyes, involuntary changes in the size of the pupils occur constantly. Smooth muscle fibres in the irises are arranged concentrically in one band and radially in another, and each is innervated by either sympathetic and parasympathetic nerve fibres. Sensory receptors in the eyes respond to light and to the proximity or distance of objects. Nerve signals travel to the brain. A response is relayed back from the brain, and one or the other set of muscles constricts to adjust pupil size.

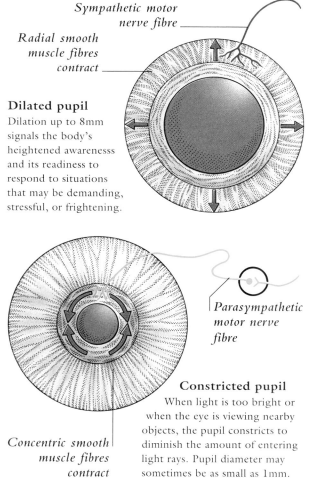

Sympathetic motor nerve fibre

Radial smooth muscle fibres contract

Dilated pupil
Dilation up to 8mm signals the body's heightened awarenesss and its readiness to respond to situations that may be demanding, stressful, or frightening.

Parasympathetic motor nerve fibre

Concentric smooth muscle fibres contract

Constricted pupil
When light is too bright or when the eye is viewing nearby objects, the pupil constricts to diminish the amount of entering light rays. Pupil diameter may sometimes be as small as 1mm.

The PRIMITIVE BRAIN

THE LIMBIC SYSTEM EVOLVED EARLY IN HUMAN ANCESTRY, and influences unconscious, instinctive behaviour similar to animal responses that relate to survival, such as the "fight-or-flight" response and reproduction. In humans, many of these innate, "primitive" behaviours are modified by the cerebral cortex. Humans plan for the future, feel hope, joy, and remorse, and their behaviour is influenced by conscious moral, social, and cultural codes.

PARTS OF THE LIMBIC SYSTEM

The components of this ring-shaped system play a complex and important role in the expression of instincts, drives, and emotions. They mediate the effects of moods on external behaviour, and influence internal changes in bodily function and their appropriate expression. The association of feelings with sensations, such as smell and sight, and the formation of memories are also influenced by the limbic system.

Cingulate gyrus

Corpus callosum

Thalamus

Location of the limbic system
The limbic system encircles the top of the brain stem and forms a border (the meaning of "limbic") linking cortical and midbrain areas with lower centres that control automatic, internal body functions.

Cingulate gyrus
This area, together with the parahippocampal gyrus and the olfactory bulbs, comprises the limbic cortex, which modifies behaviour and emotions.

Fornix
The fornix is a pathway of nerve fibres that transmits information from the hippocampus and other limbic areas to the mamillary body.

Septum pellucidum
A thin sheet of nervous tissue connects the fornix to the corpus callosum.

Column of fornix

Mamillary body
This tiny nucleus acts as a relay station, transmitting information to and from the fornix and the thalamus.

Midbrain
Limbic areas influence physical activity via the basal ganglia, the large clusters of nerve cell bodies below the cortex. Limbic midbrain areas also connect to the cortex and to the thalamus.

Pons

Olfactory bulbs
The connection of these structures with the limbic system helps explain why the sense of smell evokes strong memories and emotional responses.

Amygdala
This structure influences behaviour and activities so that they are appropriate for meeting the body's internal needs. These include feeding, sexual interest, and emotional reactions such as anger.

Parahippocampal gyrus
With other structures, this area helps modify the expression of emotions such as rage and fright.

Hippocampus
This curved band of grey matter is involved with learning, the recognition that something is new, and memory, especially of a physical, three-dimensional kind.

THE HYPOTHALAMUS

The hypothalamus is composed of numerous tiny clusters of nerve cells called nuclei. About the size of a lump of sugar, it is like a complex instrument panel that has links with the autonomic nervous, limbic, and endocrine systems. It can adjust consciousness, behaviour, and internal functions. Although its many functions are well understood, the specific roles played by every nucleus are not yet clear.

FUNCTIONS

Together with the lobes of the pituitary gland, the hypothalamic nuclei monitor and regulate the body's temperature, food intake, water-salt balance, blood flow, the sleep-wake cycle, and the activity of hormones. They also mediate the appropriate responses to emotions such as anger and fear.

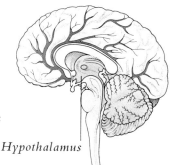

Hypothalamus

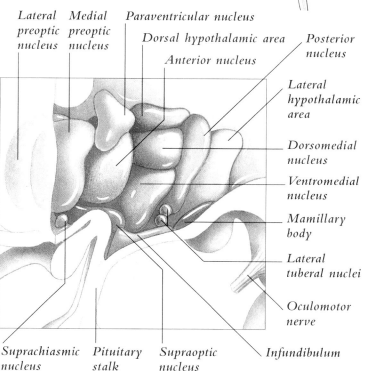

Lateral preoptic nucleus
Medial preoptic nucleus
Paraventricular nucleus
Dorsal hypothalamic area
Anterior nucleus
Posterior nucleus
Lateral hypothalamic area
Dorsomedial nucleus
Ventromedial nucleus
Mamillary body
Lateral tuberal nuclei
Oculomotor nerve
Suprachiasmic nucleus
Pituitary stalk
Supraoptic nucleus
Infundibulum

BRAIN STEM FUNCTIONS

The reticular formation, located in the brain stem, comprises at least four distinct neural systems, each with its own neurotransmitter. One of its functions is to operate an arousal system (the "reticular activating system", or RAS) that keeps the brain awake and alert. The brain stem also controls sleep, modulates spinal reflexes, maintains muscle tone and posture, and sustains breathing and heart rate.

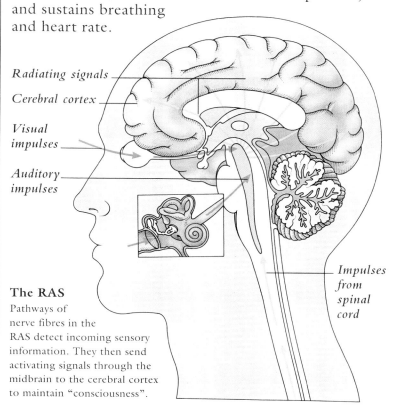

Radiating signals
Cerebral cortex
Visual impulses
Auditory impulses
Impulses from spinal cord

The RAS

Pathways of nerve fibres in the RAS detect incoming sensory information. They then send activating signals through the midbrain to the cerebral cortex to maintain "consciousness".

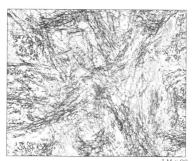

LM x 90

Nerve fibres in the pons

Tissue taken from the pons reveals the great complexity of the reticular formation. This upper part of the brain stem helps regulate breathing, and is involved in reflexes, such as pupil constriction and balance, that are mediated by the fifth, sixth, seventh, and eighth cranial nerves.

SLEEP

Nerve cells in the brain do not rest; instead, in a typical 7- or 8-hour sleep period, they carry out different activities than those that occur during waking hours. Distinctive patterns of non-rapid eye movement (NREM) as well as rapid eye movement (REM) sleep, when most dreams occur, can be detected by recording the electrical activity of the brain. As sleep deepens, body temperature drops, breathing rate slows, and blood pressure is reduced.

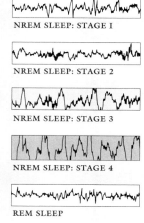

NREM SLEEP: STAGE I

NREM SLEEP: STAGE 2

NREM SLEEP: STAGE 3

NREM SLEEP: STAGE 4

REM SLEEP

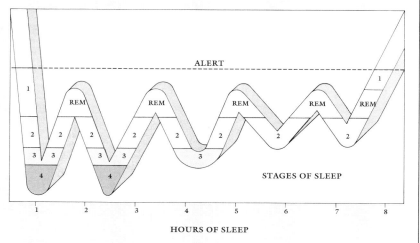

ALERT

REM REM REM REM REM

STAGES OF SLEEP

HOURS OF SLEEP

INFORMATION PROCESSING

THE INFORMATION RECEIVED FROM THE SENSES or generated by
thought is processed in many parts of the brain. Some areas process
sensory data, such as light or sound, while others issue commands
that initiate or coordinate voluntary movements. Other areas file
away important data for future use. All these areas are connected by
bundles of nerve fibres. While the functions
of the individual areas have been clearly
defined, the precise details of their
intercommunication are still not
completely understood.

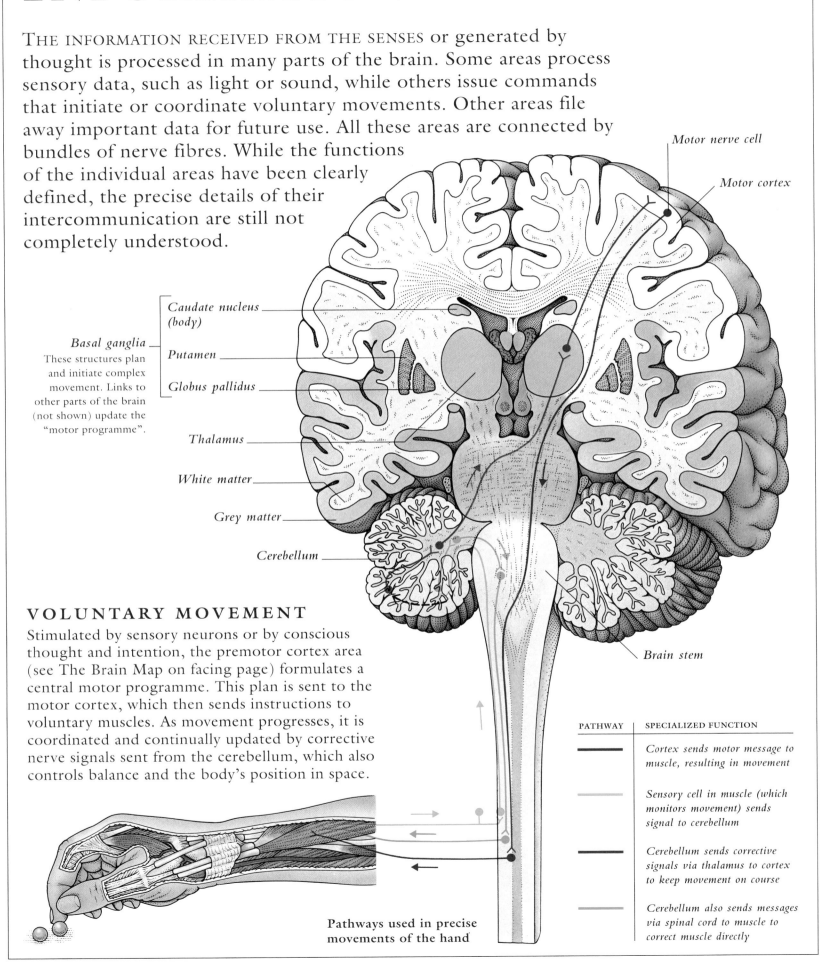

Motor nerve cell

Motor cortex

Caudate nucleus
(body)

Basal ganglia
These structures plan
and initiate complex
movement. Links to
other parts of the brain
(not shown) update the
"motor programme".

Putamen

Globus pallidus

Thalamus

White matter

Grey matter

Cerebellum

Brain stem

VOLUNTARY MOVEMENT

Stimulated by sensory neurons or by conscious
thought and intention, the premotor cortex area
(see The Brain Map on facing page) formulates a
central motor programme. This plan is sent to the
motor cortex, which then sends instructions to
voluntary muscles. As movement progresses, it is
coordinated and continually updated by corrective
nerve signals sent from the cerebellum, which also
controls balance and the body's position in space.

PATHWAY	SPECIALIZED FUNCTION
——	*Cortex sends motor message to muscle, resulting in movement*
——	*Sensory cell in muscle (which monitors movement) sends signal to cerebellum*
——	*Cerebellum sends corrective signals via thalamus to cortex to keep movement on course*
——	*Cerebellum also sends messages via spinal cord to muscle to correct muscle directly*

**Pathways used in precise
movements of the hand**

THE BRAIN MAP

Scientists mapped the cortex into specific functional areas by observing the effects of damage to or removal of certain parts of the brain, or by direct stimulation using electrodes. They also found that large parts of the cortex are taken up by "association areas". These analyze and interpret neural information received from the primary sensory areas, and help to plan and coordinate voluntary movements.

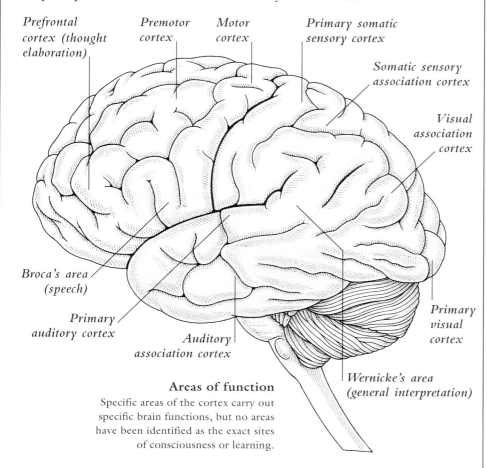

Prefrontal cortex (thought elaboration)

Premotor cortex

Motor cortex

Primary somatic sensory cortex

Somatic sensory association cortex

Visual association cortex

Broca's area (speech)

Primary auditory cortex

Auditory association cortex

Primary visual cortex

Wernicke's area (general interpretation)

Areas of function
Specific areas of the cortex carry out specific brain functions, but no areas have been identified as the exact sites of consciousness or learning.

GLUCOSE AND BRAIN ACTIVITY

An increase in glucose metabolism reliably indicates intense brain activity. A chemical that binds to glucose molecules is injected into volunteers; scans are subsequently taken as they perform various tasks or are exposed to sensory stimuli such as music or images. These scans reveal the specific areas of activity, which are shown in red in the images below.

Visual stimulation
When the eyes are closed (left) or open (centre), or when a complex scene is observed (right), the level of activity in the brain differs markedly.

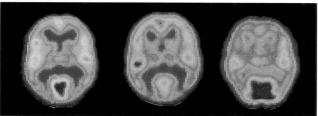

PET SCANS

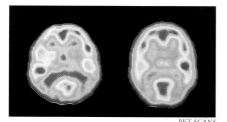

PET SCANS

Musical appreciation
When listening to music, trained musicians use the dominant, left cerebral hemisphere (left) associated with logical reasoning and sequential analysis. Untrained musicians use the right intuitive hemisphere (right), which "grasps things whole" without analysis.

MEMORY

Memories are the brain's storehouses of information, whether these are learned facts or emotionally significant events. In order to create memories, nerve cells are thought to form new protein molecules and new interconnections. No one region of the brain stores all memories because the storage site depends on the type of memory: how to type or ride a bike are memories held in motor areas, while those about music are held in the auditory areas.

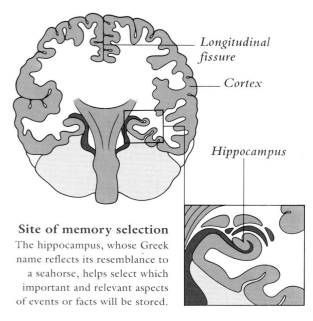

Longitudinal fissure

Cortex

Hippocampus

Site of memory selection
The hippocampus, whose Greek name reflects its resemblance to a seahorse, helps select which important and relevant aspects of events or facts will be stored.

THREE DEGREES OF MEMORY

Sensory memory, such as the brief recognition of a sound, is stored only for milliseconds. If retained and interpreted, this sensory input may become short-term memory for a few minutes. The transfer of short-term to long-term memory is known as consolidation, and requires attention, repetition, and associative ideas. How easily information is recalled depends upon how it was consolidated.

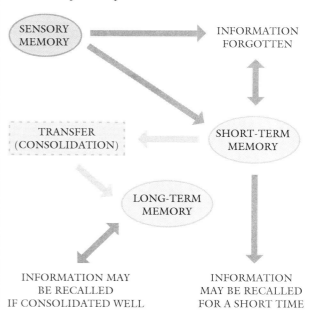

SENSORY MEMORY

INFORMATION FORGOTTEN

TRANSFER (CONSOLIDATION)

SHORT-TERM MEMORY

LONG-TERM MEMORY

INFORMATION MAY BE RECALLED IF CONSOLIDATED WELL

INFORMATION MAY BE RECALLED FOR A SHORT TIME

NEUROLOGICAL DISORDERS

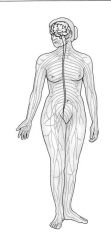

STRUCTURAL, BIOCHEMICAL, OR ELECTRICAL CHANGES in the brain and spinal cord, or the nerves leading to or from them, may cause disorders that result in paralysis, weakness, poor coordination, seizures, or loss of sensation. The introduction of scanners has brought rapid advances in diagnosis; increased understanding of brain function has generated improvements in treatment. However, some common disorders are due to conditions that are difficult to reverse. All that can be offered those affected is some relief of symptoms.

EPILEPSY

One person in 200 is affected by the repeated seizures of epilepsy. These episodes of uncontrolled, chaotic electrical activity in the brain alter consciousness and may induce involuntary movements. Often the cause is unknown, but epilepsy that first appears in adult life may be due to a brain condition such as a tumour or abscess, a head injury, stroke, or a chemical imbalance.

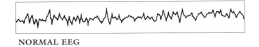

NORMAL EEG

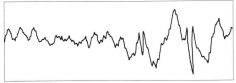

EEG DURING A SIMPLE PARTIAL SEIZURE

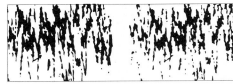

EEG DURING GRAND MAL SEIZURE

Types of seizure

In a grand mal seizure, the victim falls to the ground unconscious and makes twitching movements for as long as several minutes. In a petit mal seizure, also called an absence seizure, the victim may be unaware of the outside world for as much as half a minute but does not fall. In a partial seizure there is rarely a full loss of consciousness.

TEMPORAL LOBE EPILEPSY

This type of partial seizure affects one of the temporal lobes. Attacks may be preceded by an aura in which the victim experiences smells or sounds that others cannot detect. There may be involuntary movements during the attack, especially chewing and sucking, and a partial loss of consciousness. The attack may also cause the victim to have irrational feelings of fear or anger.

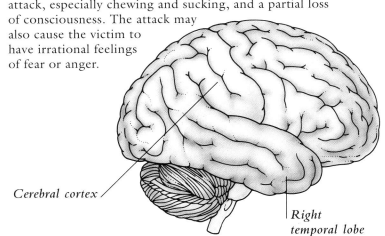

Cerebral cortex

Right temporal lobe

MULTIPLE SCLEROSIS

Multiple sclerosis (MS) is the most common disabling disorder of the nervous system affecting the young: about one in every 1000 people is affected. MS causes episodes of blurred or double vision, partial paralysis, clumsiness, and problems with walking. There may also be interference with speech or sensation. These episodes can last a few weeks and may sometimes be followed by months or years of relief from symptoms.

Sheath damage

MS is due to immune system damage to the myelin sheaths that protect nerve fibres, Macrophages, which are a type of scavenger cell, remove damaged sections of myelin, so that fibres are exposed and conduct impulses poorly or not at all.

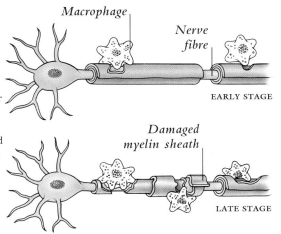

Macrophage

Nerve fibre

EARLY STAGE

Damaged myelin sheath

LATE STAGE

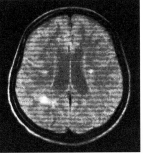

MRI SCAN

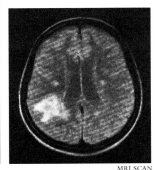

MRI SCAN

TREATMENT

Injections of corticosteroid drugs can hasten recovery during exacerbations, and physiotherapy helps relieve spastic muscle contractions. Treatment with a substance called beta interferon has been shown to prolong the intervals between relapses; other research has suggested that this treatment may help to slow the progress of the disease. Some people with MS have benefited from dietary supplements of sunflower and evening primrose oils.

Disease progression

A scan (top) taken during a study shows MS lesions as three white spots. Increased activity is shown in a scan taken 6 weeks later (bottom). Lesions usually grow as the disease progresses; this progression may be slowed by beta interferon.

PARKINSON'S DISEASE

Parkinson's disease is a degenerative condition of the brain that occurs in about one in 200 people over the age of 60. More men than women are affected. The disease causes weakness and stiffness of the muscles and interferes with speech, walking, and performance of daily tasks. Emotional responses usually prompt little change of facial expression, and there is often a tremor of the hands when they are at rest.

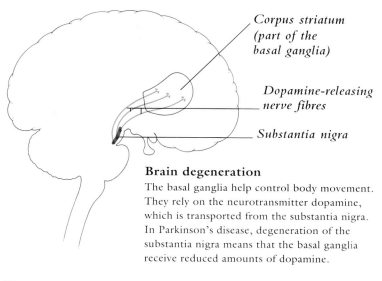

Corpus striatum (part of the basal ganglia)

Dopamine-releasing nerve fibres

Substantia nigra

Brain degeneration

The basal ganglia help control body movement. They rely on the neurotransmitter dopamine, which is transported from the substantia nigra. In Parkinson's disease, degeneration of the substantia nigra means that the basal ganglia receive reduced amounts of dopamine.

TREATMENT

The aim of treatment is to restore missing dopamine in the brain or to damp down the action of the dopamine antagonist acetylcholine. Drugs that increase dopamine levels include levodopa, selegilene, and bromocriptine. Anticholinergic drugs lower acetylcholine levels.

Normal chemical balance

In a normal brain, the levels of dopamine and acetylcholine are evenly balanced.

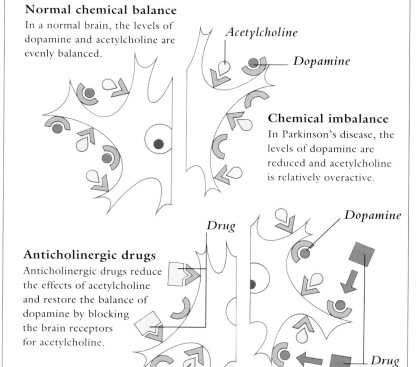

Acetylcholine

Dopamine

Chemical imbalance

In Parkinson's disease, the levels of dopamine are reduced and acetylcholine is relatively overactive.

Drug

Dopamine

Anticholinergic drugs

Anticholinergic drugs reduce the effects of acetylcholine and restore the balance of dopamine by blocking the brain receptors for acetylcholine.

Acetylcholine

Drug

Dopamine-boosting drugs

These drugs increase dopamine activity and restore a more normal balance with acetylcholine.

DEMENTIA

About a fifth of people over the age of 80 show the symptoms of dementia, including a loss of memory for recent events, neglect of appearance, and repeated questions while ignoring replies or answers. In the later stages, victims may become bedridden and also incontinent. In one rare type of Alzheimer's disease, symptoms of dementia may appear as early as age 60.

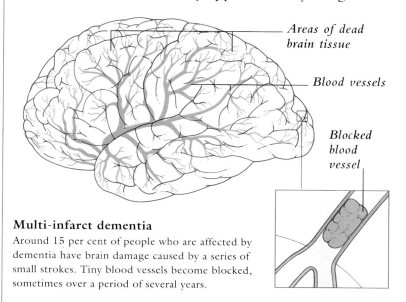

Areas of dead brain tissue

Blood vessels

Blocked blood vessel

Multi-infarct dementia

Around 15 per cent of people who are affected by dementia have brain damage caused by a series of small strokes. Tiny blood vessels become blocked, sometimes over a period of several years.

ALZHEIMER'S DISEASE

Around 55 per cent of dementia cases are the result of early or late-onset Alzheimer's disease. Each type has a different genetic cause, but in both cases brain damage occurs due to the abnormal production of the protein amyloid. No cure has been found yet, but drugs such as tacrine slow the progress of the disease in some patients.

Senile plaque

Brain tissue taken from a person afflicted with Alzheimer's disease reveals a deposit of a protein called amyloid (at centre), which is a typical feature of the disease. Another main feature is the presence of tangles of filaments within nerve cells.

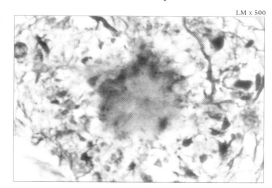

LM x 500

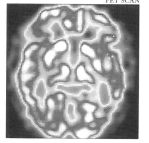

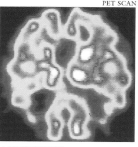

PET SCAN

PET SCAN

NORMAL

ALZHEIMER'S

Decreased brain activity

PET scanning shows how much energy is being used by brain cells. The scan of a patient with Alzheimer's shows substantially lower activity than a normal brain. Yellow represents highest activity and blue the lowest.

CEREBROVASCULAR DISORDERS

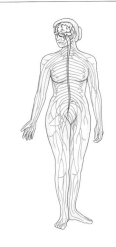

THE TERM CEREBROVASCULAR DISORDERS covers any problem that affects the blood vessels supplying the brain. Stroke is the most serious consequence of such disorders: around one-third of victims die, one-third are left with some disability, and one-third make a good recovery. Migraine is another disorder of the blood vessels but it does not cause any permanent loss of function.

THE CAUSES OF A STROKE

A stroke may be caused by a disruption to the brain's blood supply or by leakage of blood onto the brain's surface or deep within its tissue. Any disruption of blood supply to the brain starves some of the nerve cells of oxygen and nutrients. These affected cells are unable to communicate with parts of the body they serve, which results in a temporary or permanent loss of function. Leakage of blood impairs normal functioning of the brain by compressing and irritating tissue.

Blockage of tiny vessels
Prolonged high blood pressure or diabetes may damage some of the tiny blood vessels that penetrate deep within the brain. This may lead to localized blockages known as lacunar strokes that sometimes result in a form of dementia.

Thrombus
A build-up of fatty deposits within artery walls, called atherosclerosis, narrows the vessel and may encourage formation of a blood clot, or thrombus. If a thrombus blocks off an artery to the brain, a stroke follows as oxygen-starved brain tissue is damaged or even dies.

Embolus
The blockage of a cerebral artery, resulting in stroke, can be caused by a fragment of material that has travelled through the bloodstream and lodged in the vessel. Such a fragment, called an embolus, may be a piece of a clot from atherosclerotic neck arteries or from the heart lining.

Branches of the anterior cerebral artery

Posterior cerebral artery

Basilar artery

External carotid artery

Internal carotid artery

Vertebral artery

Common carotid artery

BLEEDING WITHIN BRAIN TISSUE

Bleeding within the brain, an intracerebral haemorrhage, is a main cause of stroke in older people who have hypertension. High blood pressure may put extra strain on small arteries in the brain, which causes them to balloon out and rupture.

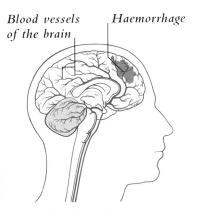

Blood vessels of the brain   *Haemorrhage*

Sudden bleeding
An intracerebral haemorrhage occurs suddenly. Headache and vomiting are common initial signs. These may be followed by progressive paralysis and a decline in consciousness.

CT SCAN

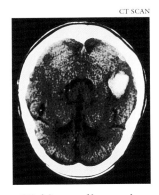

Making a diagnosis
A brain scan is essential in order to distinguish between a stroke caused by thrombosis and one caused by haemorrhage, because symptoms may be similar. Bleeding appears as a yellow patch in the image above.

STROKES IN YOUNGER PEOPLE

Whereas strokes in older people are usually associated with advanced atherosclerosis or prolonged high blood pressure, in young people they are more likely to result from the leakage of blood due to arterial defects present from birth. In the majority of such cases, leakage occurs into the subarachnoid space, the area between the pia mater and the arachnoid layers of the meninges, the protective membranes covering the brain.

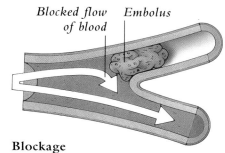

CT SCAN

Subarachnoid haemorrhage

The image seen at right reveals a subarachnoid haemorrhage (yellow) in the right frontal lobe. Bleeding was caused by the rupturing of a berry aneurysm (see below).

CONGENITAL CAUSES OF SUBARACHNOID HAEMORRHAGE

The most common congenital condition leading to subarachnoid haemorrhage is the presence of berry aneurysms. These berry-like swellings of cerebral arteries are weak points and can rupture spontaneously. Malformed connections between cerebral blood vessels, from which blood can leak, are the other important congenital cause of subarachnoid haemorrhage. Such malformations are twice as common in men as in women.

Berry aneurysm

A berry aneurysm usually forms at arterial bifurcations, often on the circle of Willis (the blood vessels at the base of the brain). Bleeding from a ruptured aneurysm can be halted by placing a clip around the neck of the aneurysm to seal it.

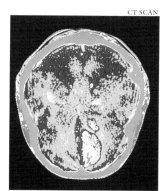

Neck of aneurysm

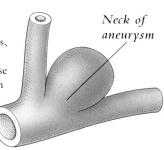

Capillaries

Arteriole

Venule

NORMAL

ABNORMAL

Arteriovenous malformation

This congenital defect is a tangle of blood vessels. Fewer capillary connections than normal exist between arterioles and venules. An increase in pressure results, which may cause blood to leak from the vessels into the subarachnoid space.

TRANSIENT ISCHAEMIC ATTACK

A transient ischaemic attack (TIA) temporarily interrupts the blood supply to the brain, resulting in stroke-like symptoms usually lasting 2 to 30 minutes but not more than 24 hours. The cause is usually an embolus, a tiny blood clot or a lipid fragment from elsewhere in the body. Up to one-third of TIA sufferers undergo a major stroke within 5 years if not treated.

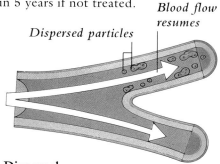

Blocked flow of blood — *Embolus*

Dispersed particles — *Blood flow resumes*

Blockage

An embolus lodging in a cerebral artery deprives part of the brain of oxygenated blood. If the front part of the brain is affected, a stroke is more likely later.

Dispersal

As normal blood flow breaks up and disperses the blood clot, oxygenated blood again reaches the starved section of the brain and symptoms disappear.

MIGRAINE

Migraine headaches are a recurring problem for 5 to 10 per cent of the population. The condition takes several different forms, with symptoms such as pain, dizziness, and visual disturbances, often accompanied by nausea and sometimes vomiting. Complicated migraine attacks can disturb brain function. The symptoms of migraine are linked with changes in the diameter of blood vessels.

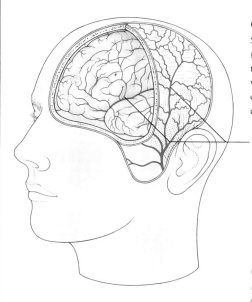

Onset of migraine attack

Some foods, red wine, stress, and drugs (such as the contraceptive pill) can be the triggers that cause the narrowing of blood vessels in the scalp and brain. This may cause the victim to see flashing lights and experience temporary areas of blindness.

Constricted blood vessels

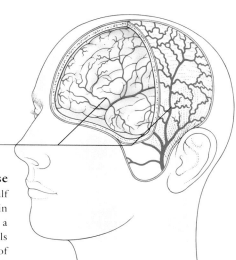

Dilated blood vessels

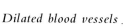

Headache phase

Severe, throbbing pain may affect half or all of the head as blood vessels in the scalp and brain widen. Serotonin, a neurotransmitter released by nerve cells in the brain, controls the diameter of blood vessels. Antimigraine drugs block the effects of serotonin in the brain.

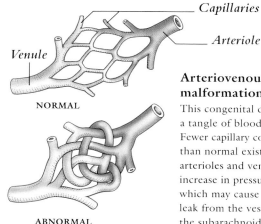

NEUROLOGICAL INFECTIONS, TUMOURS, *and* INJURIES

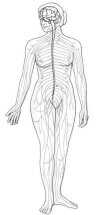

INJURIES AND DISORDERS AFFECTING THE BRAIN and nervous system can result in both physical and mental disabilities. Because the skull is a closed box, any swelling within the brain raises pressure. This can cause damage to vital nerve tissue, with some loss of bodily control and function. Spinal injuries can cause serious harm to nerve tracts, which may result in sensory loss or paralysis.

BRAIN INFECTIONS

A wide variety of viruses, bacteria, and tropical parasites can infect the brain. Some viral and parasitic brain infections are due to mosquito or other insect bites, while others develop from general infectious diseases such as mumps and measles. In many countries, immunization on a wide scale has helped to reduce the threat of viral infection affecting the brain.

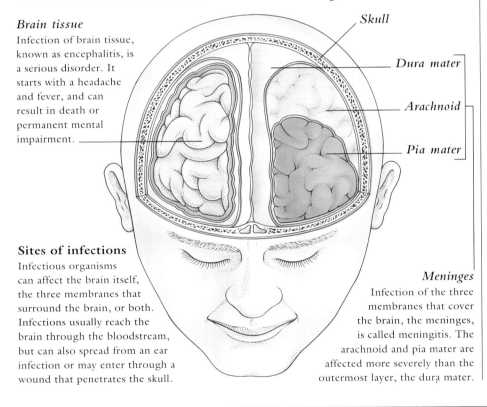

Brain tissue
Infection of brain tissue, known as encephalitis, is a serious disorder. It starts with a headache and fever, and can result in death or permanent mental impairment.

Skull

Dura mater

Arachnoid

Pia mater

Sites of infections
Infectious organisms can affect the brain itself, the three membranes that surround the brain, or both. Infections usually reach the brain through the bloodstream, but can also spread from an ear infection or may enter through a wound that penetrates the skull.

Meninges
Infection of the three membranes that cover the brain, the meninges, is called meningitis. The arachnoid and pia mater are affected more severely than the outermost layer, the dura mater.

BRAIN ABSCESSES AND TUMOURS

Both abscesses and tumours can develop inside the skull, either on the surface of the brain or within its tissue. Techniques such as CT and MRI scanning are used to identify the site of the abnormality as well as to determine its size. Certain tumours can be treated surgically; abscesses can be drained or, if recurrence is a risk, cut out, and subsequently treated with antibiotics.

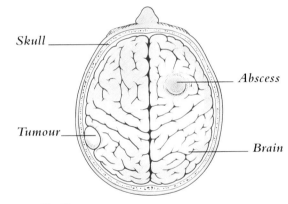

Skull

Abscess

Tumour

Brain

Similar symptoms
Abscesses and tumours both cause increased pressure inside the skull and produce similar symptoms, such as headaches, vomiting, muscle weakness, visual defects, and speech disorders.

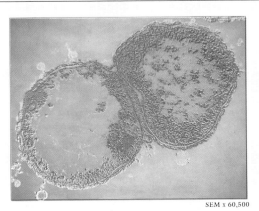

SEM x 60,500

MENINGITIS

Viral meningitis causes headache, drowsiness, and flu-like symptoms lasting a week or two, which resolve without specific treatment. It tends to occur in winter epidemics. Bacterial meningitis is much more serious and may be fatal. In parts of the world where tuberculosis is prevalent, tuberculous meningitis occurs.

Bacterial cause
Neisseria meningitidis organisms (shown left) are one cause of bacterial meningitis.

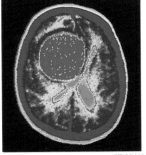

CT SCAN

Brain tumour
A tumour may be either malignant (or cancerous) or benign (non-cancerous). The large round area in the image is a glioma, a type of malignant tumour that arises from glial cells. The tumour grew slowly over a number of years.

HEAD INJURIES

Accidents and assaults causing blows or wounds to the head can have extremely serious consequences. If both the scalp and skull are penetrated, there may be damage to the brain and a high risk of infection. Such an injury must be treated urgently by a neurosurgeon to remove any foreign matter, clean the opening thoroughly, and repair the wound.

CLOSED HEAD INJURIES

Closed head injuries that do not open the skull may result from a fall or blow to the head. These injuries often cause a brief loss of consciousness and sometimes impaired brain function that may last for only a few minutes or for several hours. More serious injuries can cut or bruise the brain.

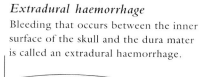

KEY

➡ *Direction of movement*

◻ *Stationary*

✦ *Blow to the head*

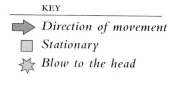

Deceleration

When a rapidly moving person is stopped suddenly, as in a fall, the brain may be injured as it smashes against the hard inner surface of the skull. It can then rebound to strike against the opposite inner skull surface.

Acceleration

If a stationary head is suddenly struck, as in boxing, the brain may be compressed against the inside of the skull near to the place of impact. The brain may then bounce off the opposite inner surface of the skull.

BLEEDING WITHIN THE SKULL

Closed head injuries can sometimes be fatal when internal bleeding occurs and is undetected. There may be no immediate symptoms, but drowsiness, a headache, confusion, as well as a noticeable change in personality may appear gradually if blood collects and forms a clot. Urgent neurosurgical treatment in hospital is needed to remove the clot, and results in immediate and dramatic relief of symptoms.

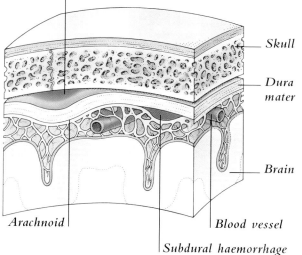

Extradural haemorrhage
Bleeding that occurs between the inner surface of the skull and the dura mater is called an extradural haemorrhage.

Skull

Dura mater

Brain

Arachnoid

Blood vessel

Subdural haemorrhage
Bleeding that occurs between the dura mater and the arachnoid is known as a subdural haemorrhage. Such bleeding may occur slowly over a long period.

PARALYSIS

Paralysis or weakness of various body areas results from damage to motor areas of the brain or neural pathways of the spinal cord. Voluntary muscle activity as well as automatic functions such as breathing may be affected, and there may be a loss of sensation. Consciousness and intellectual function are not usually affected by paralysis.

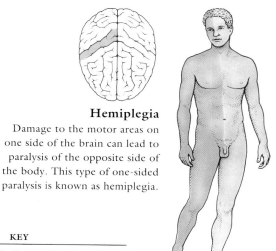

Hemiplegia

Damage to the motor areas on one side of the brain can lead to paralysis of the opposite side of the body. This type of one-sided paralysis is known as hemiplegia.

KEY

◻ *Area of body affected*

◻ *Site of damage*

Paraplegia

Damage to the middle or lower area of the spinal cord can cause paralysis of both legs and possibly part of the trunk, called paraplegia. Control of the bladder and bowel may also be affected, causing incontinence.

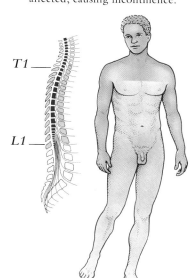

T1

L1

Quadriplegia

Damage to the spinal cord in the lower neck area can cause paralysis of the whole trunk plus arms and legs, called quadriplegia. If damage is between C1 and C2 of the spine or higher, survival is unlikely.

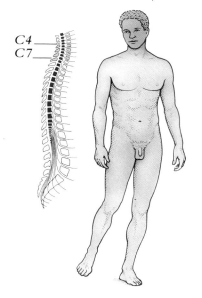

C4
C7

TOUCH, TASTE, *and* SMELL

SENSATION IS NOT ONLY OUR LINK with the outside world but also provides the body with important information about its internal environment. General sensory receptors respond to stimuli such as touch, pressure, pain, and temperature and are widespread throughout the body. Taste and smell, along with vision, hearing, and balance, are called special senses because their receptors are complex and and respond to specific stimuli at very localized sites.

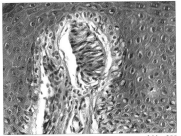

LM x 200
Meissner's corpuscle

TOUCH RECEPTORS

Touch operates by means of sensory receptors in the skin or in deeper tissues. These receptors relay signals to the spinal cord and brain stem; from there they travel to higher areas of the brain. Some receptors are enclosed in a capsule of connective tissue, while others are uncovered.

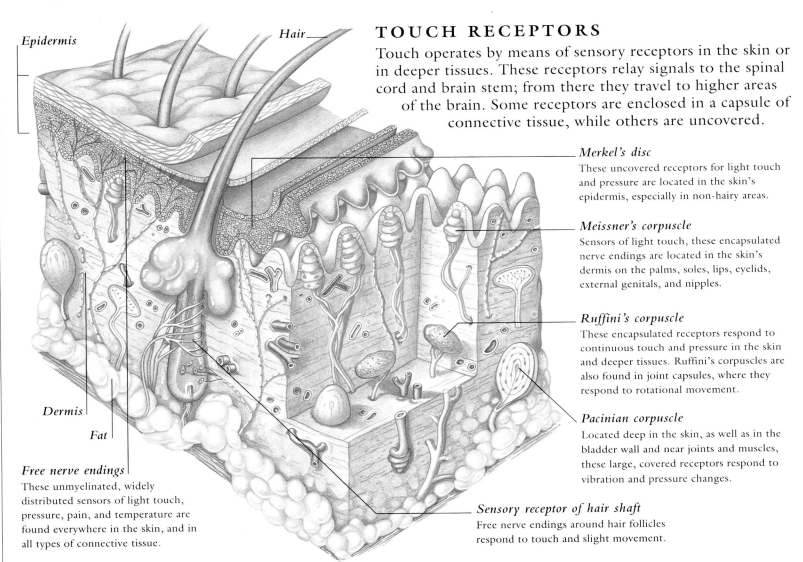

Epidermis

Hair

Dermis

Fat

Free nerve endings
These unmyelinated, widely distributed sensors of light touch, pressure, pain, and temperature are found everywhere in the skin, and in all types of connective tissue.

Merkel's disc
These uncovered receptors for light touch and pressure are located in the skin's epidermis, especially in non-hairy areas.

Meissner's corpuscle
Sensors of light touch, these encapsulated nerve endings are located in the skin's dermis on the palms, soles, lips, eyelids, external genitals, and nipples.

Ruffini's corpuscle
These encapsulated receptors respond to continuous touch and pressure in the skin and deeper tissues. Ruffini's corpuscles are also found in joint capsules, where they respond to rotational movement.

Pacinian corpuscle
Located deep in the skin, as well as in the bladder wall and near joints and muscles, these large, covered receptors respond to vibration and pressure changes.

Sensory receptor of hair shaft
Free nerve endings around hair follicles respond to touch and slight movement.

PAIN
Pain receptors are widespread, specialized free nerve endings that respond to extremes in temperature, pressure, and the chemical prostaglandin released from damaged cells. They transmit the location and intensity of the pain to the brain, and may stimulate the release of pain-blocking endorphins. Pain-relieving drugs function either by blocking prostaglandins or inhibiting pain impulses.

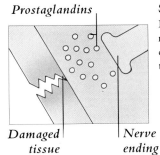

Prostaglandins

Damaged tissue

Nerve ending

Simple analgesics
Drugs such as aspirin prevent release of prostaglandins from damaged tissue, forestalling the response leading to pain.

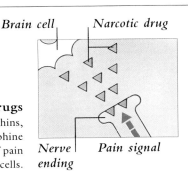

Brain cell

Narcotic drug

Narcotic drugs
Imitating body endorphins, narcotic drugs like morphine stop the transmission of pain signals between nerve cells.

Nerve ending

Pain signal

RECEPTORS FOR TASTE

Taste receptor cells, known as taste buds, are located mainly within protuberances, called papillae, on the surface of the tongue. Some taste buds are also on the palate, throat, and epiglottis. Taste buds on different parts of the tongue respond more strongly to one or other of four basic flavours – sweet, bitter, sour, and salty. More subtle taste sensations are made possible by combinations of these crude flavours along with other associated stimuli, such as odours.

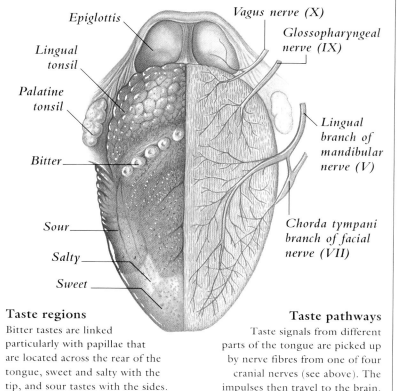

Epiglottis

Lingual tonsil

Palatine tonsil

Bitter

Sour

Salty

Sweet

Vagus nerve (X)

Glossopharyngeal nerve (IX)

Lingual branch of mandibular nerve (V)

Chorda tympani branch of facial nerve (VII)

Taste regions
Bitter tastes are linked particularly with papillae that are located across the rear of the tongue, sweet and salty with the tip, and sour tastes with the sides.

Taste pathways
Taste signals from different parts of the tongue are picked up by nerve fibres from one of four cranial nerves (see above). The impulses then travel to the brain.

TASTE BUDS

Taste buds consist of a cluster of receptor, or "taste", cells and supporting cells. Projecting from the top of a receptor cell are tiny taste hairs, which are exposed to saliva that enters through taste pores. Any substance taken into the mouth and dissolved in saliva interacts with the receptor sites on the taste hairs, generating a nerve impulse that is transmitted to the brain.

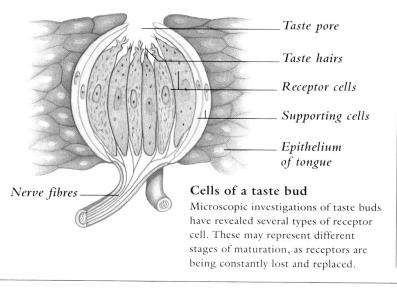

Taste pore

Taste hairs

Receptor cells

Supporting cells

Epithelium of tongue

Nerve fibres

Cells of a taste bud
Microscopic investigations of taste buds have revealed several types of receptor cell. These may represent different stages of maturation, as receptors are being constantly lost and replaced.

SMELL

The human sense of smell is much more sensitive than taste, and more than 10,000 odours can be detected. As the olfactory structures tend to deteriorate with age, children are able to distinguish more odours than adults. Most animals possess an even sharper sense of smell than humans. In addition to warning of dangers such as smoke and poisonous gases, smell makes an important contribution to the sense of taste.

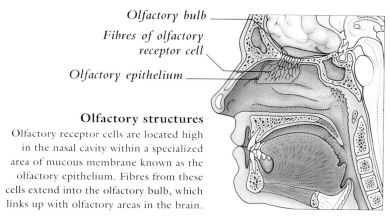

Olfactory bulb

Fibres of olfactory receptor cell

Olfactory epithelium

Olfactory structures
Olfactory receptor cells are located high in the nasal cavity within a specialized area of mucous membrane known as the olfactory epithelium. Fibres from these cells extend into the olfactory bulb, which links up with olfactory areas in the brain.

MECHANISM OF SMELL

Odour molecules entering the nose dissolve in nasal mucus and stimulate the hairlike endings (cilia) of the receptor cells, generating a nerve impulse. The impulse travels along the cells' fibres; these pass through holes in the cribriform plate of the ethmoid bone into the olfactory bulb, where they synapse with olfactory nerves.

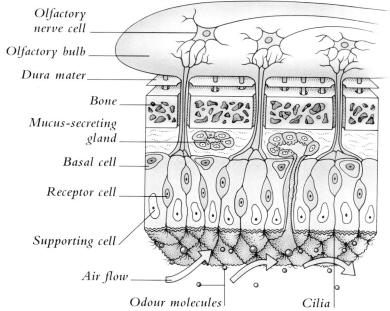

Olfactory nerve cell

Olfactory bulb

Dura mater

Bone

Mucus-secreting gland

Basal cell

Receptor cell

Supporting cell

Air flow

Odour molecules

Cilia

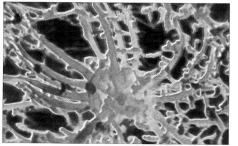

SEM x 9600

Cilia
Each olfactory receptor cell ends in a bulbous swelling called an olfactory vesicle, from which six to 20 cilia project. The image at left shows a single vesicle with numerous cilia radiating from its surface.

EAR STRUCTURE, HEARING, *and* BALANCE

THE EARS ARE ORGANS OF BOTH HEARING AND BALANCE. The structures for these sensory functions are located in separate areas of the inner ear. However, both depend on stimulation of specialized receptors called hair cells that respond to sound waves or to movement. Nerve fibres leaving the auditory and balancing structures form the vestibulocochlear nerve, which carries nerve impulses to the brain for interpretation.

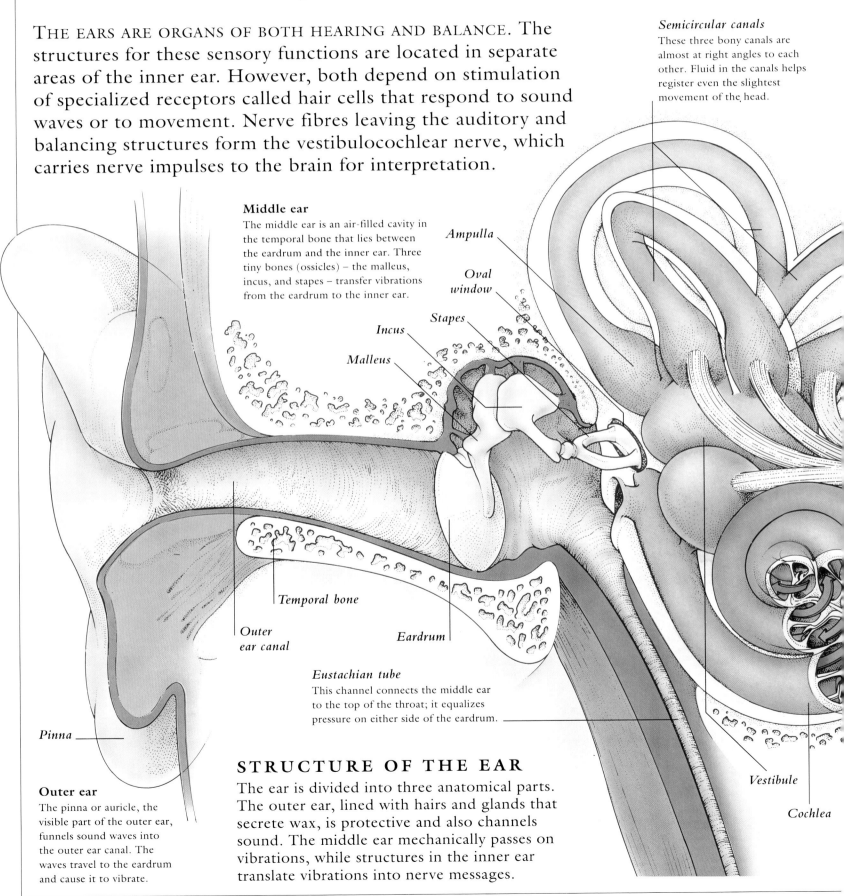

Semicircular canals
These three bony canals are almost at right angles to each other. Fluid in the canals helps register even the slightest movement of the head.

Middle ear
The middle ear is an air-filled cavity in the temporal bone that lies between the eardrum and the inner ear. Three tiny bones (ossicles) – the malleus, incus, and stapes – transfer vibrations from the eardrum to the inner ear.

Ampulla

Oval window

Stapes

Incus

Malleus

Temporal bone

Outer ear canal

Eardrum

Eustachian tube
This channel connects the middle ear to the top of the throat; it equalizes pressure on either side of the eardrum.

Pinna

Vestibule

Cochlea

Outer ear
The pinna or auricle, the visible part of the outer ear, funnels sound waves into the outer ear canal. The waves travel to the eardrum and cause it to vibrate.

STRUCTURE OF THE EAR
The ear is divided into three anatomical parts. The outer ear, lined with hairs and glands that secrete wax, is protective and also channels sound. The middle ear mechanically passes on vibrations, while structures in the inner ear translate vibrations into nerve messages.

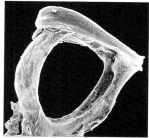

Stapes
The innermost ossicle, the stapes, is the smallest bone in the body. It closely resembles a stirrup for which it is named. It is attached to the incus by a ball-and-socket joint and, like the other two earbones, is held in place by ligaments.

SEM x 12

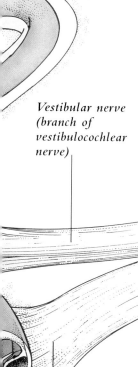

Vestibular nerve (branch of vestibulocochlear nerve)

Cochlear nerve (branch of vestibulocochlear nerve)

Inner ear
Also called the labyrinth, the inner ear consists of a complex system of membranous canals with a bony casing. The organ of hearing is located in the snail-like cochlea. The sense of balance operates from structures in the vestibule and semicircular canals.

HEARING

Sound waves entering the ear canal make the eardrum vibrate. The ossicles pass the vibrations to the oval window, a membrane at the entrance to the inner ear. When this membrane vibrates, it sets off wave-like motions in the fluid that fills the cochlea, resulting in stimulation of hair cells.

THE COCHLEA

The cochlea is subdivided into three fluid-filled chambers, which spiral in parallel around a bony core. The central channel, the cochlear duct, contains the spiral organ of Corti, the organ of hearing. Located on the basilar membrane, the spiral organ consists of supporting cells and many thousands of sensory hair cells arranged in rows.

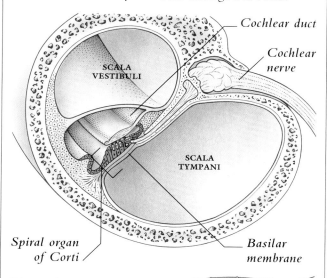

Cochlear duct

Cochlear nerve

SCALA VESTIBULI

SCALA TYMPANI

Spiral organ of Corti

Basilar membrane

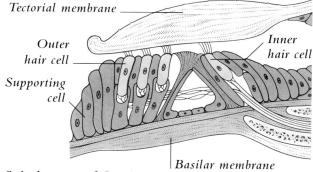

Tectorial membrane

Outer hair cell

Inner hair cell

Supporting cell

Basilar membrane

Spiral organ of Corti
From each hair cell of the spiral organ tiny sensory hairs project to make contact with the tectorial membrane above. When the basilar membrane vibrates, the hair cells are stimulated as they squash against the tectorial membrane.

Hair cells
Four rows of hair cells in the organ of Corti are shown in yellow. Each of these hair cells has up to 100 bristle-like hairs that translate mechanical movement into electrical impulses, which are transmitted directly to the brain.

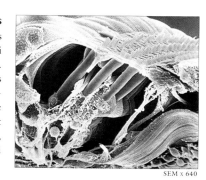

SEM x 640

BALANCE

The sense of balance relies not only on the sensory organ in the inner ear, but also on visual input and on information received from receptors in the body, especially those around joints. The information is processed by the cerebellum and cerebral cortex to enable the body to cope with changes in acceleration or direction of the head.

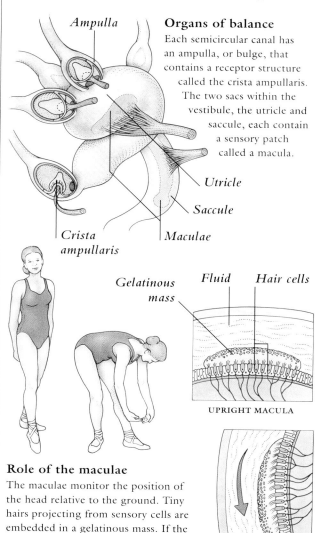

Ampulla

Organs of balance
Each semicircular canal has an ampulla, or bulge, that contains a receptor structure called the crista ampullaris. The two sacs within the vestibule, the utricle and saccule, each contain a sensory patch called a macula.

Utricle

Saccule

Crista ampullaris

Maculae

Gelatinous mass

Fluid *Hair cells*

UPRIGHT MACULA

Role of the maculae
The maculae monitor the position of the head relative to the ground. Tiny hairs projecting from sensory cells are embedded in a gelatinous mass. If the head is tipped, gravity pulls the mass down, stimulating the hair cells.

DISPLACED MACULA

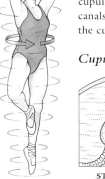

Role of the crista ampullaris
The crista ampullaris responds to rotational movements. The hair cells of each crista are embedded in a conical gelatinous mass, the cupula. When the fluid in the semicircular canals swirls during movement, it displaces the cupula, stimulating the hair cells.

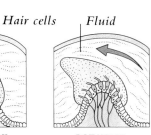

Cupula *Hair cells* *Fluid*

STATIONARY   ROTATING

EYE STRUCTURE *and* VISION

OF THE FIVE SENSES, VISION IS THE MOST SPECIALIZED and also the most complex, combining sensory reception and intellectual judgement. Light rays that enter the pupils and register on the retinas at the back of the eyes create two-dimensional images. These images are converted into electrical impulses, which are transported through the optic nerve of each eye to parts of the brain, especially the occipital lobe, where they are interpreted.

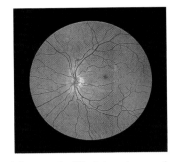

The eyeball's blood supply
The retinal artery enters the eyeball through the optic disc, known as the eye's white or "blind spot", and then branches over the retina's surface.

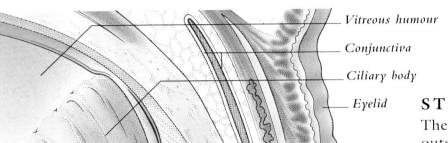

STRUCTURE OF THE EYE

The eyeball has three layers known as tunics. The outer fibrous tunic has two parts: the transparent, curved cornea, and the sclera, which is opaque, white, and helps maintain eye shape. The middle vascular tunic contains the iris, the ciliary body, and the choroid, whose blood vessels supply all the tunics. The back part of the third layer, the retina, is where light converges and images form.

THE CAVITIES OF THE EYE

The anterior and posterior chambers of the front cavity of the eye are filled with aqueous humour, a fluid providing oxgyen, glucose, and proteins. The back cavity of the eye is filled with a clear gel called vitreous humour. Produced by the ciliary body, both substances contribute to the constant internal pressure that maintains the eye's shape.

Vitreous humour
Conjunctiva
Ciliary body
Eyelid
Ligaments attached to ciliary muscle
Cornea
Lens
Iris
Choroid
Retina
Sclera

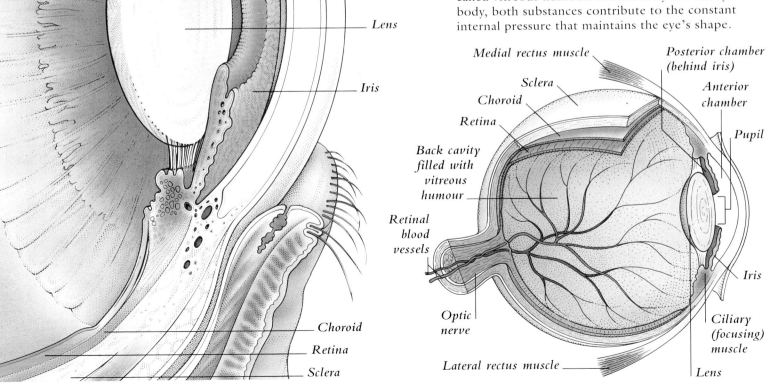

Medial rectus muscle
Posterior chamber (behind iris)
Sclera
Anterior chamber
Choroid
Retina
Pupil
Back cavity filled with vitreous humour
Retinal blood vessels
Optic nerve
Iris
Lateral rectus muscle
Ciliary (focusing) muscle
Lens

VISUAL PATHWAYS

Light passes through the cornea and lens to converge on the retina, creating an upside-down image. The medial (inner) and lateral (outer) parts of each retina transmit signals through the optic nerve; signals from the medial part of each retina intersect at the optic chiasm, which is located at the base of the brain, and cross to the opposite side of the brain. In the visual cortex, the image is turned upright and interpreted.

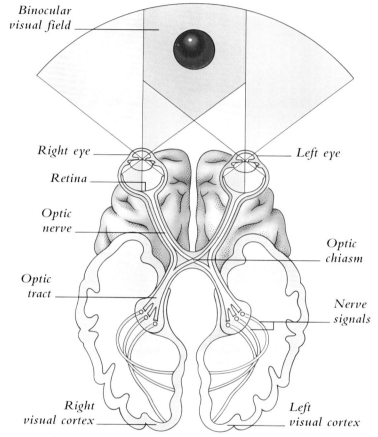

Fields of vision
Each eye sees a slightly different image, but the visual field of one eye partially overlaps the visual field of the other eye. This area of binocular vision permits depth perception – the ability to judge an object's distance.

ACCOMMODATION

The eye's ciliary muscles automatically respond to the proximity or the distance of an object by altering the shape of the lens; this changes the angle of incoming light rays and allows for sharper focus on the retina. Because the elasticity of the lens decreases as the body ages, so does the speed and power of accommodation.

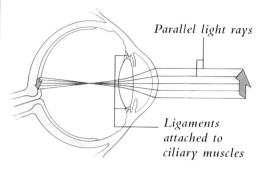

Distant object
To view an object in the distance, the ciliary muscles relax and the lens flattens and thins. Light rays are slightly refracted (bent) by the lens.

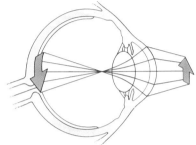

Nearby object
To view an object that is nearby, the ciliary muscles contract and the lens becomes more rounded. The point at which the image of a very close object becomes blurred is called the near point of vision; it occurs when the lens reaches its maximum curvature.

ACCESSORY STRUCTURES

The eyes depend on accessory structures that support, move, lubricate, and protect them. These include the orbital bones of the eye socket, muscles of the eyeball, eyebrows, eyelids, eyelashes as well as lacrimal (tear) glands and ducts. Vision may be impaired if any of these structures is irritated, infected, or misshapen.

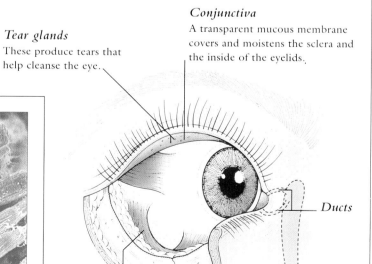

Tear glands
These produce tears that help cleanse the eye.

Conjunctiva
A transparent mucous membrane covers and moistens the sclera and the inside of the eyelids.

Ducts

Eye muscle
Six muscles (three are shown) attached to the sclera control movement.

Nasolacrimal sac
Excess tears evaporate or drain through ducts into a sac that is connected to the nasal cavity.

PHOTORECEPTIVE NEURONS

Two types of nerve cells are present in the retina. Rods contain only one light-sensitive pigment, and discern light and dark, shape, and movement. Cones, which need more light than rods to be activated, are of three types: each contains a pigment that responds to a different light wavelength (green, red, or blue). The combination of these wavelengths permits the discrimination of colour.

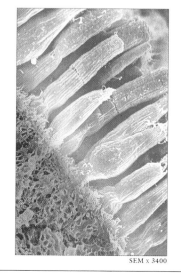

SEM x 3400

Rods and cones
Each eye has about three million cones, mainly located in the retina's macula (centre). About 100 million rods (shown here as blue) are found in the periphery.

EAR *and* EYE DISORDERS

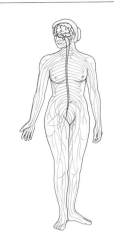

THE EARS AND THE EYES ARE VULNERABLE to many disorders, ranging from damage caused by an excess of sound and light to the natural degeneration of the senses due to age. Hearing and vision are mutually supportive, so that when one of them suffers reduced performance, the other may become more acute as a way of compensating. Some sensory disorders may be inherited. It is important to diagnose and correct ear and eye problems in young children as soon as possible because crucial learning is affected during the early years.

DEAFNESS

Conductive deafness results from impaired transmission of sound waves to the inner ear. In adults it is most commonly due to blockage by earwax. Other causes include damage to the eardrum or stiffening of the stapes bone in the middle ear, a condition called otosclerosis. Sensorineural deafness occurs when nerve impulses are poorly transmitted as a result of damage to inner ear structures or to the acoustic nerve.

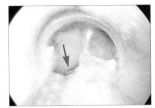

Perforated eardrum
The arrow indicates a small perforation in the eardrum. Punctures may be caused by infection, by poking objects into the ear, or by a blow.

TREATMENTS

Simple measures can be effective for treatment of conductive deafness, such as syringing of the ear for removing wax or administration of antibiotics for infections. Otosclerosis and glue ear sometimes require surgical treatment. Sensorineural deafness usually cannot be cured, but hearing aids can help by increasing the volume of sound. New cochlear implants relay signals from an external transmitter to an electrode wired into the inner ear.

Otitis media
Middle-ear infection, or otitis media, can cause temporary loss of hearing due to swelling of tissues and the accumulation of trapped fluid. It may lead to glue ear, the persistent production of sticky secretions in the middle ear.

Ear canal
Secretions in middle ear
Eardrum
Eustachian tube

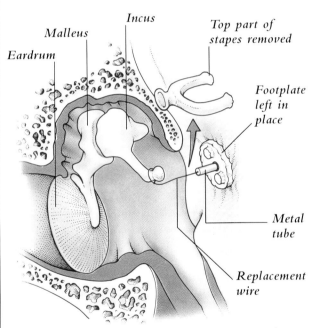

Malleus
Incus
Eardrum
Top part of stapes removed
Footplate left in place
Metal tube
Replacement wire

Stapedectomy for otosclerosis
In this operation, the top part of the stapes is removed. A laser beam is used to create a small hole in the footplate and a metal tube is inserted. A wire attached to the tube connects to the incus and transmits vibrations to the inner ear.

SENSORINEURAL DEAFNESS

Damage to inner ear structures may be present from birth. It may also be caused by some types of drugs, by prolonged exposure to loud noise, by increased fluid pressure in Meniere's disease, or by deterioration of ear structures with age.

Acoustic neuroma

This benign tumour (arrow) grows around and presses on the acoustic nerve, causing deafness. It can be removed surgically.

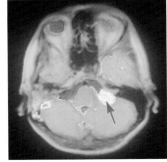

MRI SCAN OF BRAIN

Treating glue ear
Glue ear often clears up with antibiotics. If it does not, a small tube, a grommet, can be placed into a hole made in the eardrum, so that excess fluid is able to drain out and air can get in. In children, enlarged adenoids sometimes block the Eustachian tube and may need to be removed.

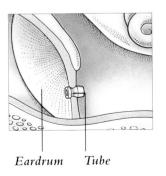

Eardrum   *Tube*

VISUAL PROBLEMS

Problems with focusing for near or far vision result from the eyeball being either too long or too short. Irregular curvature of the cornea causes astigmatism, in which parts of the visual field are blurred. Normal ageing often brings on difficulty with near vision, as the lens gradually loses its elasticity and cannot easily adjust its shape; this condition is called presbyopia.

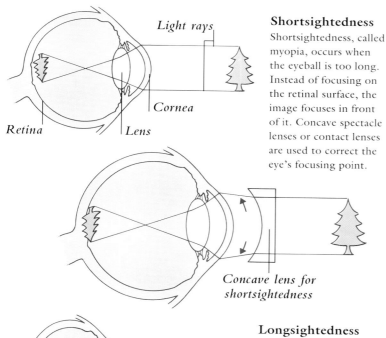

Light rays

Cornea

Retina

Lens

Shortsightedness

Shortsightedness, called myopia, occurs when the eyeball is too long. Instead of focusing on the retinal surface, the image focuses in front of it. Concave spectacle lenses or contact lenses are used to correct the eye's focusing point.

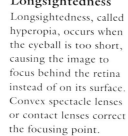

Concave lens for shortsightedness

Longsightedness

Longsightedness, called hyperopia, occurs when the eyeball is too short, causing the image to focus behind the retina instead of on its surface. Convex spectacle lenses or contact lenses correct the focusing point.

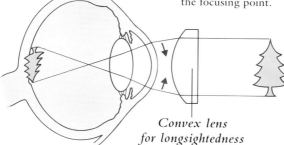

Convex lens for longsightedness

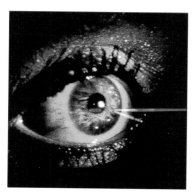

Laser surgery for shortsightedness

OPERATIONS FOR SHORTSIGHTEDNESS

Certain types of myopia and astigmatism can be treated by surgery. In radial keratotomy, a scalpel or laser can be used to make incisions in the cornea to alter the way light rays are bent. A laser can also be used to shave microscopic amounts of tissue from the front of the cornea to change the eyeball's shape. Long-term effects of both operations are unknown.

CAUSES OF BLINDNESS

In most developed countries, blindness occurs mainly later in life. Glaucoma is rare before age 40. Disease of the retina (retinopathy) can result from diabetes mellitus or hypertension, both of which occur more commonly in older people. People over 60 may be affected by macular degeneration, overlaying of the central retina with scar tissue. Opaque lenses caused by cataracts are also common in the elderly, most people over 75 being affected to some degree.

CATARACTS

The most common cause of cataracts seems to be the general ageing process. Many people are not aware that the cataracts are developing, as they cause no pain and may not interfere with vision. The changes to the lens are irreversible. Cataracts are sometimes congenital, caused when a woman has been infected with rubella during the first 3 months of pregnancy. Diabetes mellitus and exposure to radiation are other possible causes.

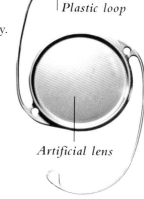

Plastic loop

Artificial lens

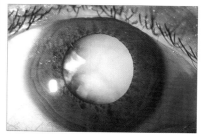

Cataract

This advanced cataract appears as a white mass behind the iris. Changes in protein fibres gradually made the lens opaque. An artificial replacement lens can restore normal vision.

Artificial lens

To treat a cataract, an incision is made in the cornea and the opaque lens is removed from its capsule. An artificial lens is then inserted and fixed in place by means of plastic loops.

GLAUCOMA

Glaucoma causes blindness as a result of damage from increasing pressure within the eye. The pressure is created by a build-up of aqueous humour, a fluid that normally drains away as fast as it is secreted. The fluid compresses blood vessels supplying the optic nerve, so that nerve fibres degenerate.

Iris   *Faulty drainage channel*

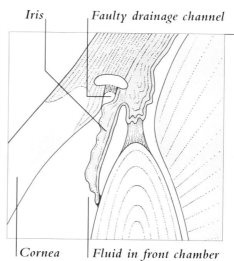

The cause

The build-up of fluid that occurs in glaucoma results from faults in the drainage channel between the back of the cornea and the iris. Drug treatment usually helps lower pressure. Surgery to open a blocked channel or create an artificial one may be needed.

Cornea   *Fluid in front chamber*

CHAPTER FIVE

C H A P T E R   5

The ENDOCRINE SYSTEM

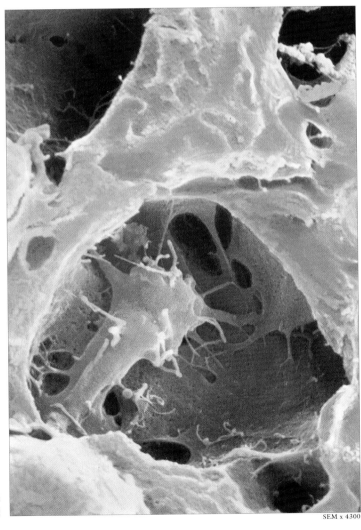

Tissue of the
pituitary gland

SEM x 4300

INTRODUCTION

Hormones are the body's internal chemical messengers. They carry the information that controls the rate at which glands and other organs work. Hormones are themselves mostly controlled by a mechanism called feedback, which is like the thermostat in a central heating system. When a gland is working harder than the body needs it to, the hormone control system switches it off; and when the body needs the gland to speed up, the system turns on the switch again. Researchers have discovered how the main endocrine (hormone-producing) glands function; some, but not all, are controlled by the pituitary gland. This master gland is located in the brain. The chemical make-up of virtually all hormones is now known, and if a gland fails, medications have been developed that will replace the missing hormones, and thus restore normal health. Another pharmaceutical innovation, the hormone blocker, can bring overactive glands under control without the need for surgery. Far-reaching social consequences have flowed from the development of the oral contraceptive pill, which is a hormone preparation that enables women to control their own fertility. Research workers are still discovering hormones, and revealing more about the subtle controls by which the body functions. These findings should lead, in time, to better and gentler treatments across the whole range of human disease.

Steroid hormones passing into a cell

Cells of the pancreas

THE ENDOCRINE SYSTEM

HORMONE PRODUCERS

THE WORD HORMONE MEANS "TO SPUR ON". Each hormone is a complex chemical substance produced and secreted directly into the bloodstream by an endocrine gland or another part of the body: the heart, for example, or a part of the gastrointestinal tract. The functions that hormones regulate include metabolism, which is the breaking down or building up of chemical elements; growth and development; sexual reproduction; and, working with the nervous system, the body's responses to stress.

HORMONE ACTION

Hormones integrate the activities of widely separated organs. Unlike the nervous system, whose effects appear rapidly but may be short-lived, the endocrine system's effects are slow to appear, longer-lasting, and usually occur at distant target sites. A special class of hormones are the prostaglandins, which produce only local effects within the same tissue. Tissues known to secrete prostaglandins include the brain and lungs.

Pineal gland
This tiny gland secretes melatonin, a hormone that controls body rhythms such as sleeping and waking and may influence sexual development.

Hypothalamus
Hormones from this cluster of nerve cells at the base of the brain are "tropic", stimulating other glands to produce their own hormones.

Parathyroid glands

Pituitary gland
Called the "master gland", this organ controls many other endocrine glands.

Thyroid gland
This gland controls metabolism, including the maintenance of body weight, the rate of energy use, and heart rate. Unlike other glands, it can store the hormones it produces.

Heart
The heart produces a hormone called atriopeptin, which reduces blood volume and blood pressure, and so helps to regulate fluid balance.

PARATHYROID GLANDS

These four glands produce a hormone that increases calcium in the blood. It acts on bones to release stored calcium, on the intestines to increase its absorption, and on the kidney to prevent its loss.

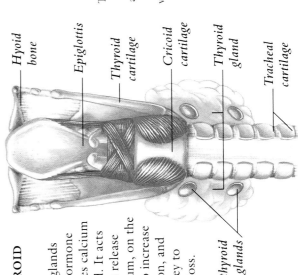

BACK VIEW

Hyoid bone

Epiglottis

Thyroid cartilage

Cricoid cartilage

Thyroid gland

Tracheal cartilage

Parathyroid glands

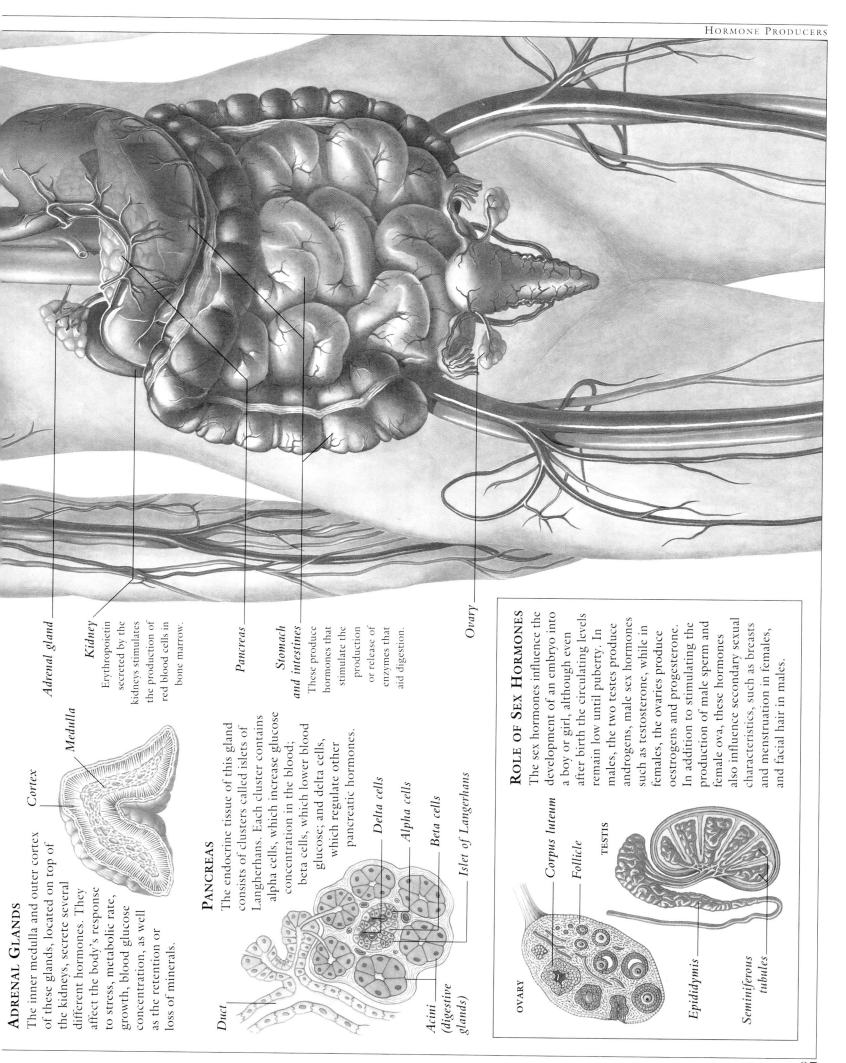

ADRENAL GLANDS

The inner medulla and outer cortex of these glands, located on top of the kidneys, secrete several different hormones. They affect the body's response to stress, metabolic rate, growth, blood glucose concentration, as well as the retention or loss of minerals.

Adrenal gland

Kidney
Erythropoietin secreted by the kidneys stimulates the production of red blood cells in bone marrow.

Pancreas

Stomach and intestines
These produce hormones that stimulate the production or release of enzymes that aid digestion.

Ovary

Cortex

Medulla

PANCREAS

The endocrine tissue of this gland consists of clusters called islets of Langherhans. Each cluster contains alpha cells, which increase glucose concentration in the blood; beta cells, which lower blood glucose; and delta cells, which regulate other pancreatic hormones.

Delta cells

Alpha cells

Beta cells

Islet of Langerhans

Duct

Acini (digestive glands)

ROLE OF SEX HORMONES

The sex hormones influence the development of an embryo into a boy or girl, although even after birth the circulating levels remain low until puberty. In males, the two testes produce androgens, male sex hormones such as testosterone, while in females, the ovaries produce oestrogens and progesterone. In addition to stimulating the production of male sperm and female ova, these hormones also influence secondary sexual characteristics, such as breasts and menstruation in females, and facial hair in males.

Corpus luteum

Follicle

TESTIS

OVARY

Epididymis

Seminiferous tubules

HORMONAL CONTROL

HORMONES REACH EVERY PART OF THE BODY, and the membrane of every cell has receptors for one or more hormones that stimulate or retard a specific body function, such as sexual development. These chemicals are controlled by specialized parts of the brain. The hypothalamus is the primary site of coordination and control of hormone production, and produces releasing, or regulatory, hormones; these travel through special blood vessels and nerve endings to the pituitary gland, the so-called "master gland".

THE MASTER GLAND

Attached to the hypothalamus by a short stalk, the pea-sized pituitary gland hangs from the base of the brain and is composed of two parts, an anterior and a posterior lobe. Some of its hormones act indirectly by stimulating target glands to release other hormones. Others have a direct effect on the function of target glands or tissue.

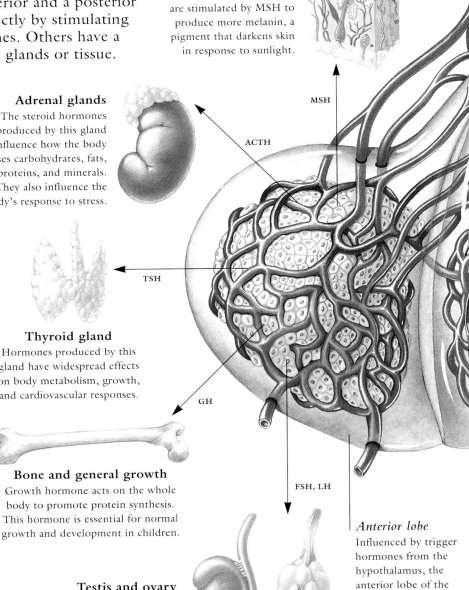

Artery

Skin

Melanocytes in skin tissue are stimulated by MSH to produce more melanin, a pigment that darkens skin in response to sunlight.

MSH

ACTH

HORMONE CONTROL MECHANISMS

Made up of molecules derived from either steroids or proteins, hormones are active only when bound to a specific receptor on or in a target cell. Hormones derived from protein bind to receptors on the outside of the cell membrane; steroid hormones pass into the cell before binding to receptors.

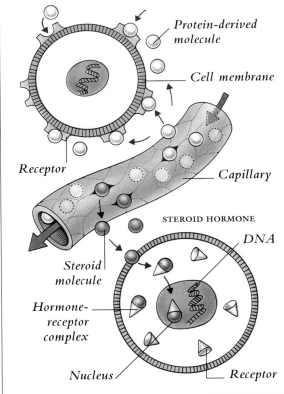

PROTEIN-DERIVED HORMONE

Protein-derived molecule

Cell membrane

Receptor

Capillary

STEROID HORMONE

DNA

Steroid molecule

Hormone-receptor complex

Nucleus

Receptor

Adrenal glands

The steroid hormones produced by this gland influence how the body uses carbohydrates, fats, proteins, and minerals. They also influence the body's response to stress.

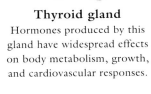

TSH

Thyroid gland

Hormones produced by this gland have widespread effects on body metabolism, growth, and cardiovascular responses.

GH

Bone and general growth

Growth hormone acts on the whole body to promote protein synthesis. This hormone is essential for normal growth and development in children.

FSH, LH

Testis and ovary

Male and female hormones released by these glands control sexual development and reproductive function.

Anterior lobe

Influenced by trigger hormones from the hypothalamus, the anterior lobe of the pituitary gland makes at least six hormones.

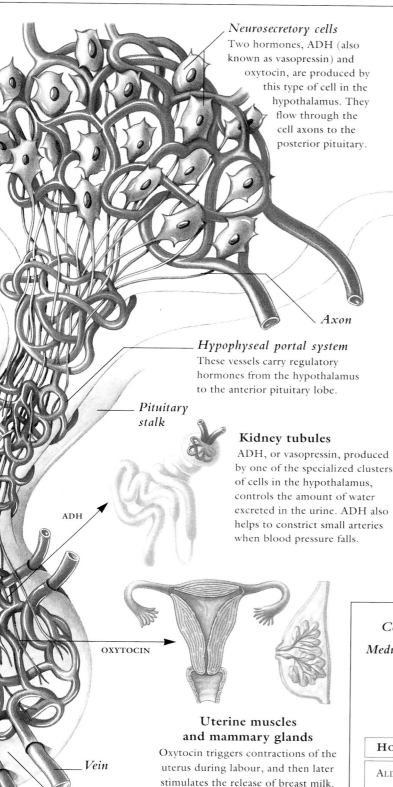

Neurosecretory cells
Two hormones, ADH (also known as vasopressin) and oxytocin, are produced by this type of cell in the hypothalamus. They flow through the cell axons to the posterior pituitary.

Axon

Hypophyseal portal system
These vessels carry regulatory hormones from the hypothalamus to the anterior pituitary lobe.

Pituitary stalk

Kidney tubules
ADH, or vasopressin, produced by one of the specialized clusters of cells in the hypothalamus, controls the amount of water excreted in the urine. ADH also helps to constrict small arteries when blood pressure falls.

ADH

OXYTOCIN

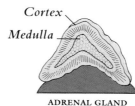

Uterine muscles and mammary glands
Oxytocin triggers contractions of the uterus during labour, and then later stimulates the release of breast milk.

Vein

Artery

Posterior lobe
Hormones from the hypothalamus are stored here and released when needed.

KEY TO PITUITARY HORMONES

ACTH	*Adrenocorticotropic hormone*
TSH	*Thyroid-stimulating hormone*
GH	*Growth hormone*
FSH	*Follicle-stimulating hormone*
LH	*Luteinizing hormone*
MSH	*Melanocyte-stimulating hormone*
ADH	*Antidiuretic hormone*

FEEDBACK MECHANISMS

A specific mechanism – "feedback" – controls hormone production, and involves the hypothalamus, the pituitary gland, and the target gland. A feedback system promotes the release of another hormone (positive feedback) or can inhibit its release (negative feedback). This involuntary mechanism maintains the body's balanced functioning.

1 Responding to levels of thyroid hormone, the hypothalamus makes TRH. This stimulates the anterior pituitary gland to release TSH. The thyroid gland is then triggered to produce its hormones.

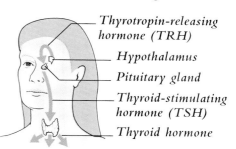

Thyrotropin-releasing hormone (TRH)

Hypothalamus

Pituitary gland

Thyroid-stimulating hormone (TSH)

Thyroid hormone

2 If thyroid hormone levels are too high, negative feedback alerts the hypothalamus so that it produces less TRH. A lower level of TRH results in a reduced level of TSH. The thyroid responds by producing less hormone.

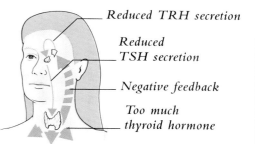

Reduced TRH secretion

Reduced TSH secretion

Negative feedback

Too much thyroid hormone

3 If thyroid hormone levels fall too low, the feedback mechanism is weakened. In response, the hypothalamus makes more TRH; TSH rises so that the levels of thyroid hormone also rise.

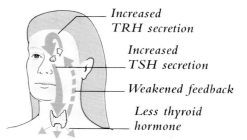

Increased TRH secretion

Increased TSH secretion

Weakened feedback

Less thyroid hormone

ADRENAL HORMONES

Cortex

Medulla

ADRENAL GLAND

The adrenal cortex has three zones, each of which produces its own hormones. The inner medulla is almost a separate endocrine gland: it produces hormones, but its nerve fibres also link it with the sympathetic nervous system and are involved in the "fight-or-flight" response.

HORMONES OF THE ADRENAL CORTEX AND ADRENAL MEDULLA	
ALDOSTERONE	Secreted by the outermost zone of the adrenal cortex, this hormone inhibits the amount of sodium excreted in the urine and helps maintain blood volume and blood pressure.
CORTISOL	The middle layer of the cortex produces this hormone. It controls how the body utilizes fat, protein, carbohydrates, and minerals, and helps to reduce inflammation.
GONADO-CORTICOIDS	Produced by the inner layer of the adrenal cortex, these sex hormones have only a slight effect on the sex organs. They influence sperm production in males, while in females they mainly influence the distribution of body hair.
ADRENALINE AND NORADRENALINE	These hormones from the adrenal medulla affect the body during stress. Noradrenaline raises heart rate and blood pressure, and adrenaline stimulates carbohydrate metabolism.

CHAPTER 6

The CARDIOVASCULAR SYSTEM

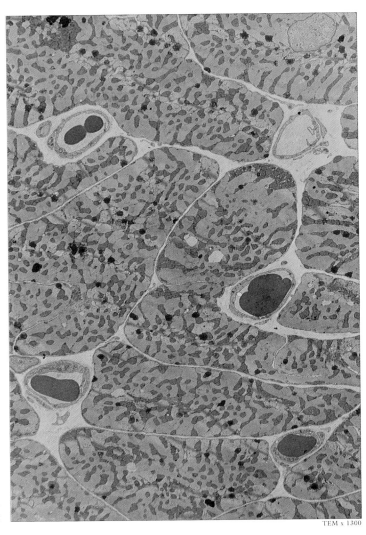

Myocardium, a special
type of muscle tissue
unique to the heart

TEM x 1300

INTRODUCTION

For most of us the heart has a special meaning, being linked with emotions and virtues such as love and courage. In fact, it is simply a pump. The assumed link between the heart and the emotions dates back to ancient times, when the pumping function of the heart was not well understood. The ancient Greeks and Romans believed that the arteries transported air rather than blood. Some two thousand years later, the English physician William Harvey discovered that the blood is pumped by the heart through two circuits, which carry it to and from the lungs and around the entire body. Heart disease has always been a major cause of death, but during the twentieth century the pattern has changed. In the early 1900s, the most common type of heart disease was valve damage caused by rheumatic fever in children and young adults; now, however, heart valve disease is rare in those under the age of 60. Today coronary heart disease is the leading cause of death in industrialized countries in people over age 35. Links between this disease and smoking, excessive cholesterol associated with high-fat diets, high blood pressure, and insufficient exercise are all well established. Available treatments include drugs, surgery, and even heart transplantation, but the key to preventing coronary heart disease is simply maintaining a healthy lifestyle.

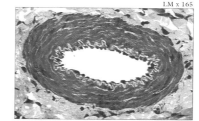

LM x 165

Cross-section of the aorta

Pathways of impulses from the heart's pacemaker

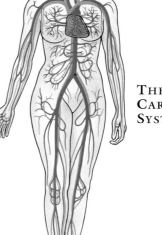

THE CARDIOVASCULAR SYSTEM

The HEART and CIRCULATION

BLOOD IS PUMPED OUT FROM THE HEART through tough, elastic tubes called arteries. Vessels from the right side of the heart initiate the pulmonary circulatory system, which carries blood to the lungs for replenishment with fresh oxygen. The aorta, the single main artery from the heart, branches to form the systemic circulation, which takes oxygen to all body tissues. Another network of veins returns blood to the heart. Linking the smallest arteries and veins are tiny vessels called capillaries. This highly intricate system is about 150,000 kilometres long (approximately 90,000 miles).

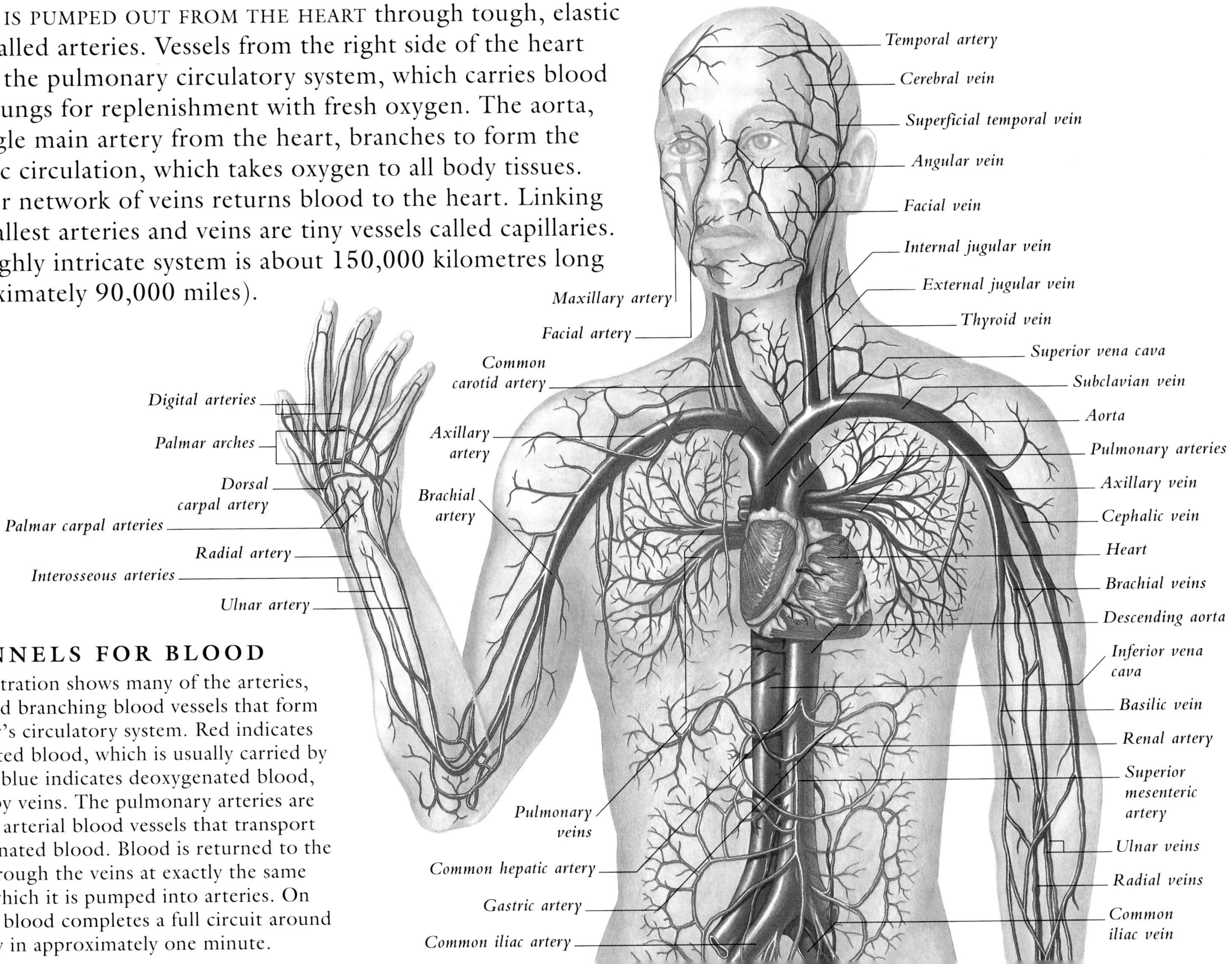

CHANNELS FOR BLOOD

The illustration shows many of the arteries, veins, and branching blood vessels that form the body's circulatory system. Red indicates oxygenated blood, which is usually carried by arteries; blue indicates deoxygenated blood, carried by veins. The pulmonary arteries are the only arterial blood vessels that transport deoxygenated blood. Blood is returned to the heart through the veins at exactly the same rate at which it is pumped into arteries. On average, blood completes a full circuit around the body in approximately one minute.

Temporal artery
Cerebral vein
Superficial temporal vein
Angular vein
Facial vein
Internal jugular vein
External jugular vein
Thyroid vein
Superior vena cava
Subclavian vein
Aorta
Pulmonary arteries
Axillary vein
Cephalic vein
Heart
Brachial veins
Descending aorta
Inferior vena cava
Basilic vein
Renal artery
Superior mesenteric artery
Ulnar veins
Radial veins
Common iliac vein

Maxillary artery
Facial artery
Common carotid artery
Axillary artery
Brachial artery
Pulmonary veins
Common hepatic artery
Gastric artery
Common iliac artery

Digital arteries
Palmar arches
Dorsal carpal artery
Radial artery
Ulnar artery
Palmar carpal arteries
Interosseous arteries

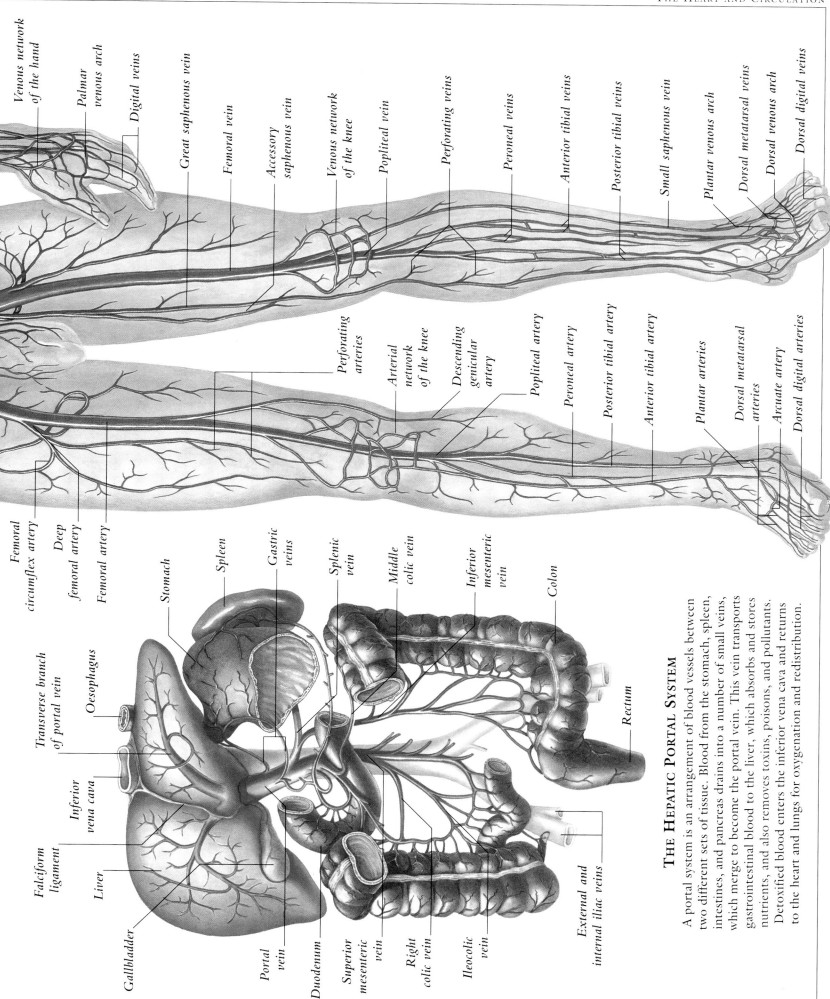

Venous network of the hand

Palmar venous arch

Digital veins

Great saphenous vein

Femoral vein

Accessory saphenous vein

Venous network of the knee

Popliteal vein

Perforating veins

Peroneal veins

Anterior tibial veins

Posterior tibial veins

Small saphenous vein

Plantar venous arch

Dorsal metatarsal veins

Dorsal venous arch

Dorsal digital veins

Perforating arteries

Arterial network of the knee

Descending genicular artery

Popliteal artery

Peroneal artery

Posterior tibial artery

Anterior tibial artery

Plantar arteries

Dorsal metatarsal arteries

Arcuate artery

Dorsal digital arteries

Femoral circumflex artery

Deep femoral artery

Femoral artery

Stomach

Spleen

Gastric veins

Splenic vein

Middle colic vein

Inferior mesenteric vein

Colon

Transverse branch of portal vein

Oesophagus

Rectum

Inferior vena cava

Falciform ligament

Liver

Gallbladder

Portal vein

Duodenum

Superior mesenteric vein

Right colic vein

Ileocolic vein

External and internal iliac veins

THE HEPATIC PORTAL SYSTEM

A portal system is an arrangement of blood vessels between two different sets of tissue. Blood from the stomach, spleen, intestines, and pancreas drains into a number of small veins, which merge to become the portal vein. This vein transports gastrointestinal blood to the liver, which absorbs and stores nutrients, and also removes toxins, poisons, and pollutants. Detoxified blood enters the inferior vena cava and returns to the heart and lungs for oxygenation and redistribution.

HEART STRUCTURE

THE HEART IS A POWERFUL MUSCLE about the size of a grapefruit. Located just left of the centre of the chest, it operates as two coordinated pumps, sending blood continuously around the body. This circulation carries oxygen and nutrients to all organs and tissues and also removes harmful wastes. A specialized type of muscle called myocardium is found only in the heart.

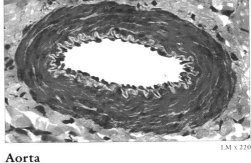

L.M x 220

Aorta
This cross-section shows the aorta, the largest blood vessel in the body, with an inner diameter of about 2.5cm (1in). The aorta arches out from the left ventricle, carrying blood with essential fresh oxygen to every other part of the body.

HEART STRUCTURE

The heart has four chambers: two upper chambers called atria, and two thicker-walled lower chambers known as ventricles. A strong muscular wall, the septum, divides the two sides of the heart. The four heart valves are crucial for allowing blood to pass in and out of the heart chambers in only one direction.

Aorta

Superior vena cava
This large vein carries used blood from the head and arms into the right atrium.

Pulmonary veins
Newly oxygenated blood from the lungs returns to the left atrium via the four pulmonary veins; oxygenated blood is not carried in veins anywhere else in the body.

Right atrium

Endocardium
This smooth membrane lines the inside of the heart. It also lines the heart valves.

Pulmonary valve

Tricuspid valve

Inferior vena cava
Deoxygenated blood returns from the lower body and legs and enters the right atrium through the inferior vena cava.

Right ventricle

Pulmonary artery
The pulmonary artery branches after leaving the right ventricle, each branch carrying deoxygenated blood to one lung. It is the only artery that carries deoxygenated blood.

Pulmonary veins

Left atrium

Aortic valve

Mitral valve

Septum
A thick muscle wall divides the heart into two distinct halves.

Pericardium
The pericardium is a tough, fibrous sac surrounding the entire surface of the heart. It has an inner, fluid-filled, cushioning membrane.

Myocardium
The heart's interconnected muscle fibres (cells) enable it to contract automatically.

Left ventricle

TWO PUMPS IN ONE

Used blood from body tissues enters the right side of the heart and is pumped out to the lungs. Passage of blood through the lungs, the pulmonary circulation, enables blood to pick up oxygen. The refreshed blood returns to the left side of the heart and is pumped out again to the body tissues. The blood's circuit through body tissues is called the systemic circulation. When the body is at rest, the entire circuit around the lungs and body takes only about one minute, with the heart pumping out about 5 to 7L (10 to 15pt) of blood.

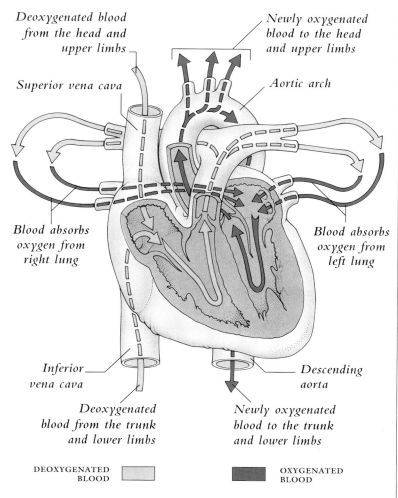

Deoxygenated blood from the head and upper limbs

Newly oxygenated blood to the head and upper limbs

Superior vena cava

Aortic arch

Blood absorbs oxygen from right lung

Blood absorbs oxygen from left lung

Inferior vena cava

Descending aorta

Deoxygenated blood from the trunk and lower limbs

Newly oxygenated blood to the trunk and lower limbs

DEOXYGENATED BLOOD

OXYGENATED BLOOD

BLOOD SUPPLY TO THE HEART

Because the heart needs a generous supply of oxygen, it needs a correspondingly large supply of blood; only the brain requires more. Blood that flows through the chambers of the heart cannot seep through to reach the muscle cells, so the heart muscle has a separate network of blood vessels called the coronary system.

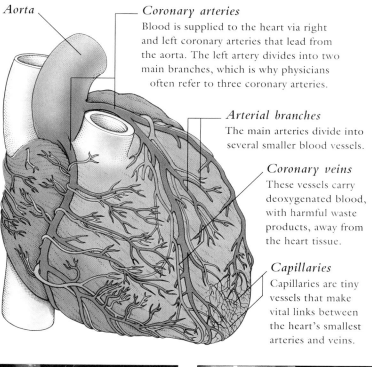

Aorta

Coronary arteries
Blood is supplied to the heart via right and left coronary arteries that lead from the aorta. The left artery divides into two main branches, which is why physicians often refer to three coronary arteries.

Arterial branches
The main arteries divide into several smaller blood vessels.

Coronary veins
These vessels carry deoxygenated blood, with harmful waste products, away from the heart tissue.

Capillaries
Capillaries are tiny vessels that make vital links between the heart's smallest arteries and veins.

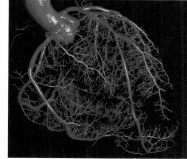

Resin cast of coronary arteries

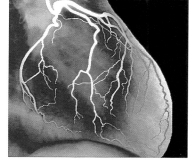

Angiogram of coronary arteries

CARDIAC SKELETON

A set of four tough fibrous rings, or cuffs, known as the cardiac skeleton, provides the points of attachment for the four heart valves and for the heart muscle. The illustration shows the muscle fibres of the left and right ventricles, which make up the bulk of the heart. The wraparound arrangement of the muscle fibres enables the ventricles to squirt blood out of the heart, just as a closing fist squirts water from a balloon.

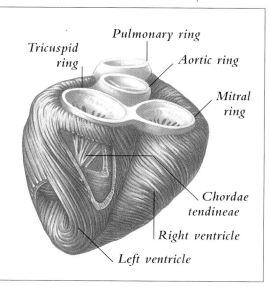

Tricuspid ring

Pulmonary ring

Aortic ring

Mitral ring

Chordae tendineae

Right ventricle

Left ventricle

BLOOD COLLECTION

The pattern formed by coronary veins closely mirrors that of the coronary arteries. Most of them drain into the coronary sinus, a large vein at the back of the heart. From this vein, the blood flows into the right atrium. Some small veins empty directly into the right atrium.

Right pulmonary veins

Left pulmonary veins

Coronary sinus

Coronary veins

HEART FUNCTION

As a DYNAMIC PUMP, the heart forces blood around an impressive network of blood vessels that would circle the Earth two-and-a-half times. The real power comes from the ventricles, with their thick muscular walls which contract so that blood surges out into the arteries. The pumping action of the heart is repeated automatically, with the rate of beating and the amount of blood that is pumped out varying according to the body's level of stress and exertion.

ECG recording
Electrocardiography (ECG) detects the flow of electrical impulses throughout the heart. Colour-coding relates the tracing to various stages in the passage of the impulses (see below and also page 116).

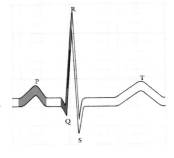

ELECTRICAL PATHWAYS

Regular, rhythmic beating of the heart is maintained by electrical impulses that originate in the sinoatrial node, which is the body's natural pacemaker. Impulses spread through the atria, stimulating contraction, to the atrioventricular node. After a slight pause at this node, the impulses pass along special conducting muscle fibres through the ventricles, causing them to contract. Any variation from this normal sequence may indicate the possibility of a heart disorder.

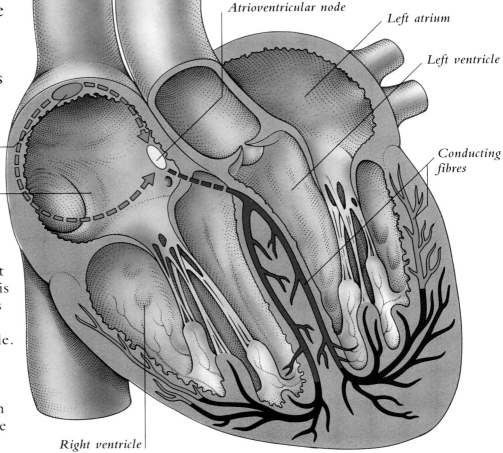

Atrioventricular node

Left atrium

Left ventricle

Conducting fibres

Sinoatrial node

Right atrium

Right ventricle

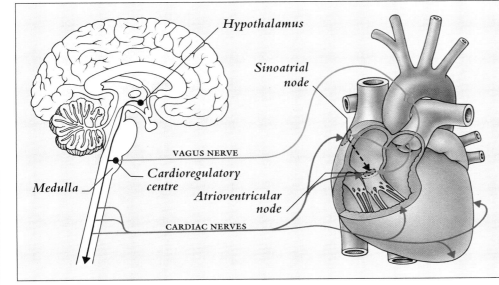

Hypothalamus

Sinoatrial node

VAGUS NERVE

Medulla

Cardioregulatory centre

Atrioventricular node

CARDIAC NERVES

NERVOUS SYSTEM CONTROL

Without control by nerves, the heart would beat about 100 times per minute. However, parasympathetic nerves, especially the vagus nerve, set a resting rate of about 70 by means of impulses to the cardioregulatory centre in the medulla. During exercise or stress, the sympathetic cardiac nerves, controlled by the hypothalamus, are signalled to speed the heart rate. This provides more oxygenated blood to muscles. The heart rate also increases when hormones are released by the adrenal glands.

■ PARASYMPATHETIC NERVES

■ SYMPATHETIC NERVES

THE HEART VALVES

Four valves allow the blood to move through the heart chambers in only one direction. They consist of two or three half-moon flaps, or cusps, of fibrous tissue that attach to the heart walls. The cusps separate when the blood is flowing correctly but close into a tight seal to prevent any backward movement. Opening and closing of the heart valves occurs in reaction to a change in pressure on either side as blood surges through.

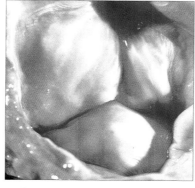

Pulmonary valve
Blood flows through the pulmonary valve from the right ventricle into the pulmonary artery. This three-cusped valve is essential to prevent backflow of blood when the ventricle, after its vigorous contraction, relaxes again.

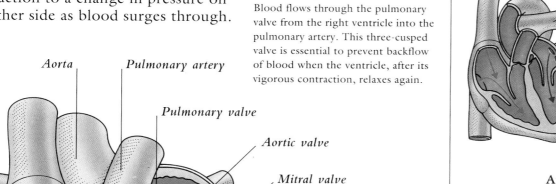

Aorta   *Pulmonary artery*

Pulmonary valve

Aortic valve

Mitral valve

Tricuspid valve

Chordae tendineae

Location of valves
The tricuspid and mitral valves are located between the upper and lower chambers on the right and the left sides of the heart, respectively. The pulmonary and aortic valves are placed at the exits from the ventricles into the pulmonary artery and the aorta.

Valve cusps
These thin, fibrous cusps of the valves are covered by a smooth membrane called endocardium and reinforced by dense connective tissue. The pulmonary, aortic, and tricuspid valves have three cusps. The mitral valve has two cusps.

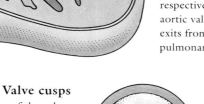

TWO CUSPS   THREE CUSPS

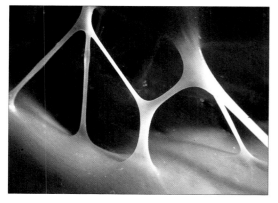

Chordae tendineae
Fibrous strands known as chordae tendineae fasten the tricuspid and mitral valves to the ventricular walls. These cords prevent the valves from being pushed upward by the forceful pressure of flowing blood. The aortic and pulmonary valves are less likely to be pushed out by pressure and so do not need such fastenings.

HEARTBEAT CYCLE

Three separate and distinct phases make up the carefully timed, sequential beating of the heart. The relaxing and refilling of blood during the first stage is followed by stages of contracting and squeezing. The whole cycle takes, on average, only about four-fifths of a second; during vigorous exercise, however, or in times of stress, this speed may more than double.

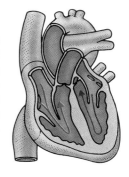

Diastole
In the first phase of the cycle, deoxygenated blood enters the right atrium and oxygenated blood enters the left atrium. The blood then flows through into the ventricles. By the end of this phase, the ventricles are filled to about 80 per cent of capacity.

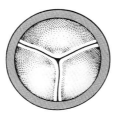

Atrial systole
Impulses from the sinoatrial node initiate the next phase of the cycle, during which the atria contract. This squeezes any blood remaining in the atria into the ventricles.

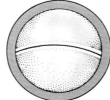

Ventricular systole
During the third phase of the heartbeat sequence, the ventricles contract. Valves at the exits of the ventricles open and blood is forced into the pulmonary artery and the aorta. As this phase ends, diastole starts again.

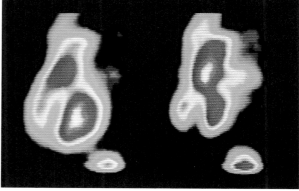

RADIONUCLIDE SCANS

Relaxation and contraction
The scans shown above were produced by using a gamma camera to detect radioactively tagged red blood cells. They show how the distribution of blood (red and yellow areas) in the heart varies at different stages of the pumping cycle. On the left, the heart is relaxed and filling with blood. On the right, the heart is squeezing blood out.

BLOOD VESSELS *and* BLOOD

A COMPLEX CIRCULATORY SYSTEM ENABLES BLOOD to perform its many different functions. Blood transports oxygen, nutrients, and waste products excreted from cells; it helps to regulate the body's water content, temperature, and acid-alkali balance; and its specialized cells and proteins protect against blood loss resulting from injury, and against infection.

BLOOD TRANSPORT

Without oxygen, all cells in the body would quickly die. Oxygenated blood from the lungs circulates through muscular, thick-walled arteries, such as the one shown at right, into progressively smaller vessels called arterioles. These vessels connect with the venous system through capillaries.

VEIN STRUCTURE

Deoxygenated blood returning to the heart through the veins is at low pressure. Its movement is helped by a succession of one-way valves that prevent backflow.

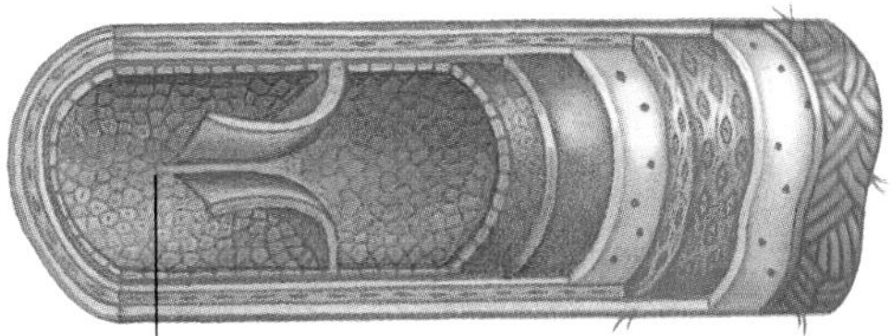

Valve flaps

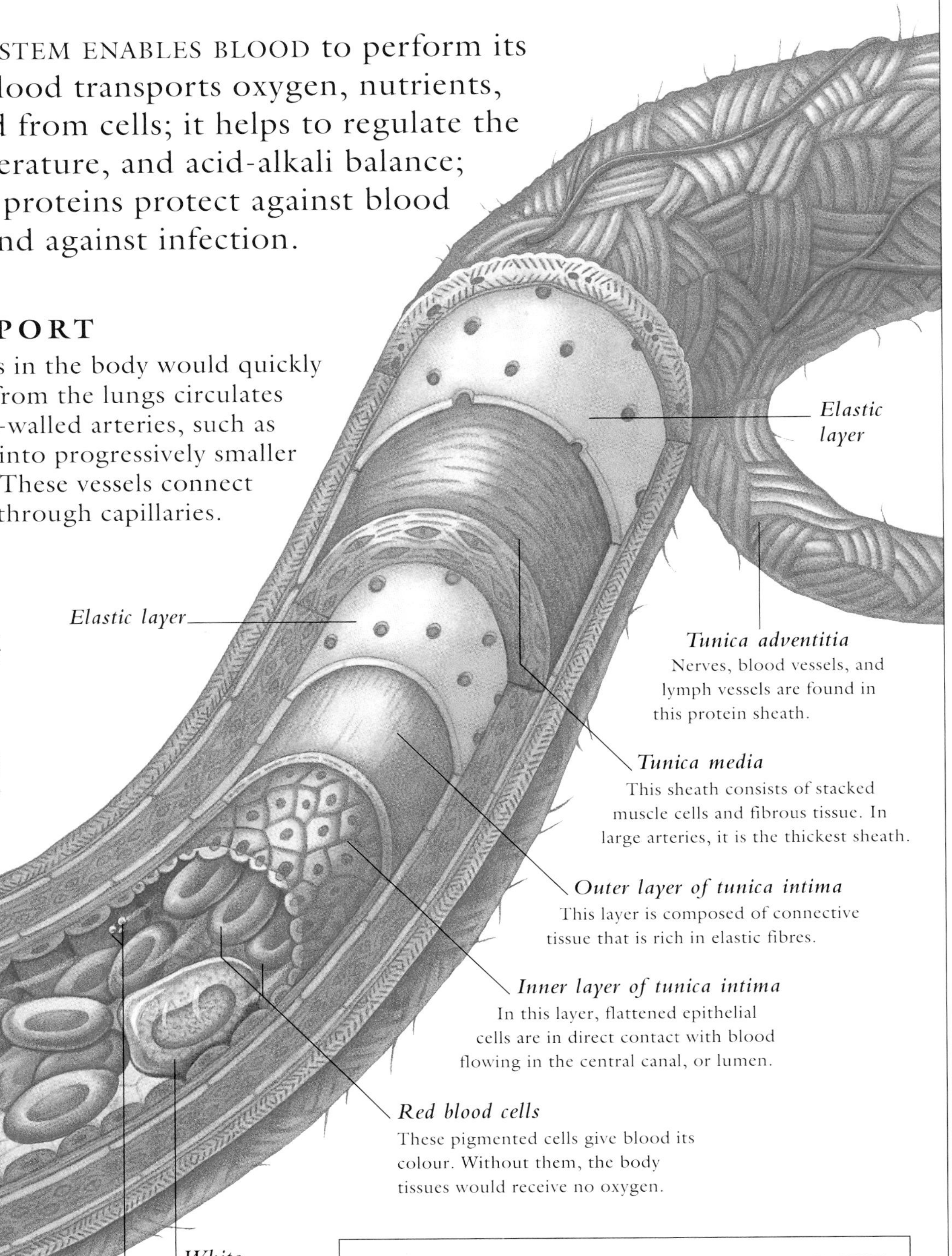

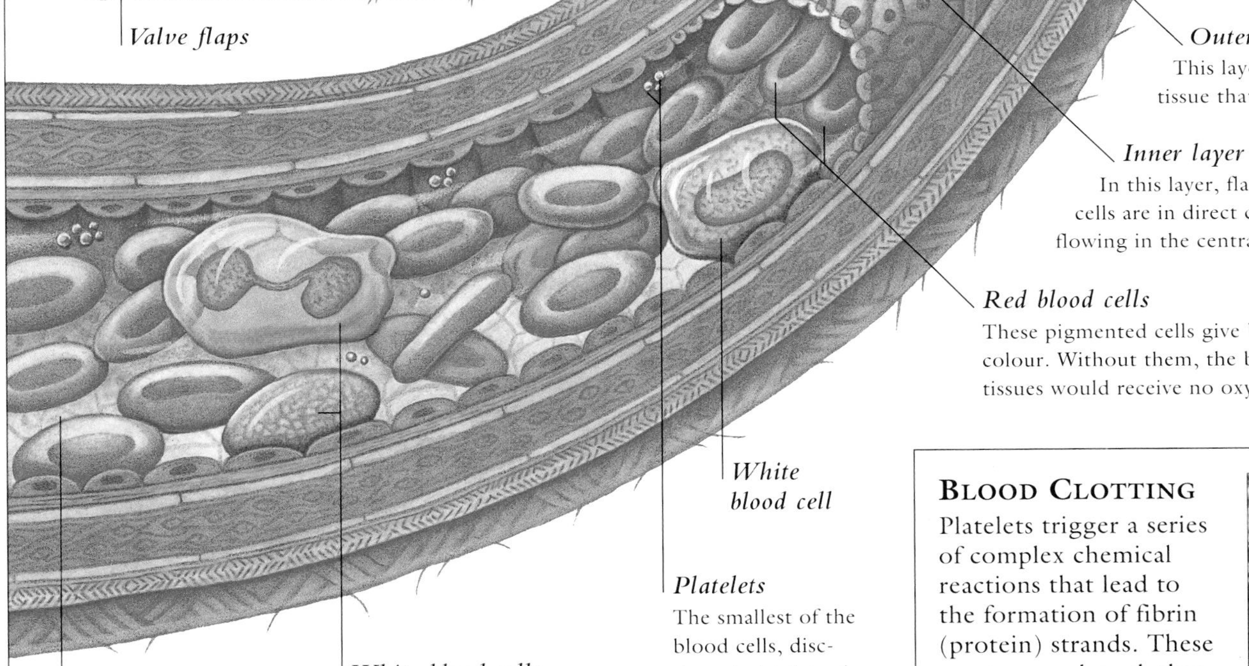

Elastic layer

Elastic layer

Tunica adventitia
Nerves, blood vessels, and lymph vessels are found in this protein sheath.

Tunica media
This sheath consists of stacked muscle cells and fibrous tissue. In large arteries, it is the thickest sheath.

Outer layer of tunica intima
This layer is composed of connective tissue that is rich in elastic fibres.

Inner layer of tunica intima
In this layer, flattened epithelial cells are in direct contact with blood flowing in the central canal, or lumen.

Red blood cells
These pigmented cells give blood its colour. Without them, the body tissues would receive no oxygen.

White blood cell

Platelets
The smallest of the blood cells, disc-shaped platelets play an essential role in stopping the flow of blood after injury to the body's tissues.

Plasma
More than half of blood is a straw-coloured liquid, which contains nutrients, minerals, water, and proteins.

White blood cells
The main function of these variously shaped cells, which are grouped under the name of leucocytes, is to defend the body against infection.

BLOOD CLOTTING
Platelets trigger a series of complex chemical reactions that lead to the formation of fibrin (protein) strands. These create a meshwork that traps red blood cells to form a blood clot.

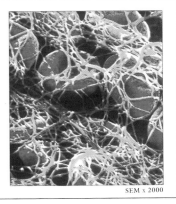

Red blood cells in fibrin strands

SEM x 2000

THE CAPILLARY NETWORK

The two circulatory routes, arterial and venous, are linked by capillaries. These extremely small blood vessels interconnect to form networks, the density of which varies with the type of tissue activity: the heart, for example, has a dense capillary network, while that in the skin is less complex. Blood flow in these vessels is slower than in the arteries so that the exchange of oxygen and nutrients can occur.

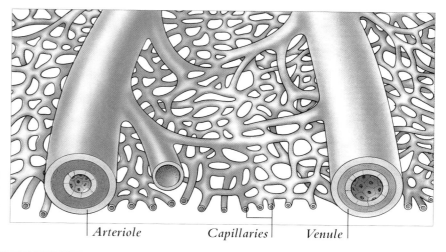

Site of exchange
The thin capillary walls are punctuated by tiny spaces so that nutrient- and oxygen-bearing fluid flows out onto tissue cells and waste products such as carbon dioxide move back into the vessels.

Arteriole   *Capillaries*   *Venule*

RED BLOOD CELL PRODUCTION

The lifespan of oxyxgen-bearing red blood cells, or erythrocytes, is only 80 to 120 days. Every second, two million of them die, but these are replaced at the same rate by new ones generated in the body's red bone marrow in a process called erythropoiesis. This ensures that a constant and appropriate supply of essential oxygen is available for cell life and function.

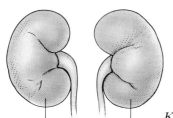

The role of the kidneys
If the kidneys are receiving only low amounts of oxygen, some of their cells stimulate the activation of a hormone known as erythropoietin.

Kidneys

Site of production
Erythropoietin travels to the red bone marrow, and stimulates increased production of erythrocytes.

Erythropoietin

Bone marrow

Production of red blood cells

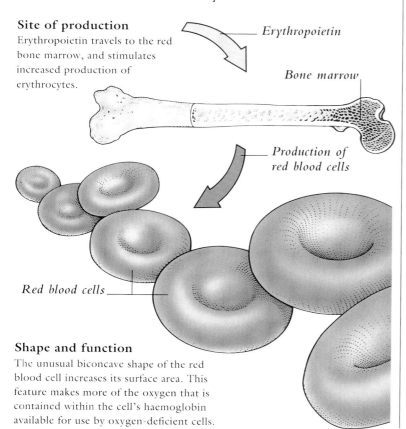

Red blood cells

Shape and function
The unusual biconcave shape of the red blood cell increases its surface area. This feature makes more of the oxygen that is contained within the cell's haemoglobin available for use by oxygen-deficient cells.

HAEMOGLOBIN AND OXYGEN

Haemoglobin in the red blood cells is composed of haeme, an iron-bearing red pigment, and of globin, ribbon-like protein chains. Oxygen from the lungs' tiny air sacs enters the red blood cells and combines with the iron to form oxyhaemoglobin. In this form, oxygen is transported through the body. It is then released in the capillaries and passes into the fluid that bathes surrounding tissues. Deoxygenated cells take up this vital element and use it to produce energy.

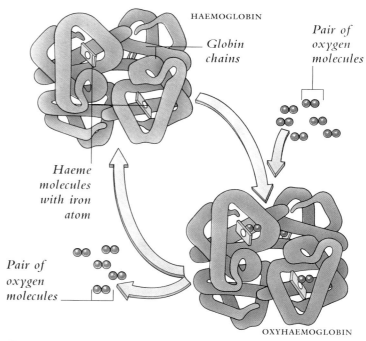

HAEMOGLOBIN

Globin chains

Pair of oxygen molecules

Haeme molecules with iron atom

Pair of oxygen molecules

OXYHAEMOGLOBIN

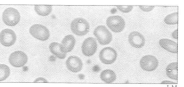

Normal blood
Molecules of haemoglobin, the oxygen-receptive pigment, give blood its red colour, as seen in this smear of normal red blood cells.

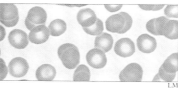

Iron-deficiency anaemia
In anaemia, red blood cells are few in number, pale due to lack of haemoglobin, and contain less oxygen than normal cells.

CORONARY HEART DISEASE

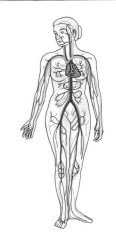

ANY HEART DISORDER DUE TO A RESTRICTED SUPPLY of blood to the heart muscle is called coronary heart disease. The most common manifestations are angina pectoris (gripping chest pains usually brought on by exertion) and myocardial infarction, also called a heart attack, which is the death of an area of heart muscle caused by a more serious deprivation of blood.

ATHEROSCLEROSIS

Coronary heart disease is commonly caused by narrowing of the coronary arteries by atherosclerosis, which is the build-up of fatty deposists in the lining of the arteries. The process that leads to atherosclerosis begins with the accumulation of excess fats and cholesterol in the blood. These substances infiltrate the lining of arteries at sites of microscopic damage, forming deposits called atheroma.

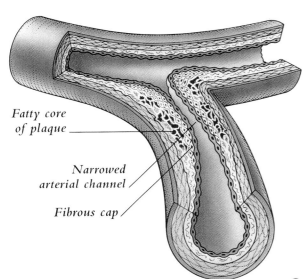

Fatty core
of plaque

Narrowed
arterial channel

Fibrous cap

Build-up of plaque
Deposits of atheroma gradually build up to form masses known as plaques. Consisting of a fatty core topped by a fibrous cap, plaques thicken arterial walls, narrowing the inner channel and impeding blood flow. If blood turbulence roughens the surface of the plaque, platelets and blood cells can collect, creating a blood clot that may block the artery completely.

Sites of atherosclerosis
Atherosclerosis can occur anywhere in the main coronary arteries or in smaller branches, but plaque usually builds up at stress points in the artery such as branch junctions.

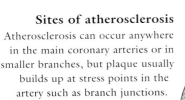

Right coronary artery

Aorta

Left main
coronary artery

Left
circumflex
artery

Left
anterior
descending
artery

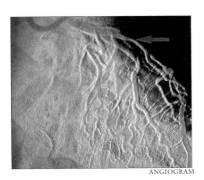

ANGIOGRAM

A narrowed artery
This image clearly shows the effects of atherosclerosis. Sections of the left coronary artery, seen at top right, are severely narrowed and only a minimal amount of blood flows through.

RISK FACTORS

Smoking, insufficient exercise, a diet high in saturated fats, being overweight, high blood pressure, and diabetes are the main risk factors that contribute to coronary heart disease. The stresses people face and how well they cope may also play a role.

NATIONAL PATTERNS

Rates of death from coronary heart disease vary markedly among different countries. The richer, more industrialized countries have higher rates, but these have declined since the 1960s (except in Eastern Europe) as a result of better medical treatments as well as increased awareness of the influence of lifestyle on health. Men generally have rates three to six times higher than women, although this gap is narrowing.

CORONARY HEART DISEASE DEATHS* (MEN)			
COUNTRY	1960–64	1970–74	1985–89
US	333.6	316.1	165.7
UK	272.1	259.2	218.3
FINLAND	335.2	314.5	248.3
ITALY	172.0	123.9	91.5
JAPAN	72.4	48.7	32.6
AUSTRALIA	317.4	309.1	179.7
URUGUAY	167.4	187.8	111.6
COSTA RICA	79.3	76.1	133.8

*PER 100,000 POPULATION

CORONARY HEART DISEASE DEATHS* (WOMEN)			
COUNTRY	1960–64	1970–74	1985–89
US	168.5	156.3	83.2
UK	137.7	108.5	95.2
FINLAND	158.6	115.3	97.9
ITALY	119.1	65.9	38.3
JAPAN	50.6	27.6	17.8
AUSTRALIA	154.9	143.3	87.1
URUGUAY	93.0	105.9	56.6
COSTA RICA	65.6	57.2	75.8

*PER 100,000 POPULATION

ANGINA

Chest pains that come on with exertion are a warning sign that the cardiac muscle is not receiving enough blood for the effort being expended. An angina attack typically begins with a gripping or pressure-like pain behind the breastbone that sometimes radiates into the neck and jaw and then down into the arms. The pain usually subsides rapidly with rest. Less exertion is needed to trigger an attack if a person is exposed to cold, feels strong emotions, or has eaten a heavy meal.

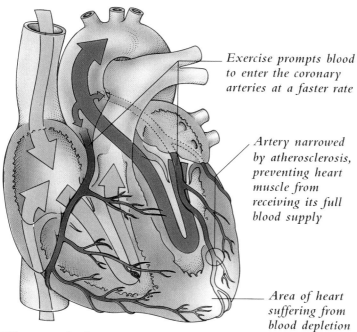

Exercise prompts blood to enter the coronary arteries at a faster rate

Artery narrowed by atherosclerosis, preventing heart muscle from receiving its full blood supply

Area of heart suffering from blood depletion

Effects on the heart
When blood supply is insufficient, the heart does not receive the oxygen and glucose it needs. The heart tries to create energy by alternative chemical processes, but produces waste products that the reduced blood supply cannot remove adequately. Pain is the result.

DRUG TREATMENT

Drugs used to treat angina act by widening the coronary arteries, thus improving blood flow. They also lower blood pressure and slow the heart so that the work of the heart muscle can be reduced. Nitrate drugs, beta-blockers, and calcium-channel blockers are frequently prescribed.

Narrowed blood vessels

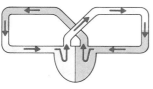

Resistance to blood flow makes heart work harder

Before drugs
Narrowed arteries starve the heart muscle of the oxygen and glucose it needs to produce energy during exertion.

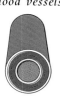

Widened blood vessels

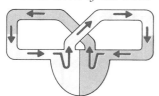

Less resistance to blood flow reduces work of the heart

After drugs
Nitrate drugs relax the blood vessel walls, causing them to widen. This helps improve the flow of blood and also the supply of nutrients.

HEART ATTACK

A heart attack usually occurs suddenly, with little or no warning. Chest pain may be like that of angina, but is usually more severe and not necessarily brought on by exertion or relieved by rest. A victim may also sweat, feel weak, and even lose consciousness. If the attack leads to complete stoppage of the heart, known as cardiac arrest, death may follow.

Blocked blood supply
When a coronary artery becomes blocked, and remains blocked, the heart muscle it supplies dies. The severity of a heart attack depends on the amount of muscle affected and the health of other coronary arteries.

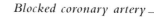

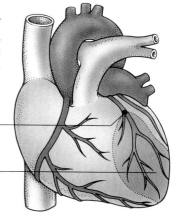

Blocked coronary artery

Damaged heart muscle

MEASURING ENZYME ACTIVITY

Proteins called enzymes regulate the body's chemical reactions. Tissue damage during a heart attack results in the release of certain enzymes into the bloodstream. Measuring enzyme activity helps reveal the extent of damage to the heart.

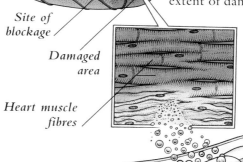

Site of blockage

Damaged area

Heart muscle fibres

Enzyme release
Enzymes from heart muscle fibres pass into capillaries and travel through coronary veins into the circulation.

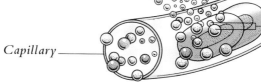

Capillary

A number of different enzymes are released

DRUG TREATMENT

Doctors prescribe a number of different drugs to help keep blood flowing freely. Thrombolytic drugs act to break down recent clots, while antiplatelet drugs and anticoagulants are useful for maintaining normal circulation of the blood and preventing clots from forming.

Thrombolytics
Clots form when strands of fibrin enmesh blood cells. Thrombolytic drugs cause the normally inactive substance plasminogen to change into plasmin, which breaks down fibrin and dissolves clots.

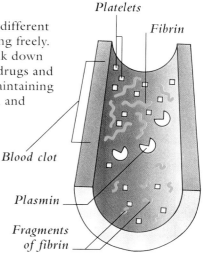

Platelets

Fibrin

Blood clot

Plasmin

Fragments of fibrin

SURGERY *for* CORONARY HEART DISEASE

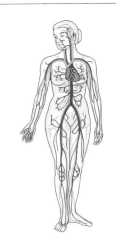

A NARROWED OR BLOCKED BLOOD VESSEL CAN BE DEALT with chemically by drugs, or surgically by clearing or bypassing the blockage. Coronary artery bypass requires the temporary use of a heart-lung machine, which permits stoppage of the heart. The more recent technique of balloon angioplasty uses an inflatable catheter, for which a heart-lung machine is not needed.

BALLOON ANGIOPLASTY

Balloon angioplasty is particularly suited for patients in whom only one artery is critically narrowed. It is also preferable to bypass surgery in elderly patients, or those with associated lung disease. The technique uses a catheter to inflate a balloon at the site of the blockage, squashing and cracking the plaque to create a wider channel. It is a brief operation, after which the patient needs only a short convalescence period.

1 An incision is made in the patient's arm (or leg), and through this a guide wire is pushed into the brachial (or femoral) artery. Using X-ray or ultrasound guidance, the wire is then threaded into the affected coronary artery (via the aorta) to the blockage.

Aorta

Coronary artery

Guide wire

Brachial artery

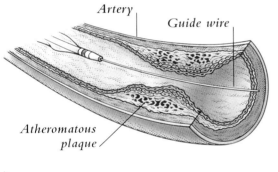

Artery

Guide wire

Atheromatous plaque

2 At the blockage, the wire is carefully manoeuvred between the plaque accretions. Threaded on the guide wire, the catheter is pushed until the balloon at its tip is in place at the site of the obstruction.

Supply tube *Artery* *Inflated balloon*

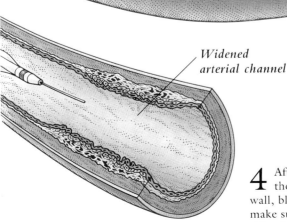

Widened arterial channel

3 A pump outside the body forces air or liquid along the catheter and into the balloon, inflating it to up to eight times atmospheric pressure. Pressure is maintained for up to 60 seconds, then released. This procedure is repeated several times.

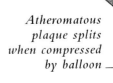

Atheromatous plaque splits when compressed by balloon

4 After inflations have squeezed the plaque against the arterial wall, blood pressure is checked to make sure that it is equal on either side of the site of obstruction. The balloon catheter is then withdrawn.

LASER CATHETERS

In a developing laser technique, the surgeon introduces a catheter to the blockage site, using an associated fibreoptic channel to position a laser-beam emitter. A small balloon is inflated to cut off blood supply momentarily while a burst of the laser beam breaks up the plaque. A vacuum device sucks out the fragments.

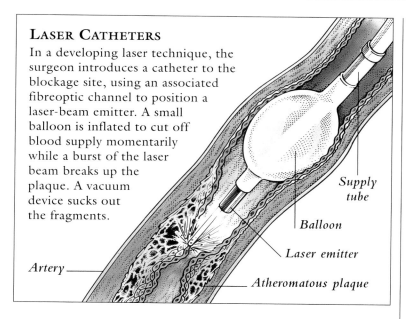

Artery

Supply tube

Balloon

Laser emitter

Atheromatous plaque

CORONARY ANGIOGRAMS

Angiography is a technique that shows the outline of arteries. Radiopaque dye, a contrast medium, is introduced via a catheter into the coronary arteries, and a series of X-ray pictures is then taken to record the dye's progress. The technique is often used to examine the coronary arteries in order to check on the success of balloon angioplasty. The angiograms below were taken before and after the operation.

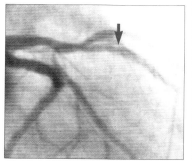

NARROWED ARTERY

WIDENED ARTERY

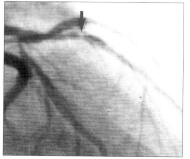

Balloon catheters

The balloons used in balloon angioplasty have to be tiny, strong, and flexible. They are uninflated when introduced into blood vessels in order to minimize friction and have to withstand great pressure when inflated. Liquid has replaced air as an inflation medium, enabling greater force to be exerted against the arterial wall.

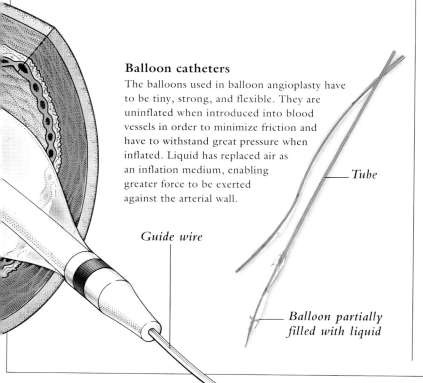

Guide wire

Tube

Balloon partially filled with liquid

CORONARY ARTERY BYPASS

Bypass surgery is the most common procedure used to treat critically narrowed or blocked coronary arteries, and uncontrollable angina. The operation involves use of a section of one or more of the patient's arteries or veins, usually the saphenous vein, to bypass the blocked section. A heart-lung machine temporarily takes over the functions of both organs, thus enabling the surgeon to work on a non-beating heart during the critical phase of the operation.

Site of chest incision

Saphenous vein

1 After the patient has been given general anaesthesia, the chest is opened by making a central incision down the breastbone. To expose the heart, the pericardium is then opened. Incisions made in the leg allow a part of the saphenous vein to be removed.

Connections to the heart-lung machine

Clamp

Aorta

2 The patient's blood is pumped, filtered, and oxygenated by using the heart-lung machine. Clamps cut off the heart from the circulation, and a solution that paralyzes the heart and stops it from beating is injected. The surgeon grafts the vein between the aorta and the affected artery beyond the obstruction.

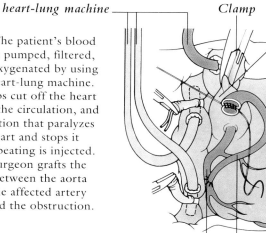

Narrowed coronary artery

Length of vein

Right coronary artery

Aorta

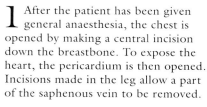

3 More than one bypass can be carried out at the same time. A triple bypass is seen at left. After grafting, the clamps are removed; if the heart does not beat on its own, electrical stimulation is used. The heart-lung machine is disconnected.

Left circumflex artery

Blockages

Blockage

Left anterior descending artery

HEART STRUCTURE DISORDERS

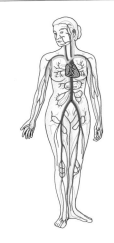

HEART STRUCTURE DISORDERS ARE COMMON, and can affect people of any age. These disorders may be congenital or acquired through infections that affect heart muscle, such as rheumatic fever or endocarditis. In some cases, they result from diseases, such as syphilis, that arise elsewhere in the body. Artificial valves and microsurgical techniques can repair many disorders.

HEART VALVE DISORDERS

Effective pumping by the heart depends on all four valves operating properly. There are two main types of disorder that may affect one or more of the valves. Stenosis, a condition in which a valve outlet is too narrow, may be congenital or due to rheumatic fever or sometimes ageing. Incompetence, or insufficiency, is a condition in which the cusps of the valve do not meet and the valve fails to close properly. It may be due to coronary heart disease or an infection.

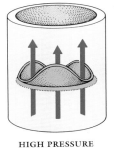

LOWER PRESSURE

HIGH PRESSURE

Normal aortic valve
As the ventricles contract, high pressure forces the valve open, allowing blood through (left). When the ventricles relax and fill with blood, the pressure is higher on the other side of the valve so that the valve closes tightly. This prevents blood from flowing backward (right).

HIGH PRESSURE

LOWER PRESSURE

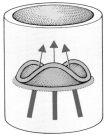

LOWER PRESSURE

HIGH PRESSURE

Stenosis
A narrowed valve allows less blood through, so the heart must pump harder to maintain blood flow.

Incompetence
The leakage of blood back into the ventricles can occur when the cusps of a valve fail to close completely.

HIGH PRESSURE

LOWER PRESSURE

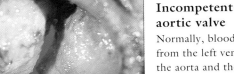

Incompetent aortic valve
Normally, blood is pumped from the left ventricle into the aorta and then out to the rest of the body. When the aortic valve leaks, blood flows back into the heart. The left ventricle strains to pump this blood pool, and its muscle wall thickens.

HEART MURMURS

Normally, blood flow in the heart cannot be heard. A murmur commonly results from turbulent blood flow through a defective valve. So-called "innocent" heart murmurs may occur in childhood or can be associated with increased cardiac output that occurs in anaemia or pregnancy. They are intermittent and fainter than those associated with structural abnormalities.

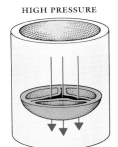

Areas of turbulence

Audible defects
Murmurs are produced by blood that rushes around and through the cusps of a stenosed valve, or blood that leaks back through an incompetent valve and collides with onrushing blood.

Pulmonary valve stenosis

Mitral valve incompetence

REPLACEMENT VALVES

Valves made from metal and plastic may use a caged-ball or tilting disc mechanism. Both are long-lasting but tend to cause blood clots, so patients may need anticoagulant drugs. Valves made from animal or human tissues are less durable but do not cause clots.

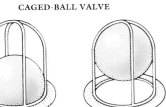

CAGED-BALL VALVE

Closed   *Open*

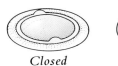

TILTING DISC VALVE

Closed   *Open*

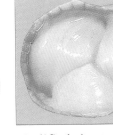

Modified tissue valve
Tissue valves may be taken from a pig (shown above), a human after death, or may be made of tendons from a patient's own body.

CONGENITAL DEFECTS

If a woman contracts a viral infection (particularly rubella) during early pregnancy, the fetal heart may fail to develop normally. Congenital defects can also occur if a pregnant woman has diabetes that is not well controlled, or if the child has Down's syndrome (caused by a chromosomal abnormality). Ultrasound screening has made it possible to recognize and plan for the treatment of some heart defects before birth.

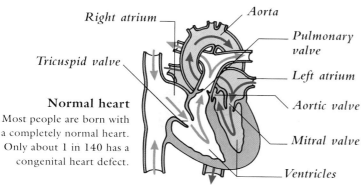

Right atrium
Aorta
Pulmonary valve
Tricuspid valve
Left atrium
Aortic valve
Mitral valve
Ventricles

Normal heart
Most people are born with a completely normal heart. Only about 1 in 140 has a congenital heart defect.

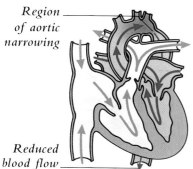

Region of aortic narrowing

Reduced blood flow

Coarctation of the aorta
In this defect a short section of the aorta is narrowed, which results in reduced blood flow to the lower body. An infant may be pale and find it difficult to breathe or eat. Urgent corrective surgery is usually needed.

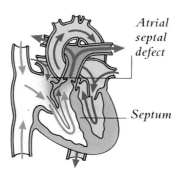

Atrial septal defect

Septum

Atrial septal defect
A hole in the septum, the wall that separates the atria, allows too much blood to flow to the lungs. Often occurring in children with Down's syndrome, these defects may need surgery when a child is age 4 or 5.

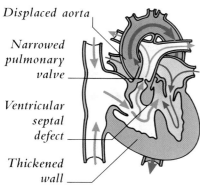

Displaced aorta

Narrowed pulmonary valve

Ventricular septal defect

Thickened wall

Tetralogy of Fallot
This is a combination of four structural defects: a hole in the septum between the ventricles, a thickened right ventricular wall, a displaced aorta, and a narrowed pulmonary valve. Symptoms are cyanosis (a distinctive bluish cast to the skin) and breathlessness.

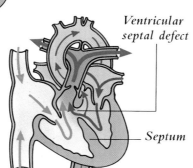

Ventricular septal defect

Septum

Ventricular septal defect
A hole in the septum separating the ventricles means that blood from the left ventricle pumps into the right. Too much blood is pumped at high pressure into the lungs. Although a small hole may often close as a child grows, larger holes require surgery.

SURGICAL REPAIR OF A VENTRICULAR SEPTAL DEFECT

Although about 60 per cent of ventricular septal defects heal on their own, others are life-threatening and need surgical repair. The size of the septal hole will affect the child's symptoms, which may include a heart murmur, cyanosis (a bluish cast to the skin), as well as breathing difficulties due to high pressure in the lungs. Surgical repair is usually performed before a child is 2 years old.

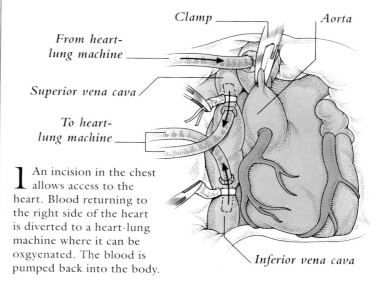

Clamp
Aorta
From heart-lung machine
Superior vena cava
To heart-lung machine
Inferior vena cava

1 An incision in the chest allows access to the heart. Blood returning to the right side of the heart is diverted to a heart-lung machine where it can be oxygenated. The blood is pumped back into the body.

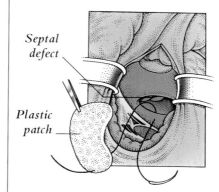

Septal defect

Plastic patch

2 The pumping of the heart is stopped and its chambers emptied of blood. An incision is made in the wall of the right ventricle. The surgeon stitches a small plastic patch over the septal defect, and then stitches the incision in the ventricle wall tightly together. After the heart has been restarted, the patient is taken off the heart-lung machine.

3 Closing the hole restores normal circulation so that contractions of the left ventricle pump blood throughout the body and contractions of the right ventricle pump blood to the lungs. After the operation, the patient's symptoms and quality of life improve markedly.

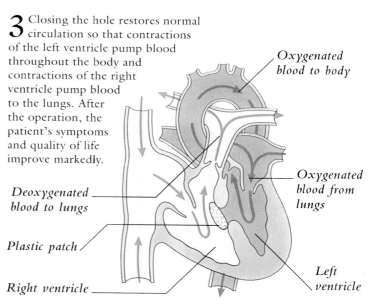

Oxygenated blood to body

Oxygenated blood from lungs

Deoxygenated blood to lungs

Plastic patch

Right ventricle

Left ventricle

HEART RATE *and* RHYTHM DISORDERS

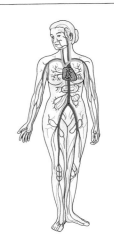

A NORMAL HEART BEATS STEADILY about 60 to 100 times per minute, although this rate rises during exercise or stress. If the rhythm becomes erratic, or the rate becomes unusually slow or fast, the condition is known as an arrhythmia. The most common cause of such disorders is coronary heart disease; however, a congenital abnormality in heart structure may be a contributory factor.

DIAGNOSING THE CAUSE

Heartbeat occurs when electrical impulses are initiated by "pacemaker" cells that are located at the top of the heart. These impulses spread through the atria, and then travel along conducting fibres to the ventricles, continually stimulating contractions. An irregular pattern or abnormal rate will usually produce symptoms such as dizziness and fainting, palpitations, breathing difficulties, and chest pain.

Recording an ECG

An electrocardiogram (ECG) detects the site and type of arrhythmia. Electrodes placed on the chest, the wrists, and the ankles connect via wires to a machine. A tracing of the heartbeat is produced.

Reading an ECG

Each deflection represents a stage in the passage of impulses through the heart.

P: *Atria contract*
Q: *Impulses start to pass along conducting fibres*
R: *Ventricles contract (positive charge)*
S: *Negative charge*
T: *Ventricles return to resting state*

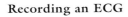

|◄ 0.2 SEC ►|

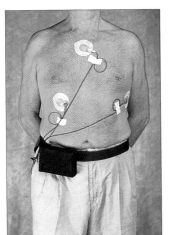

AMBULATORY ECG

Because an ECG is performed for a brief period of time only, a normal reading may be obtained even when an arrhythmia exists. Intermittent abnormalities in heartbeat may be detected by a Holter monitor worn over a 24-hour period. The patient also records when any symptoms, such as dizziness or pain, occur.

Wearing a Holter monitor

The patient continues with normal activities while wearing a Holter monitor on a belt around the waist.

ABNORMAL PATTERNS

Arrhythmias are grouped into tachycardias, in which the heart beats faster than 100 times per minute, or bradycardias, in which the rate drops below 60 beats per minute. Patterns can also be classified by rhythm (regular, irregular), the part of the heart where the impulse originates, and the part of the heart that is affected. Common causes of arrhythmias include coronary heart disease, stress, caffeine, and some types of medication.

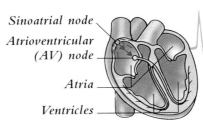

Sinoatrial node
Atrioventricular (AV) node
Atria
Ventricles

Sinus tachycardia

This regular but rapid pattern (over 100 beats per minute) can occur during exercise, a fever, or stress, or as a response to stimulants such as caffeine.

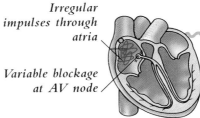

Irregular impulses through atria
Variable blockage at AV node

Atrial fibrillation

Random and extremely rapid atrial contractions (between 300 and 500 beats per minute) trigger an irregular pattern of ventricular contractions.

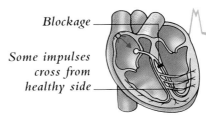

Blockage
Some impulses cross from healthy side

Bundle-branch block

Damage to a branch of the heart's bundle of conducting fibres impedes the passage of impulses. Rate slows if right and left branches are blocked.

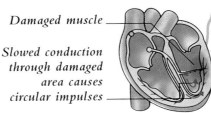

Damaged muscle
Slowed conduction through damaged area causes circular impulses

Ventricular tachycardia

Damaged heart muscle causes abnormal electrical activity. This triggers very rapid but ineffective ventricular contractions (more than 140 beats per minute).

REGULATING HEART RHYTHM

Arrhythmias are commonly caused by an inadequate blood flow to the cells that stimulate cardiac contractions. This may be treated by defibrillation, in which an electric shock is passed through the heart, or by drugs. If these prove not to be effective, several types of pacemaker are available to regulate the heart's action and correct abnormal patterns.

PACEMAKERS

A pacemaker is a battery-operated device that can send timed electrical impulses to the heart to make it contract regularly. There are several types: some supply constant impulses at a predetermined rate, while others are activated only when the heart is not beating normally. Insertion of a pacemaker is usually carried out under local anaesthesia.

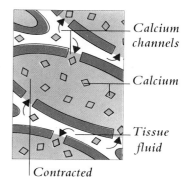

Dual-chamber
With this device, the atria and the ventricles are served by separate wires that adjust heart rhythm automatically.

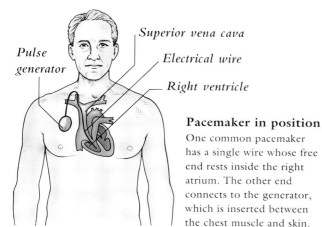

Pulse generator
Superior vena cava
Electrical wire
Right ventricle

Pacemaker in position
One common pacemaker has a single wire whose free end rests inside the right atrium. The other end connects to the generator, which is inserted between the chest muscle and skin.

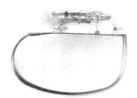

Programmable
This type of pacemaker can be programmed by sending electromagnetic signals through the skin.

IMPLANTABLE DEFIBRILLATORS

To stabilize ventricular tachycardia, a potentially fatal arrhythmia, an implantable defibrillator may be used. The device is a small electric generator that has three wires. When it detects a racing heartbeat, an electric shock is produced. This stops the heart for a split second so that the sinoatrial node can restart normal heart rate.

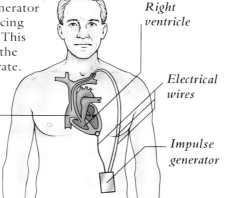

Right ventricle
Electrical wires
Impulse generator

Abdominal generator
After a generator has been inserted under the abdominal skin, wires are connected to the left lower heart surface and then fed into the right atrium and ventricle.

Right atrium

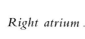

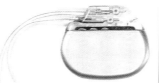

EMERGENCY DEFIBRILLATION
A heart attack sometimes brings on a severe ventricular fibrillation, which must be treated urgently. Two metal paddles are placed on the patient's chest and deliver an electric shock to the heart. The two round electrodes shown here connect to an ECG machine in order to monitor heart activity.

CALCIUM-CHANNEL BLOCKERS

These drugs slow the passage of impulses through heart muscle and so help to correct some types of arrhythmia. Their effect results from their action in stopping the flow of calcium into the heart muscle fibres. Although calcium-channel blockers can have dramatic results in improving an arrhythmia, they cannot cure the underlying disorder.

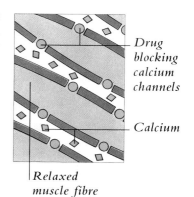

Before treatment
Calcium flows freely from the fluid that bathes cells through the membranes of cardiac muscle fibres. The calcium combines with a protein within the fibre, triggering muscle contraction.

Calcium channels
Calcium
Tissue fluid
Contracted muscle fibre

After treatment
The flow of calcium through the cardiac muscle membranes is blocked by the action of the drug. Muscle fibres relax, inhibiting passage of impulses through the heart and slowing heart rate.

Drug blocking calcium channels
Calcium
Relaxed muscle fibre

CARDIAC GLYCOSIDES

Produced originally from the leaves of the foxglove plant and commonly known as digitalis drugs, the cardiac glycosides lengthen the conduction time of nerve impulses through the heart muscle; they also make contractions of the ventricles stronger.

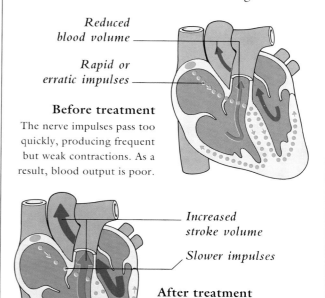

Reduced blood volume
Rapid or erratic impulses

Before treatment
The nerve impulses pass too quickly, producing frequent but weak contractions. As a result, blood output is poor.

Increased stroke volume
Slower impulses

After treatment
The drug slows down impulses through the heart, strengthens contractions, and increases the output of blood per heartbeat.

HEART MUSCLE DISEASE *and* HEART FAILURE

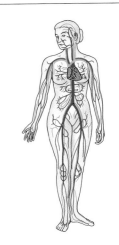

HEART PROBLEMS ARE MOST OFTEN the result of hypertension, a congenital defect, or coronary heart disease. Sometimes, however, they are caused by a disease of the heart muscle itself, or of the sac-like pericardium surrounding the heart. All these disorders, if they are long-standing or severe, can lead to heart failure and reduce the heart's ability to pump blood to the body.

HEART MUSCLE DISEASE

Inflammation of the heart muscle, called myocarditis, is usually caused by a viral infection, but may also be the result of rheumatic fever or exposure to radiation, drugs, or chemicals. Many patients recover without treatment. Non-inflammatory heart muscle disease, known as cardiomyopathy, may result from a genetic disorder, a vitamin or mineral deficiency, or excessive alcohol; the three main types are shown below.

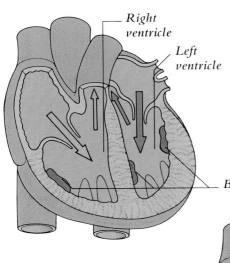

Right ventricle

Left ventricle

Blood clots

Dilated cardiomyopathy

Dilation (widening) of the ventricles causes the heart to contract less forcefully. As a result, not enough blood is ejected with each heartbeat and less oxygen reaches the body tissues. In some cases, blood clots may form on the inner walls of the heart.

Hypertrophic cardiomyopathy

This type of cardiomyopathy is usually inherited, although its cause is still not known. Overgrowth of heart muscle fibres causes thickening, especially in the left ventricle and the septum.

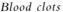

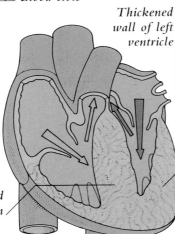

Thickened wall of left ventricle

Thickened septum

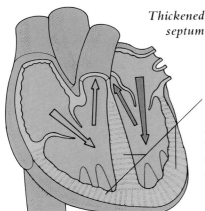

Rigid ventricular walls

Restrictive cardiomyopathy

The walls of the ventricles become abnormally rigid and do not allow for normal filling. This disease is caused by scar tissue on the inner lining of the heart, or by deposits of iron or protein in the heart.

PERICARDITIS

Inflammation of the pericardium – the membranous bag that completely surrounds the heart – is usually due to a viral infection or a heart attack. It may also occur as a complication of rheumatic fever, cancer, an autoimmune disease, kidney failure, or injury to the pericardium from a penetrating wound. Symptoms of breathlessness, fever, and fatigue may be relieved by anti-inflammatory drugs or, in some cases, surgery.

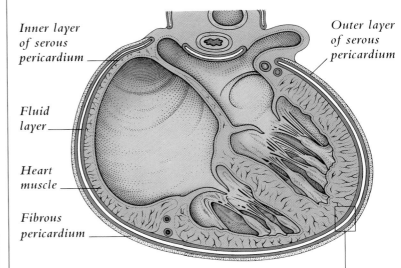

Inner layer of serous pericardium

Fluid layer

Heart muscle

Fibrous pericardium

Outer layer of serous pericardium

Structure of pericardium

The membrane of the pericardium has two layers. The outer layer, the fibrous pericardium, is tough and inelastic. The serous pericardium is the inner layer, and has two sheets separated by a thin film of lubricating fluid secreted by the inner sheet.

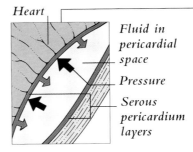

Heart

Fluid in pericardial space

Pressure

Serous pericardium layers

Pericardial effusion

An inflamed serous pericardium may produce too much fluid, which can compress the heart and interfere with pumping.

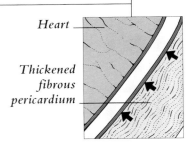

Heart

Thickened fibrous pericardium

Constrictive pericarditis

Inflammation sometimes scars the pericardium, causing it to thicken and shrink. The heart may not be able to fill between contractions.

HEART FAILURE

Heart failure, also known as ventricular failure, does not mean that the heart cannot beat: it means that it cannot pump blood effectively to the lungs and body tissues. Symptoms of the disease include coughing, fatigue, oedema (fluid in tissues), and breathlessness, and are related to which side of the heart is affected. Drugs to strengthen heart contractions, widen blood vessels, and prevent fluid build-up may be prescribed.

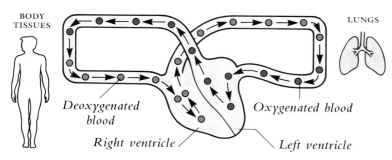

BODY TISSUES

LUNGS

Deoxygenated blood

Oxygenated blood

Right ventricle

Left ventricle

Normal circulation
Both sides of the heart normally pump out the same amount of blood after each beat, and take in the same amount as they pump out. There is no blood congestion anywhere in the circulation.

RIGHT-SIDED HEART FAILURE

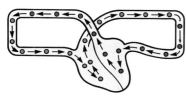

1 A diseased right side of the heart, possibly due to a valve defect or a respiratory disorder, is unable to pump blood to the lungs as fast as it returns from the body through the veins.

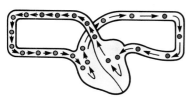

2 Blood begins to pool in the right side of the heart. The veins, continuing their attempt to return blood, become congested.

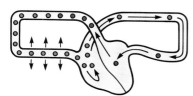

3 Increased congestion causes raised pressure in the veins, which forces fluid out through the capillary walls. Tissues in the ankles and sometimes the lower back swell as fluid accumulates.

LEFT-SIDED HEART FAILURE

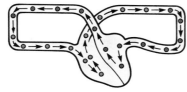

1 The left side of the heart may fail to pump blood out to the body as fast as it returns from the lungs through the pulmonary veins. This may be due to a heart structure defect or an arrhythmia.

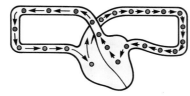

2 Blood that cannot re-enter the circulation begins to back up into the pulmonary veins and the lungs, causing congestion.

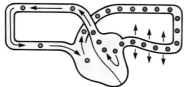

3 The pressure from increasing congestion causes fluid to collect in the lungs, preventing efficient transfer of oxygen to the blood. This leads to coughing, breathlessness, and fatigue.

HEART TRANSPLANTATION

This major operation is usually reserved for people under the age of 55 whose progressive heart failure has not been successfully treated by medications or previous surgery. The main risks are infection and the recipient's rejection of the donor heart. To prevent rejection from occurring, immunosuppressant drugs are given before the operation; these must be taken for the rest of the patient's life, and may have serious side-effects.

1 The patient is anaesthetized, and the surgeon makes an incision in the patient's chest. The sternum, or breastbone, is split apart, and the pericardial membranes are cut open to expose the defective heart.

Site of incision

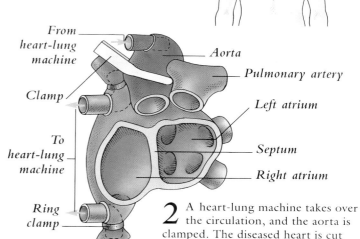

From heart-lung machine

Aorta

Pulmonary artery

Clamp

Left atrium

To heart-lung machine

Septum

Right atrium

Ring clamp

2 A heart-lung machine takes over the circulation, and the aorta is clamped. The diseased heart is cut away from the aorta, the front walls of the two atria, and the pulmonary artery. The heart is then removed.

3 The back walls of the atria remain in place, and the donor heart is stitched to their free edges as well as to the septal wall (not seen in this illustration).

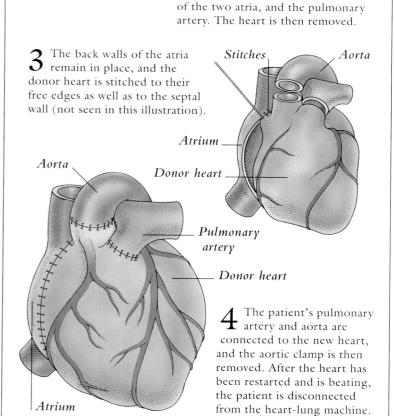

Stitches

Aorta

Atrium

Donor heart

Aorta

Pulmonary artery

Donor heart

Atrium

4 The patient's pulmonary artery and aorta are connected to the new heart, and the aortic clamp is then removed. After the heart has been restarted and is beating, the patient is disconnected from the heart-lung machine.

CIRCULATORY DISORDERS

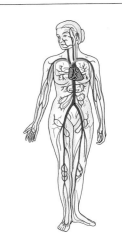

BLOOD FLOW MAY BE IMPEDED OR BLOCKED as it travels through arteries and veins. Normally, blood flow varies in response to exercise, digestion, and changes in external temperature, all of which influence the diameter of blood vessels. However, these responses can be impaired by structural defects such as weakened or thickened arterial walls or malfunctioning valves. Blood flow may also be hindered by obstructions: blood clots or fatty deposits. Treatment is required to forestall strokes or heart attacks.

THROMBOSIS

When a blood vessel is cut or damaged, a clot forms to prevent blood loss. A blood clot can form in an intact vessel, especially if an artery contains fatty deposits or if an artery or vein is inflamed. These clots, known as thrombi, cause pain and loss of function in the area served by the vessel, and can also be life-threatening.

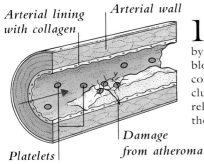

Arterial lining with collagen
Arterial wall
Platelets
Damage from atheroma

1 When a blood vessel wall is damaged, for example by atheroma, platelets in the blood come into contact with collagen. This makes them clump together and start to release chemicals that begin the process of blood clotting.

2 The released chemicals help convert fibrinogen, a soluble blood protein, into strands of insoluble fibrin. These strands trap platelets and blood cells to form a clot.

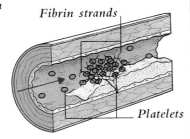

Fibrin strands
Platelets

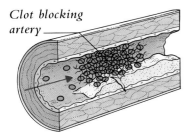

Clot blocking artery

3 Blood flow slows down as the fibrin enmeshes more platelets. The clot increases in size and may eventually block the artery. Particles may break away to become emboli.

ANTICOAGULANTS

Anticoagulant drugs such as warfarin and heparin slow down the chemical processes that lead to the formation of blood clots. They may be given to people whose blood has an increased tendency to clot, such as those with atherosclerosis or who have just had surgery. These drugs do not dissolve clots, but they stop further growth, and prevent new clots forming.

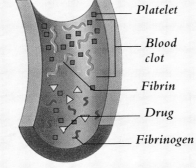

Platelet
Blood clot
Fibrin
Drug
Fibrinogen

EMBOLISM

An embolism occurs when particles of material travel in the bloodstream and lodge in some site away from their point of origin. These fragments may be parts of a thrombus, or a whole thrombus that has detached from its original site. Emboli may also be composed of atheromatous debris, cholesterol crystals, air, or fat from the marrow of fractured bones. If drugs do not inhibit or dissolve clots, surgery may be needed.

Pulmonary embolism
An embolus may travel from the veins of the leg or pelvis, through the heart, to a pulmonary artery. It may lodge there, thus creating an obstruction that deprives lung tissue of vital oxygen. Known as a pulmonary embolism, this condition is life-threatening.

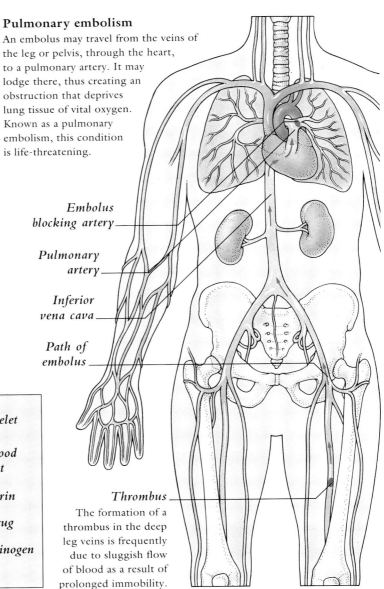

Embolus blocking artery
Pulmonary artery
Inferior vena cava
Path of embolus

Thrombus
The formation of a thrombus in the deep leg veins is frequently due to sluggish flow of blood as a result of prolonged immobility.

ANEURYSM

An aneurysm is an abnormal swelling in a weakened arterial wall. The defect may be due to disease or an injury, or it may be congenital. Although aneurysms may occur anywhere in the body, they most often affect the aorta. In older people, they develop more frequently in the abdominal aorta, at a point just below the kidneys. They are usually treated surgically.

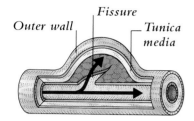

Outer wall *Fissure* *Tunica media*

Dissecting aneurysm

A fissure, or split, in the inner lining of an arterial wall allows blood to seep through and press against the tunica media (middle wall) and the outer arterial wall. The artery swells and its walls thin and may burst.

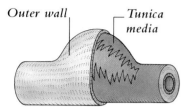

Outer wall *Tunica media*

Common aneurysm

A common aneurysm forms when muscle fibres of the tunica media are weak. When blood flows through an affected area, the arterial wall may bulge and sometimes even rupture.

OPERATION

VARICOSE VEINS

Defective valves in deep, lower-leg veins can cause blood to drain backward and pool in the superficial veins nearest the skin surface. These veins may then become swollen, twisted, and painful, leading to skin ulcers or swelling of the feet. Surgery may be needed.

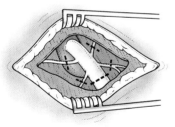

1 A small incision is made in the groin. This exposes the great saphenous vein and its four branches. All are tied and then cut to stop blood flow.

2 A wire is inserted into a hole created in the vein. The wire is then guided down the leg to either the calf or the ankle, where it is brought out through a small incision.

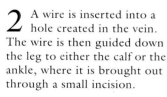

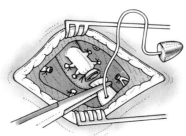

3 The wire has a specially designed, thick top end. This is tied securely to the vein, and the groin incision is closed.

4 The vein is "stripped", or removed, by pulling on the wire exiting from the lower incision. The incision is closed and the leg bandaged.

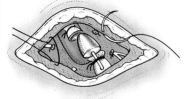

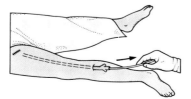

HYPERTENSION

Blood pressure is the force with which blood flows through the arteries. Hypertension is persistent, abnormally elevated blood pressure. Although it may cause no symptoms, this condition increases the risk of stroke, heart attack, and other circulatory diseases. Blood pressure is recorded in millimetres of mercury (mmHg) using a device called a sphygmomanometer.

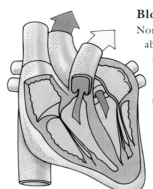

Blood pressure readings

Normal blood pressure in healthy young adults is about 110/75mmHg. The first number is the systolic pressure, taken just after the ventricles contract (when pressure is at its greatest). The second is the diastolic pressure, taken when the ventricles relax (when pressure is lowest).

SYSTOLE: VENTRICLES CONTRACT AND FORCE BLOOD OUT

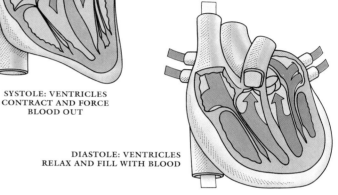

DIASTOLE: VENTRICLES RELAX AND FILL WITH BLOOD

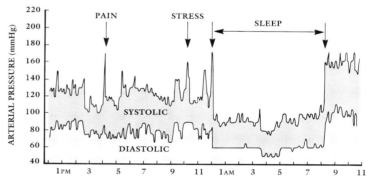

Variations in a 24-hour period

The chart above shows how blood pressure varies greatly in response to various stimuli, such as pain or stress. Variations of this kind are normal.

TREATMENT

Low-sodium, low-fat diets and lifestyle changes to reduce stress are recommended, and diuretics may be prescribed. By inhibiting the reabsorption of water and salt, diuretics increase urine excretion. Less water in the blood reduces the workload of the heart, thus lowering blood pressure.

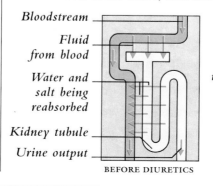

Bloodstream
Fluid from blood
Water and salt being reabsorbed
Kidney tubule
Urine output

BEFORE DIURETICS

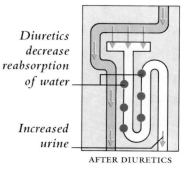

Diuretics decrease reabsorption of water
Increased urine

AFTER DIURETICS

CHAPTER SEVEN

C H A P T E R   7

The
IMMUNE
SYSTEM

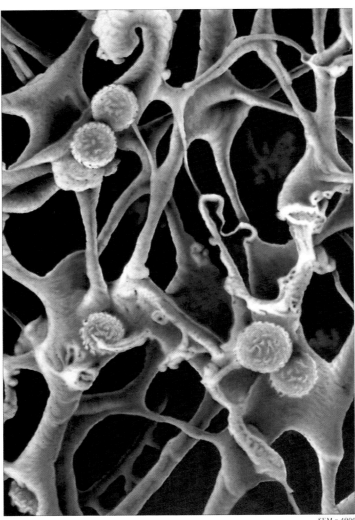

Lymphatic tissue from
inside a lymph node

SEM x 4900

INTRODUCTION

The body has its very own security force – the immune system, which patrols the body and guards it against invasion from outside and subversion from within. A newborn baby is protected by the antibodies supplied by its mother, partly in breast milk. Soon after birth, the immune defences take up their lifelong task of recognizing invading disease organisms, such as parasites and bacteria. Certain cells of the immune system, the B and T lymphocytes, have memories, which enable them to respond quickly to any infection they have previously encountered. Immunization is a way of stimulating the body to form more of these defence memories; it plays a crucial role in controlling infectious diseases, such as poliomyelitis and diphtheria. The internal surveillance system is also alert to abnormal cell division within body tissues, and a healthy immune system will eliminate potential cancers at an early stage. Impairment of the immune system by ageing, or by diseases such as AIDS, inhibits this response, increasing the risk of malignancy. Some medications, such as the steroid drugs that are given to some patients suffering from chronic diseases, can do harm to the immune system. Malfunctioning of the immune system may also cause it to turn in upon itself, leading to one of the autoimmune disorders, such as rheumatoid arthritis, in which the body attacks its own tissues.

A bacterium

Virus particles escape after attacking a cell

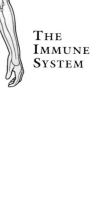

THE IMMUNE SYSTEM

DEFENCES AGAINST INFECTION

A HEALTHY BODY CAN DEFEND ITSELF against most invading organisms that may cause infection or disease. There are two types of defence, innate and adaptive. Innate defences include mechanical barriers, such as the skin, and chemical defences such as an antibacterial enzyme in tears. The adaptive system is based on specialized white blood cells called lymphocytes, which respond to invasion of the body by microorganisms. B cells produce chemicals called antibodies, which circulate in the blood and attack specific disease-causing organisms; T cells attack the organisms directly. These cells can retain a memory of earlier infections and respond quickly to further attacks.

LYMPH AND LYMPH VESSELS

Lymph is a clear, watery liquid that begins as fluid flowing between cells. This so-called interstitial fluid is not called lymph until it drains into the network of lymph capillaries located in the tissue spaces. From lymph capillaries, lymph flows into larger vessels called lymphatics (seen at right), which are studded with filters called nodes. Lymph is not pumped, but is moved when lymph vessels are compressed by surrounding muscles as they contract during movement.

Supratrochlear node

Thoracic duct

Subclavian veins
Lymph drains from the upper right part of the body into the right subclavian vein, while lymph from the rest of the body collects in the thoracic duct, draining from here into the left subclavian vein.

Spleen
Some types of lymphocyte mature in and are then stored in the spleen, the largest of the lymph organs.

Stomach
Acid and enzymes secreted here destroy ingested organisms.

Peyer's patch
Clusters of lymph tissue, called Peyer's patches, are found in the lower part of the small intestine.

Lacrimal glands
These glands produce tears that contain a protective enzyme.

Adenoid

Tonsils
These two glands and the adenoids produce antibodies against ingested or inhaled organisms.

Salivary glands

Thymus
Stem cells are produced in bone marrow. They then migrate to the thymus, increase in number, and develop into T cells.

Axillary nodes

Cisterna chyli
Lymphatics from the lower body converge to form this vessel.

Lateral aortic nodes

Common iliac nodes

Open valve governs direction of flow

Interstitial fluid enters

LYMPH CAPILLARY

Valve closed

Overlapping epithelial cells

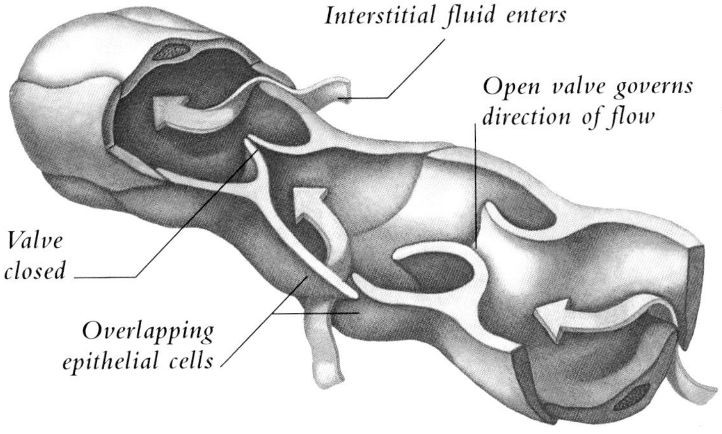

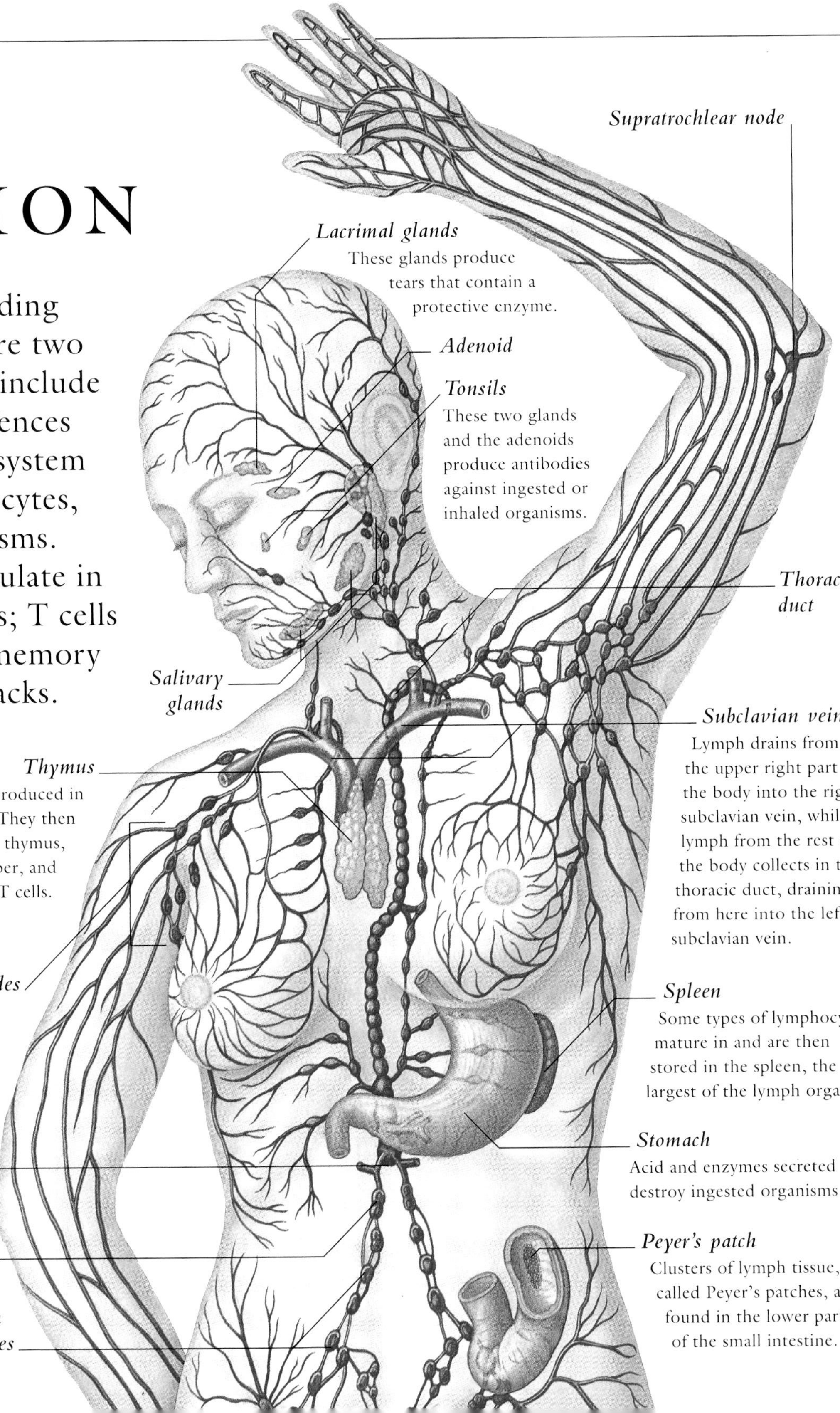

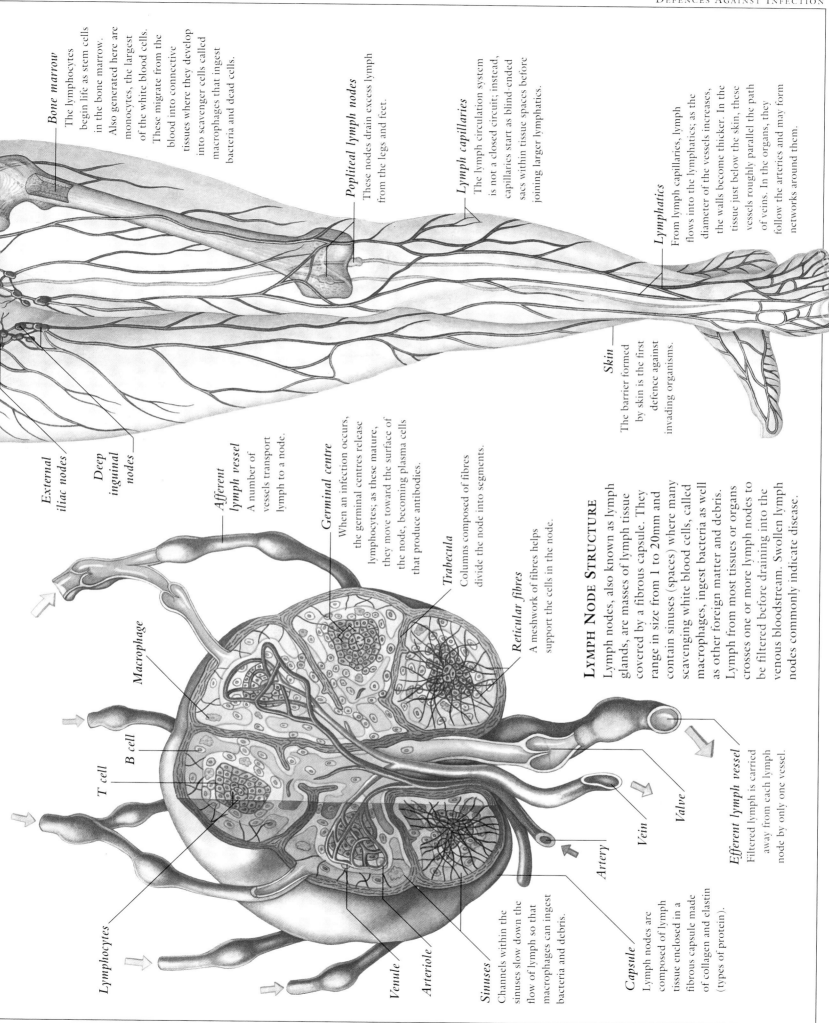

Bone marrow
The lymphocytes begin life as stem cells in the bone marrow. Also generated here are monocytes, the largest of the white blood cells. These migrate from the blood into connective tissues where they develop into scavenger cells called macrophages that ingest bacteria and dead cells.

Popliteal lymph nodes
These nodes drain excess lymph from the legs and feet.

Lymph capillaries
The lymph circulation system is not a closed circuit; instead, capillaries start as blind-ended sacs within tissue spaces before joining larger lymphatics.

Lymphatics
From lymph capillaries, lymph flows into the lymphatics; as the diameter of the vessels increases, the walls become thicker. In the tissue just below the skin, these vessels roughly parallel the path of veins. In the organs, they follow the arteries and may form networks around them.

Skin
The barrier formed by skin is the first defence against invading organisms.

External iliac nodes

Deep inguinal nodes

Afferent lymph vessel
A number of vessels transport lymph to a node.

Germinal centre
When an infection occurs, the germinal centres release lymphocytes; as these mature, they move toward the surface of the node, becoming plasma cells that produce antibodies.

Trabecula
Columns composed of fibres divide the node into segments.

Reticular fibres
A meshwork of fibres helps support the cells in the node.

LYMPH NODE STRUCTURE

Lymph nodes, also known as lymph glands, are masses of lymph tissue covered by a fibrous capsule. They range in size from 1 to 20mm and contain sinuses (spaces) where many scavenging white blood cells, called macrophages, ingest bacteria as well as other foreign matter and debris. Lymph from most tissues or organs crosses one or more lymph nodes to be filtered before draining into the venous bloodstream. Swollen lymph nodes commonly indicate disease.

Macrophage

T cell

B cell

Lymphocytes

Sinuses
Channels within the sinuses slow down the flow of lymph so that macrophages can ingest bacteria and debris.

Capsule
Lymph nodes are composed of lymph tissue enclosed in a fibrous capsule made of collagen and elastin (types of protein).

Venule

Arteriole

Artery

Vein

Valve

Efferent lymph vessel
Filtered lymph is carried away from each lymph node by only one vessel.

INFLAMMATORY *and* IMMUNE RESPONSES

IF INVADING INFECTIOUS ORGANISMS BREACH THE SKIN or are not killed by surface chemicals such as enzymes contained in tears or saliva, the inflammatory and immune responses of the body spring into action. Pain, swelling, and fever may may be signs of the battle against infection as several types of white blood cell try to prevent infection from spreading.

INFLAMMATORY RESPONSE

Some disease organisms may trigger an inflammatory response in affected tissues. This type of defence is non-specific: it is not specially tailored to destroy a specific organism, but attacks all invading organisms in the same way. It increases blood flow and brings special cells called neutrophils to the area (seen here are bronchi) to ingest and destroy the organisms.

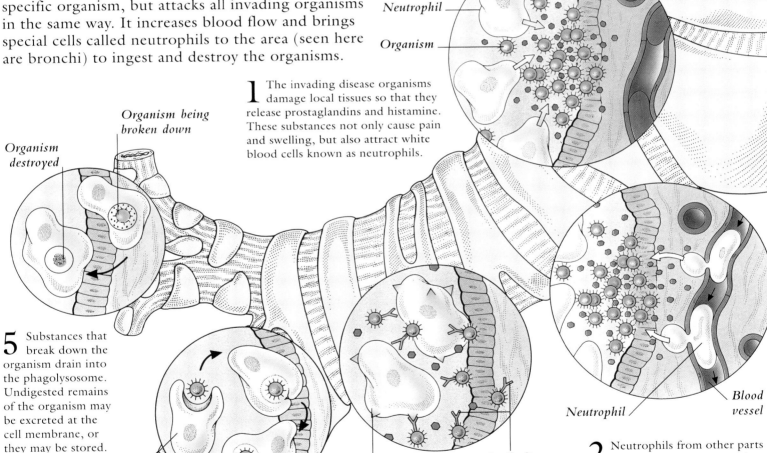

Bronchial lining

Prostaglandin

Neutrophil

Organism

Organism being broken down

Organism destroyed

Blood vessel

Neutrophil

Receptor   *Antibodies*

Neutrophil ingesting organism

Phagolysosome

1 The invading disease organisms damage local tissues so that they release prostaglandins and histamine. These substances not only cause pain and swelling, but also attract white blood cells known as neutrophils.

5 Substances that break down the organism drain into the phagolysosome. Undigested remains of the organism may be excreted at the cell membrane, or they may be stored.

2 Neutrophils from other parts of the body are attracted by toxins (poisons) produced by the organisms as well as by histamine and prostaglandins. Neutrophils squeeze through tiny spaces in the blood vessel walls in order to reach the site of the injured tissues.

3 Antibodies are specifically created proteins that attach to the invading organisms. The newly arrived neutrophils have receptors so that they recognize the antibodies. Both the antibody and the disease organism then attach to the neutrophils.

4 The neutrophils form pseudopods, or "false feet", that engulf the organism. After it has been ingested, the organism is isolated within a phagolysosome, a small, spherical organelle (a type of cell subunit). This process is known as phagocytosis.

SPECIFIC IMMUNE RESPONSES

The rapid, non-specific inflammatory response may prevent the spread of infection. If infection persists or spreads, however, two types of specific defence, either an antibody or a cellular defence, may be activated. These defences are called immune responses; they depend on the action of white blood cells, the B and T lymphocytes, and provide protection against future infections.

ANTIBODY DEFENCES

B lymphocytes recognize foreign proteins from disease organisms, called antigens, that are different from natural body proteins. Antigens trigger B cells to multiply. Some develop into plasma cells, which secrete antibodies – special proteins that attack and destroy only the antigens.

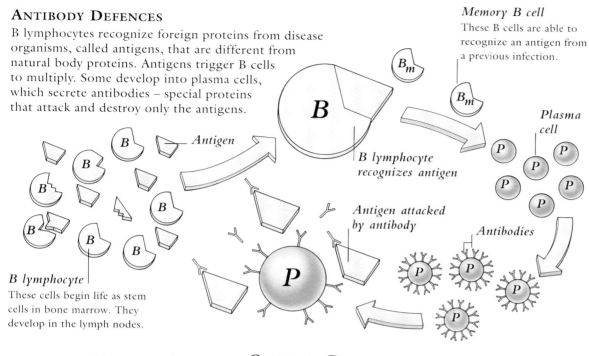

B lymphocyte
These cells begin life as stem cells in bone marrow. They develop in the lymph nodes.

Antigen

B lymphocyte recognizes antigen

Antigen attacked by antibody

Memory B cell
These B cells are able to recognize an antigen from a previous infection.

Plasma cell

Antibodies

CELLULAR DEFENCES

T lymphocytes develop inside the thymus gland. "Killer" T cells react to the remains of destroyed specific antigens, attacking them, as well as any infected cells, with powerful proteins called lymphokines. "Helper" T cells activate B and T cells, while "suppressor" T cells inhibit the response of other cells to the invading antigens.

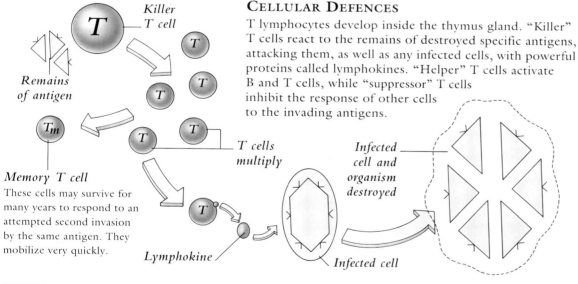

Killer T cell

Remains of antigen

Memory T cell
These cells may survive for many years to respond to an attempted second invasion by the same antigen. They mobilize very quickly.

T cells multiply

Lymphokine

Infected cell

Infected cell and organism destroyed

COMPLEMENT SYSTEM

Circulating in the blood are at least 25 inactive proteins. These "complement" proteins are activated by antibodies or certain lymphokines. They help to destroy bacteria, neutralize their toxins, and clear away antigen/antibody complexes.

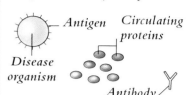

Antigen   *Circulating proteins*

Disease organism

Antibody

1 In response to the antigens manufactured by a disease organism, such as a virus or a bacterium, the immune system produces specific antibodies.

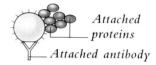

Attached proteins

Attached antibody

2 Antibodies become attached to the antigens, resulting in antigen/antibody complexes that trigger a cascade of complement proteins. These proteins also attach to the disease organism.

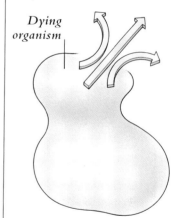

Dying organism

3 The proteins penetrate the cell membrane of the disease organism, which bursts and dies as intracellular fluid rushes in.

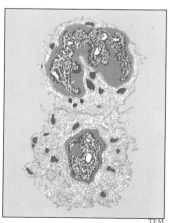

A T cell in action
The activated cytotoxic ("killer") T lymphocyte at the top of the image has become attached to an infected target cell after having recognized antigens on its surface. In addition to attacking specific antigens, T cells attack cancer cells, thus slowing tumour growth.

TEM

LOCAL AND SYSTEMIC INFECTION

Battles against infection are often simply local skirmishes, such as a swelling in one of the lymph nodes or a slightly infected wound. If local defences are breached, a global response to spreading infection occurs, signs of which may be fever or a high white blood cell count.

An abscess: isolated war zone
Pus is a collection of damaged cells, destroyed bacteria, and dead neutrophils. An abscess is formed when a membrane surrounds pus.

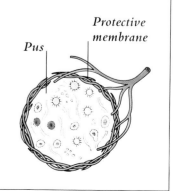

Pus   *Protective membrane*

INFECTIOUS ORGANISMS *and* IMMUNIZATION

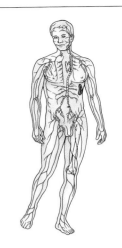

THE HUMAN BODY IS CONSTANTLY INFECTED by organisms: bacteria, viruses, fungi, and protozoa. Some organisms are beneficial, such as the intestinal bacteria that aid digestion. Others are harmful and cause illnesses that range from mild colds to life-threatening tetanus. The immune system produces antibodies to fight infections, some of which help to prevent re-infection.

BACTERIA

Bacteria that are present in soil, water, and air can cause serious illnesses such as pneumonia, tetanus, and syphilis. Fortunately, antibiotics are effective against most bacteria; they work by destroying the bacterial cell wall. As well as antibiotics, vaccines are available to combat some bacterial infections, such as tetanus and *Haemophilus influenzae* B.

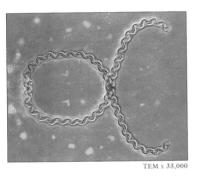

TEM x 33,000

Structure of bacteria
Bacteria are single-celled organisms whose shapes vary greatly. Shown on the far left is a spiral-shaped spirochete, while on the near left an oval-shaped bacillus is seen. Coccal bacteria (not seen) are round.

Flagella help organism to move

HOW BACTERIA DAMAGE TISSUE

Some bacteria adhere to and invade tissue cells, such as the dysentery-causing *Shigella*. Others produce poisonous substances known as toxins. Some toxins are very dangerous: 3kg of botulinum could kill all the people in the world.

1 Toxins may alter certain chemical reactions in cells so that normal cell function is disrupted or the cell dies. One example is the diphtheria toxin, which damages heart muscle by inhibiting protein synthesis.

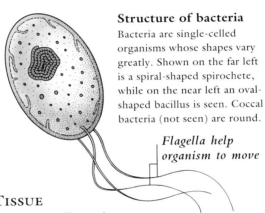

Bacteria *Body cells*

Toxins *Damaged or dying cells*

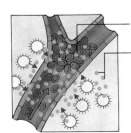

— *Clot in blood vessel*

— *Toxins from bacteria*

2 Some toxins cause blood to clot in small blood vessels. Areas of tissue supplied by these vessels may be deprived of blood and damaged.

3 Toxins can damage the cell walls of blood vessels so that there is leakage. This fluid loss causes blood pressure to decrease. Eventually, the heart is unable to transport adequate amounts of blood to the brain.

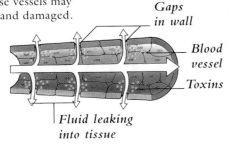

Gaps in wall

Blood vessel

Toxins

Fluid leaking into tissue

RESISTANCE TO ANTIBIOTICS

Since the introduction of penicillin in 1940, many bacteria have developed intricate ways of resisting antibiotics. The most effective mechanism is the rapid transfer of plasmids – small packages of the cell's DNA, its genetic material – between bacterial populations. Plasmids may contain resistant genes: the bacteria that receive these plasmids also inherit the resistant genes, and therefore develop the same resistance that the donor bacterium had.

The role of plasmids
Plasmids signal bacteria to produce enzymes that can inactivate drugs. They may also stimulate a bacterium to alter its receptor sites (where antibiotics normally bind).

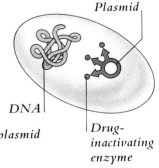

Plasmid

DNA

Drug-inactivating enzyme

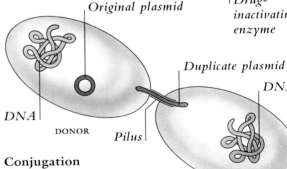

Original plasmid

Duplicate plasmid

DNA

DNA

DONOR

Pilus

RECIPIENT

Conjugation
Plasmid transfer takes place during a process known as conjugation. The plasmid duplicates itself in a "donor" bacterium. This copy passes through a tube, the pilus, to the "recipient" cell.

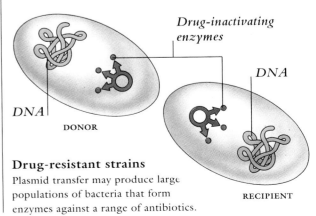

Drug-inactivating enzymes

DNA

DNA

DONOR

RECIPIENT

Drug-resistant strains
Plasmid transfer may produce large populations of bacteria that form enzymes against a range of antibiotics.

VIRUSES

Billions of viruses can cover a pinhead, and infections from these tiny germs can cause a wide range of diseases, including colds, polio, and AIDS. Unlike bacteria, viruses cannot be killed by antibiotics. Instead, the body must produce specific antibodies to combat each virus.

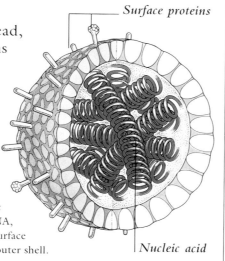

Surface proteins

Nucleic acid

Typical structure

Each virus has a core of nucleic acid, composed of DNA or RNA, and one or two protein shells. Surface proteins, or antigens, stud the outer shell.

HOW VIRAL DISEASES OCCUR

Because viruses have very few genes, they cannot reproduce by themselves, nor can they process nutrients independently. To live and reproduce, viruses must invade host cells, which either die or function abnormally. Certain viruses provoke the immune system to destroy normal cells.

Viral nucleic acid

HUMAN CELL

Invading virus

1 Before a virus invades a host cell, its surface proteins must attach to specific receptor sites on the surface. After attaching itself, part or all of the virus penetrates the host cell and sheds its protein shell to release its nucleic acid.

Cytoplasm

Nucleus

Cell membrane

Replicated virus particles

2 The nucleic acid makes copies of itself, using the host cell's raw materials, and sometimes its enzymes, to do so. Replicated nucleic acid generates new virus particles.

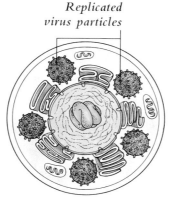

DYING CELL

3 The cell swells with new virus particles and may burst and die. When the cell bursts, the virus particles are released; these subsequently infect other cells. However, not all viruses destroy cells as they leave. Instead, some, such as herpesviruses, form buds and take away part of the host cell's membrane with them. They are known as enveloped viruses.

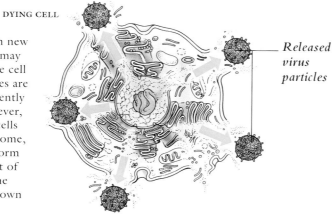

Released virus particles

ANTIGENIC SHIFT IN INFLUENZA

The three types of influenza viruses are designated as A, B, and C. Each can change its structure. The antibodies that were able to defend the body against a previous viral structure may be ineffective against a new one, and re-infection may occur. This change in structure, called the antigenic shift, occurs in the surface proteins (antigens) where antibodies attach.

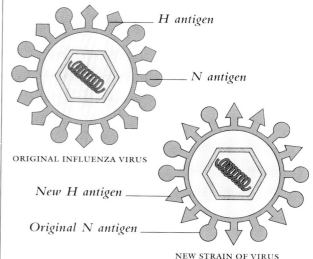

H antigen

N antigen

ORIGINAL INFLUENZA VIRUS

New H antigen

Original N antigen

NEW STRAIN OF VIRUS

TYPES OF VIRUS

Depending on the main constituent of the genetic material, viruses can be broadly classified as RNA viruses or DNA viruses. Further classification is governed by the size, shape, and symmetry of the virus. The most common families are listed below.

FAMILY		TYPE AND DISEASES
Adenoviruses		DNA viruses. Cause infections of the tonsils, respiratory tract, and eyes (such as conjunctivitis).
Papovaviruses		DNA viruses. Initiate benign, or non-cancerous, tumours such as warts on the hands and feet.
Herpesviruses		DNA viruses. Cause cold sores, genital herpes, chickenpox, shingles, and glandular fever.
Coronaviruses		RNA viruses. Named for their resemblance to the sun, they cause the common cold.
Picornaviruses		RNA viruses. Cause myocarditis, polio, viral hepatitis, and one form of meningitis.
Retroviruses		RNA viruses that can convert DNA into RNA. They cause AIDS and a type of leukaemia.
Reoviruses		RNA viruses. Cause respiratory infections; a group (rotaviruses) causes gastroenteritis.
Orthomyxo-viruses		RNA viruses. Cause influenza, symptoms of which include fever, cough, and a sore throat.
Paramyxo-viruses		RNA viruses. Cause mumps, measles, rubella and respiratory infections such as croup.

PROTOZOA

Protozoa are primitive, single-celled animals, some of which are parasites that sometimes cause serious disease in humans. Malaria and toxoplasmosis are caused by protozoal parasites, and affect over a third of the world's people. Parasites employ various mechanisms for evading the body's immune system. The *Leishmania* parasite, for example, which is responsible for causing a disease called kala-azar, lives and multiplies within phagocytes, blood cells that normally engulf microorganisms.

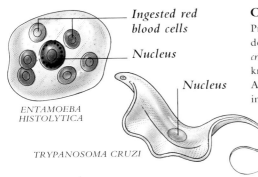

Ingested red blood cells

Nucleus

ENTAMOEBA HISTOLYTICA

Nucleus

Flagellum

TRYPANOSOMA CRUZI

Characteristics of protozoa

Protozoa have no cell wall and a large well-defined nucleus. Many, such as *Trypanosoma cruzi*, have one or more tail-like appendages known as flagella, which aid movement. Amoebae, such as *Entamoeba histolytica*, can ingest red blood cells and food particles.

MALARIA

Four types of *Plasmodia* protozoan can cause malaria. Spread by the bite of the female *Anopheles* mosquito, most of these have a similar life cycle (shown below) and produce chills and fever. One type, *Plasmodium falciparum*, affects vital organs such as the kidneys and brain, and can be fatal within hours if it is not treated immediately. Because resistance to antimalarial drugs is increasing, scientists are trying to develop vaccines.

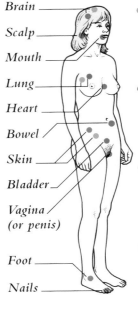

TEM x 5000

Two *P. falciparum* in a red blood cell

Female Anopheles *mosquito bites, injecting saliva that contains sporozoites, the infective form of malaria parasites*

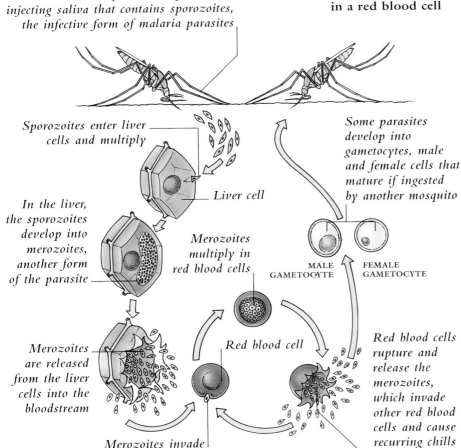

Sporozoites enter liver cells and multiply

Liver cell

In the liver, the sporozoites develop into merozoites, another form of the parasite

Merozoites are released from the liver cells into the bloodstream

Merozoites invade red blood cells

Red blood cell

Merozoites multiply in red blood cells

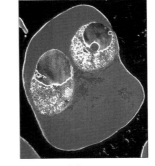

MALE GAMETOCYTE

FEMALE GAMETOCYTE

Some parasites develop into gametocytes, male and female cells that mature if ingested by another mosquito

Red blood cells rupture and release the merozoites, which invade other red blood cells and cause recurring chills and fever

FUNGI

Fungi are simple organisms that scavenge dead or rotting tissue. Some types infect humans, causing either harmless superficial diseases of the skin, hair, nails, or mucous membranes, or possibly fatal infections of certain vital organs, such as the lungs.

Brain

Scalp

Mouth

Lung

Heart

Bowel

Skin

Bladder

Vagina (or penis)

Foot

Nails

● *Cryptococcosis*
This infection causes meningitis and pneumonia, and can affect the skin and bones.

● *Aspergillosis*
This is a fungal infection that may spread through ventilation systems and affect the lungs.

● *Dermatophytosis*
This skin infection, also called tinea, most commonly affects the scalp, feet, or nails.

● *Candidiasis*
Candida infect the mouth and genitals, and occur in the heart, bowel, bladder, and brain.

Histoplasmosis

Histoplasmosis is associated with soil contaminated by bird droppings. Fungal spores may be inhaled by humans and can cause pneumonia. Spores can spread to and infect other organs, such as the heart.

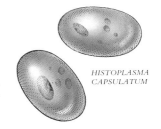

HISTOPLASMA CAPSULATUM

TREATMENT

Fungal infections respond in a variety of ways to antifungal drugs. Superficial infections like thrush (oral candidiasis) respond to local applications of antifungal drugs. Deep infections in people with lowered immunity are difficult to cure, and often require prolonged therapy with more toxic drugs.

Before drug

Fungal cells, which are harder to treat than bacteria, closely resemble human cells. Drugs have to differentiate between the two cells so that human cells remain unharmed.

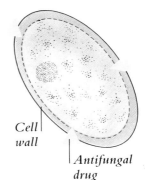

Cell wall

Antifungal drug

Cell contents leak out

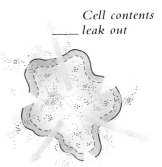

After drug

Most antifungal drugs form channels in the membrane of the fungal cell through which vital cell contents can leak out, causing cell death.

DIAGNOSIS

Diagnosis of infectious diseases is usually confirmed in the laboratory by techniques like microscopy or culture. Many bacteria are colourless, and require special staining techniques. With Gram's stain, different types of bacteria take up different dyes.

Culture

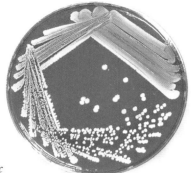

Certain bacteria or fungi are identified when specimens are cultured by growing them on plates until colonies are visible. Viruses are cultured on live cells or eggs.

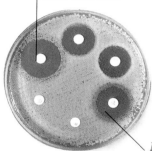

Saturated disc

Antibiotic sensitivity

To find the best treatment, bacterial colonies may be transferred onto plates that contain discs saturated with different antibiotics. No bacteria grow around the most effective antibiotic.

No growth

TESTS FOR VIRUSES

Viruses are too small to see with a light microscope. Instead, infections caused by viruses are diagnosed indirectly by their effects on cells. Certain viruses alter the surface of cultured cells, causing them to agglutinate, or stick together.

Single layer of cells

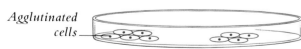

Blood sample

1 A single layer of tissue cells is cultured on a prepared plate. A specimen, such as blood from an infected person, is added to the plate.

Agglutinated cells

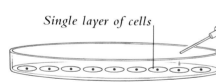

2 The presence of a virus can be identified in several ways. In this case, the virus has caused the single layer of tissue cells to clump together.

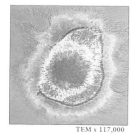

TEM x 117,000

A virus that agglutinates

Like many viruses, herpes simplex is identified by agglutination, and not by means of microscopy. The high-magnification image on the left reveals the virus's protein coat (seen in orange) surrounded by an irregular membrane.

IMMUNIZATION

Some infectious diseases are common and can recur in the same person. Others occur only once in a lifetime because the immune system can remember the organism and resist subsequent infections. To prevent an epidemic of a serious infectious disease, such as polio, immunization artificially creates a "memory" before the disease has been acquired.

ACTIVE IMMUNIZATION

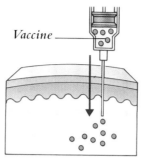
Vaccine

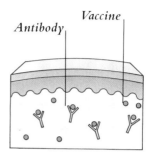
Antibody — *Vaccine*

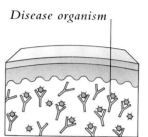
Disease organism

1 A vaccine with dead or harmless forms of an organism is injected into a healthy person.

2 The vaccine stimulates the immune system to produce antibodies, which remember the organism.

3 In any subsequent infection, these antibodies recognize and stop the organism.

PASSIVE IMMUNIZATION

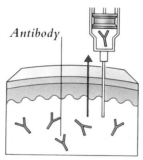
Antibody

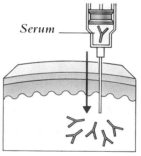
Serum

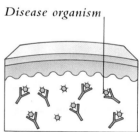
Disease organism

1 Blood with antibodies is taken from humans or animals who have had the infection recently.

2 Blood containing antibodies is separated to form serum, which is then purified and injected.

3 Antibodies either attack a current infection or provide short-term protection.

GENETICALLY ENGINEERED VIRUSES

Genetic engineering is a term that describes a technique to alter the genetic material (DNA) of an organism by inserting the genes from another organism. Viral genes are inserted into the DNA of other organisms. When these organisms multiply, the large amounts of replicated viral material are used as vaccines.

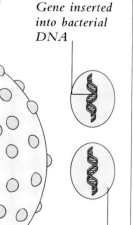

Gene inserted into bacterial DNA

Surface antigen gene from DNA

Replicated bacterium

Surface antigen

Hepatitis B vaccine

The gene of the surface antigen (protein) of the hepatitis B virus is inserted into the DNA of a bacterial cell. This cell produces antigens that are injected to stimulate an immune response.

IMMUNE SYSTEM DISORDERS

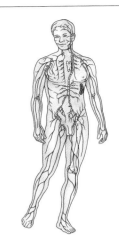

THE IMMUNE SYSTEM PROVIDES THE BODY WITH DEFENCES against infections as well as against cancers, injuries, and damage by poisonous and corrosive chemicals. There are two types of immune system disorders. In allergies and autoimmune diseases, the immune system overreacts; in immunodeficiency diseases, the defence systems are too weak to cope with threats to health.

THE ALLERGIC RESPONSE

Allergy is an inappropriate response by the immune system to a substance that, for most people, is usually harmless. These substances, known as allergens, may be inhaled or swallowed, or they may come into direct contact with the eyes or skin. They may then provoke allergic responses, such as hay fever, asthma, or rashes. Some people are allergic to eggs, milk, and grains.

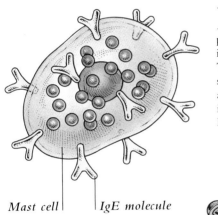

1 Allergens can provoke the immune system to produce an antibody called immunoglobulin E (IgE). The IgE molecules coat the surface of mast cells, which are located in the skin and in the lining of the stomach, lungs, and upper airways.

Mast cell *IgE molecule*

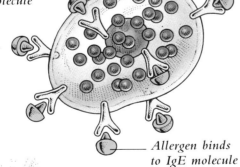

2 In an allergic person, subsequent exposure to allergens, which may be ingested or inhaled, causes them to bind to the IgE molecules. This is known as cross-linking.

Allergen binds to IgE molecule

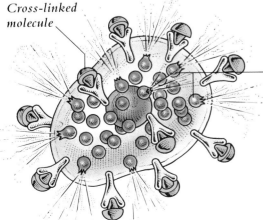

Cross-linked molecule

Granules release histamine and prostaglandins

3 Cross-linking causes granules located inside the mast cell to release the inflammatory substances histamine and prostaglandins, which trigger types of allergic response.

AUTOIMMUNE DISORDERS

Sometimes the immune system forms antibodies not against invaders such as bacteria, but against some of the body's own tissues. The mistaken attack may be directed against a particular organ, such as the thyroid gland, or it may cause a more general illness (see the table below). These diseases become more common in middle age and affect women more often than men.

Vitiligo

Melanocytes are cells that produce a skin-darkening pigment called melanin. Vitiligo, thought to be an autoimmune disorder, is due to an absence of these cells. As a result, there are multiple irregular areas of depigmentation in the skin.

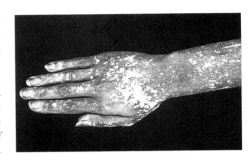

DISORDER	DESCRIPTION
ADDISON'S DISEASE	Damaged adrenal glands result in low blood pressure and weakness, lowering the body's ability to respond to stress.
INSULIN-DEPENDENT DIABETES MELLITUS	Clusters of pancreatic cells called islets of Langerhans cannot produce sufficient insulin, which causes high blood glucose levels.
HAEMOLYTIC ANAEMIA	This autoimmune form of anaemia shortens the lifespan of red blood cells, causing loss of energy, pallor, headaches, and breathlessness.
GRAVES' DISEASE	The thyroid becomes overactive and may become enlarged, forming a goitre. There is loss of weight, restlessness, and tremor.
MULTIPLE SCLEROSIS	Damage to nerve fibre coverings causes muscle weakness, disordered sensations, and problems with speech and vision.
MYASTHENIA GRAVIS	Damage to the junctions between nerves and muscles causes muscle weakness and fatigue, especially noticeable in muscles of the face.
SYSTEMIC LUPUS ERYTHEMATOSUS	Damaged connective tissue causes progressive loss of function in the kidneys, lungs, and joints. A distinctive rash appears on the face.

AIDS

Acquired immune deficiency syndrome, or AIDS, is caused by the human immunodeficiency virus (HIV). The virus destroys one type of white blood cell, the CD$_4$ lymphocyte. As the number of cells declines, the immune system becomes less effective, and death may occur approximately 10 years after infection. HIV is spread by sexual intercourse and contaminated blood.

SEM x 16,000

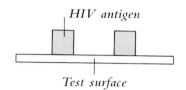

An infected lymphocyte

Small, spherical HIV particles are shown in green on the surface of a CD$_4$ "helper" lymphocyte. HIV compromises the body's immune system by destroying the CD$_4$ lymphocytes within which it lives.

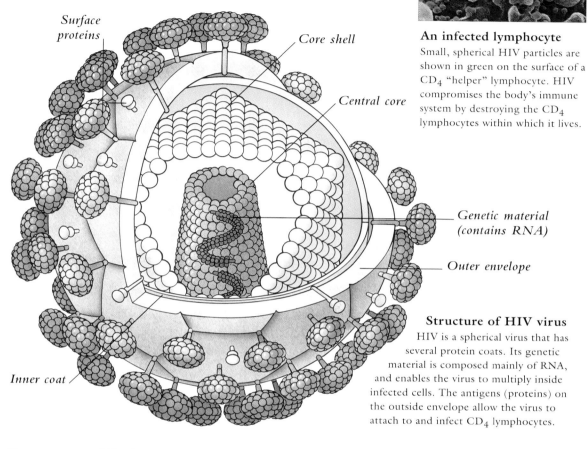

Surface proteins

Core shell

Central core

Genetic material (contains RNA)

Outer envelope

Inner coat

Structure of HIV virus

HIV is a spherical virus that has several protein coats. Its genetic material is composed mainly of RNA, and enables the virus to multiply inside infected cells. The antigens (proteins) on the outside envelope allow the virus to attach to and infect CD$_4$ lymphocytes.

EFFECTS OF AIDS

Many infected people have no symptoms for many years, and are known as "asymptomatic carriers". In later stages, they lose weight and develop night sweats, fevers, and diarrhoea. In full-blown AIDS, infected people become susceptible to a variety of infections and to certain cancers.

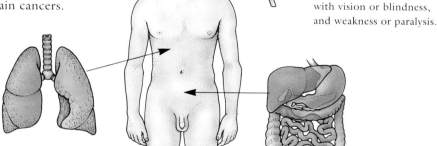

Nervous system

If HIV infection spreads to the brain and nervous system, it causes mental disturbances, problems with vision or blindness, and weakness or paralysis.

Lungs

Someone whose immune system has been damaged by HIV often develops lung infections. One type commonly associated with the disease is *Pneumocystis carinii* pneumonia, or PCP.

Skin

Kaposi's sarcoma is the cancer most often associated with AIDS. Brown or blue patches and nodules appear on the skin. These gradually spread to all parts of the body surface and also affect the internal organs.

Digestive system

Persistent diarrhoea is one of the most common features of AIDS. It is caused by infection of the gastrointestinal tract with parasites, for example *Giardia* and *Cryptosporidia*, and with fungi, especially *Candida*.

ELISA TEST

A blood test for HIV infection looks for the antibodies to the virus, which are easy to detect. The technique employed is the enzyme-linked immunosorbent assay, or ELISA. If antibodies are found, a confirmatory test, the Western Blot, is done. If both test results are positive, the person is HIV-positive.

HIV antigen

Test surface

1 Antigens, or surface proteins, from the AIDS virus are first spread on a prepared test surface or on the inside of a test tube.

HIV antibody

HIV antigen

2 The test surface is exposed to blood serum. If any HIV antibodies are present, they will bind to the HIV antigens.

Enzyme

HIV antibody

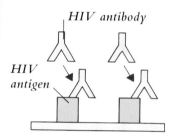

3 The test surface is washed. A special chemical linked to the enzyme peroxidase, which is known to bind to HIV antibodies, is added to the test surface. The surface is then washed again.

Reagent

Enzyme

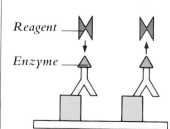

4 A reagent – a substance that is used to analyze biological substances – is added to the test surface. Any HIV antibodies will change the reagent's colour; the result would then be positive.

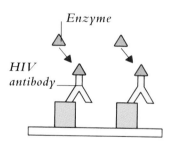

CHAPTER EIGHT

C H A P T E R   8

The RESPIRATORY SYSTEM

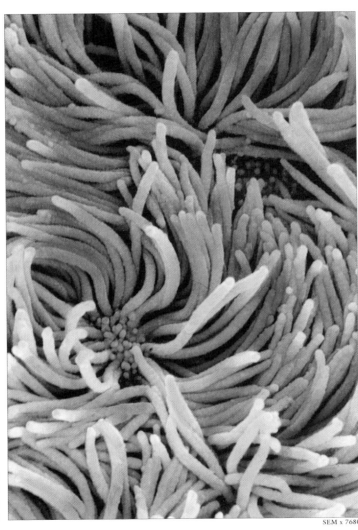

Cilia, tiny hairs projecting from the mucous lining of the respiratory tract

SEM x 7680

INTRODUCTION

Our lungs are second only to the heart in their work rate: each lung expands and contracts between 12 and 80 times a minute to supply the body with the oxygen it needs and, just as importantly, to expel carbon dioxide. The air is sometimes contaminated by chemicals and usually contains dust, pollen, bacteria, and viruses. So it is not surprising that, in industrialized countries, respiratory disorders are the most common reason for seeing a doctor. As has occurred in other areas of medicine, the investigation of patients with lung disorders has been transformed by the invention of fibreoptic endoscopes. These enable doctors to inspect

A narrowed airway due to asthma

the interior of the breathing organs in great detail. Doctors are also able to measure the effectiveness of the lungs very precisely by carrying out tests in a respiratory laboratory. In spite of these decisive advances, the list of important respiratory illnesses is long. Bronchitis due to smoking is the most frequent cause of serious respiratory illness, and lung cancer (which is also usually caused by smoking) remains another leading cause of adult mortality. Pneumonia is often a cause of death in the elderly, while tuberculosis may be about to pose a renewed threat to people of all ages. The number of children suffering from asthma has doubled in the past two decades, although the reason for this is not known.

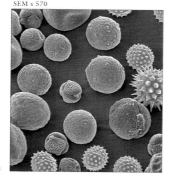
SEM x 570

Pollen grains

THE RESPIRATORY SYSTEM

The BODY'S GASEOUS EXCHANGE SYSTEM

TO FUNCTION, BODY CELLS REQUIRE OXYGEN. The respiratory system, which consists of air passages, pulmonary vessels, and the lungs, as well as breathing muscles, supplies fresh oxygen to the blood so that it can be distributed to the rest of the body tissues. It also removes carbon dioxide, a waste product of body processes. Air moves into and out of the lungs as a result of pressure changes brought about by contraction and relaxation of the diaphragm and other breathing muscles. Normal breathing is mainly an involuntary process, controlled by respiratory centres in the brain stem.

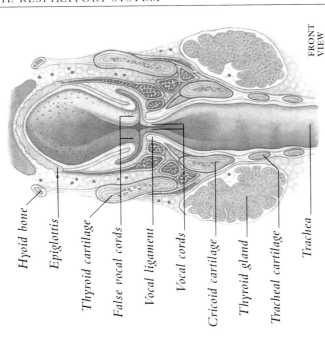

FRONT VIEW

Hyoid bone

Epiglottis

Thyroid cartilage

False vocal cords

Vocal ligament

Vocal cords

Cricoid cartilage

Thyroid gland

Tracheal cartilage

Trachea

THE LARYNX

The larynx plays an essential role in human speech. During sound production, the vocal cords close together and vibrate as air expelled from the lungs passes between them. The false vocal cords have no role in sound production, but close off the larynx when food is swallowed.

Paranasal sinuses
Air spaces within the skull make it lighter. Sounds echo in these spaces, creating vocal resonance.

Brain stem

Nasopharynx

Oropharynx

Laryngopharynx

Pharynx
The pharynx, or throat, has three parts. The upper part allows the passage of only air; lower parts permit the passage of foods and fluids.

Epiglottis
This flap of cartilage stops food from entering the trachea.

Nasal cavity
A sticky mucous membrane lines the nasal cavity and traps dust particles; its surface hairs, called cilia, move them toward the nose to be sneezed out. A similar membrane lines the larynx and the trachea; it moves particles toward the oropharynx to be swallowed.

Nose hairs
Hairs at the entrance to the nose trap large inhaled particles.

AIR PASSAGES

As air is inhaled and passes through the nasal passages, it is filtered, heated, and humidified. The filtering process continues as air flows down through the throat, larynx, trachea, and bronchi to the lungs. Each lung contains a tree of branching tubes that end in tiny air sacs, or alveoli, where gases diffuse into and out of the bloodstream in tiny vessels.

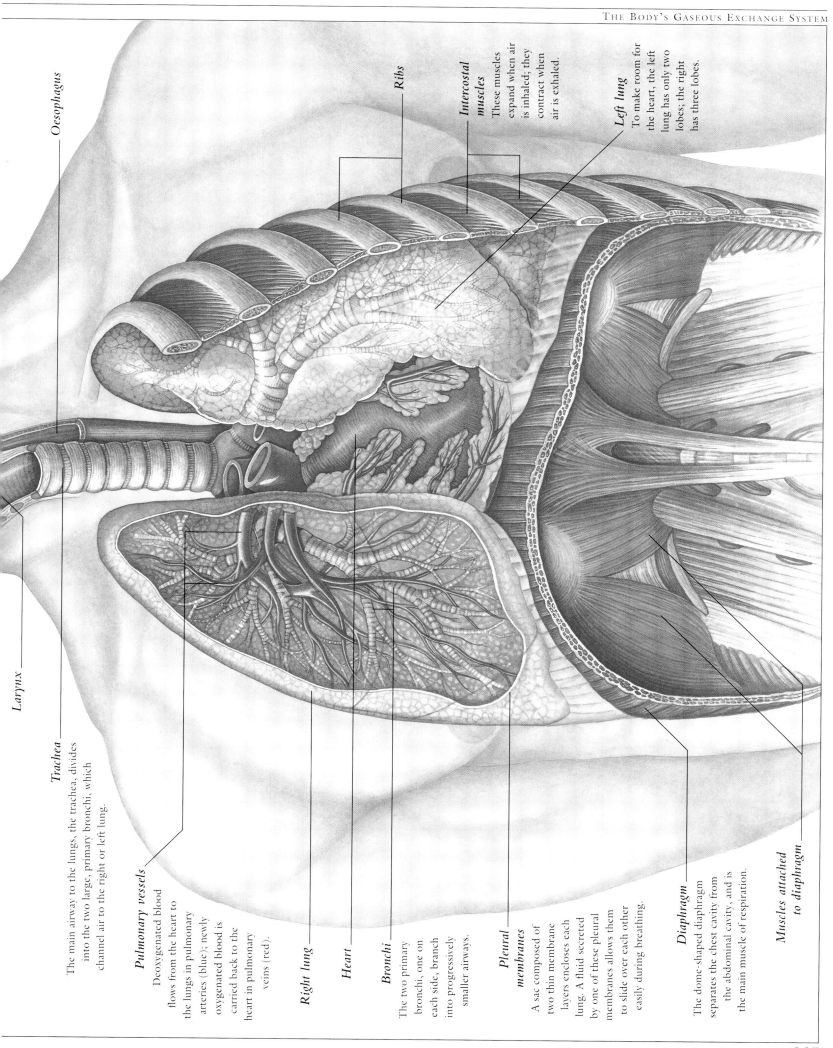

Oesophagus

Ribs

Intercostal muscles
These muscles expand when air is inhaled; they contract when air is exhaled.

Left lung
To make room for the heart, the left lung has only two lobes; the right has three lobes.

Larynx

Trachea
The main airway to the lungs, the trachea, divides into the two large, primary bronchi, which channel air to the right or left lung.

Pulmonary vessels
Deoxygenated blood flows from the heart to the lungs in pulmonary arteries (blue); newly oxygenated blood is carried back to the heart in pulmonary veins (red).

Right lung

Heart

Bronchi
The two primary bronchi, one on each side, branch into progressively smaller airways.

Pleural membranes
A sac composed of two thin membrane layers encloses each lung. A fluid secreted by one of these pleural membranes allows them to slide over each other easily during breathing.

Diaphragm
The dome-shaped diaphragm separates the chest cavity from the abdominal cavity, and is the main muscle of respiration.

Muscles attached to diaphragm

The LUNGS

THE TWO SPONGE-LIKE LUNGS FILL MOST OF THE CHEST CAVITY and are protected by the flexible rib cage. Together they form one of the body's largest organs. Their essential function, which is shared with the circulatory system, is gas exchange and the distribution of oxygen. The surface area of tissue involved in the exchange of oxygen and carbon dioxide is vast: about 40 times greater than the body's outer surface.

LUNG STRUCTURE

Each lung is cone-shaped, with a slightly concave base that rests on the diaphragm. Air enters the lungs via a complex of air passages that begins at the trachea below the larynx. The trachea bifurcates to form two primary, or main, bronchi, which enter each lung at the hilum. The branches continue to subdivide into increasingly smaller branches until they distribute air to the alveoli.

THE BRONCHIAL TREE

The intricate network of air passages that supply the lungs looks rather like an inverted tree, with the trachea forming the trunk. The photograph below shows a resin cast of this bronchial tree; each colour indicates an individual segment of the lung. Because each segment is aerated by a tertiary, or segmental, bronchus, it is possible to remove a single segment surgically.

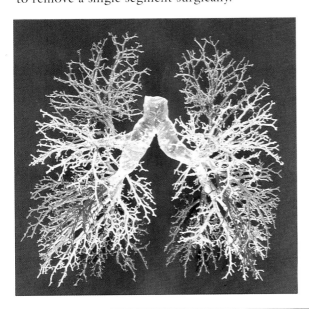

Trachea

Hilum

Right primary bronchus

Lobes of the lung
The right lung is separated by surface fissures into three lobes, while the smaller left lung is divided into only two lobes. Each lobe is subdivided into segments.

Ribs

Tertiary bronchus
These branches of the five lobar (secondary) bronchi are also called segmental bronchi because each one aerates an individual segment within each lobe. They may subdivide further into 50 to 80 terminal bronchioles.

Secondary bronchus
The five secondary, or lobar, bronchi are branches of the primary bronchus. Each supplies an individual lobe of the lung.

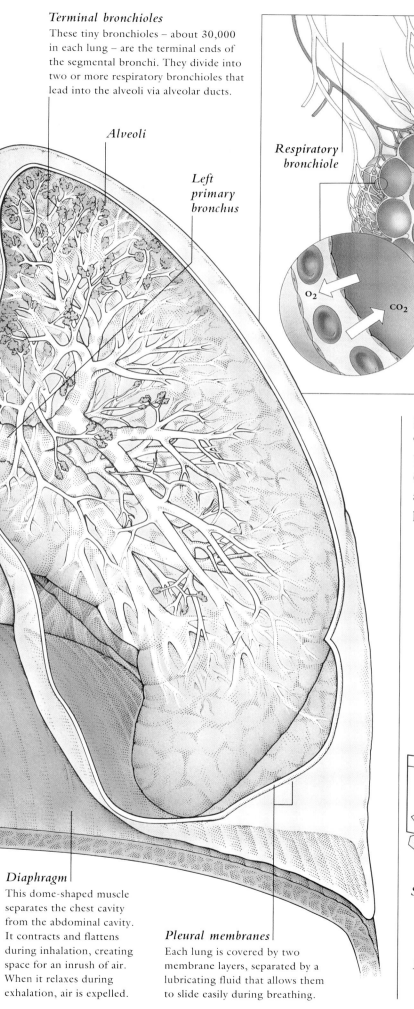

Terminal bronchioles
These tiny bronchioles – about 30,000 in each lung – are the terminal ends of the segmental bronchi. They divide into two or more respiratory bronchioles that lead into the alveoli via alveolar ducts.

Alveoli

Left primary bronchus

Diaphragm
This dome-shaped muscle separates the chest cavity from the abdominal cavity. It contracts and flattens during inhalation, creating space for an inrush of air. When it relaxes during exhalation, air is expelled.

Pleural membranes
Each lung is covered by two membrane layers, separated by a lubricating fluid that allows them to slide easily during breathing.

Respiratory bronchiole

ALVEOLI: BALLOON-LIKE SACS

The air sacs of the lungs, called alveoli, are elastic, thin-walled structures that are fed via ducts by respiratory bronchioles. Some white blood cells known as macrophages are always present on the inner surface of each alveolus; they ingest and destroy airborne irritants such as bacteria, chemicals, and dust. If a lung disorder destroys the alveolar sacs, there is less surface area for gas exchange, and breathlessness occurs.

Alveolus

Capillary network

Sites of exchange
Oxygen passes into the blood by diffusing through the alveolar walls into the surrounding capillary network. Carbon dioxide, a waste product, diffuses from blood into the alveoli; from there it is exhaled.

O_2

CO_2

SURFACTANT

The lungs remain partly inflated even after exhalation because of an essential fluid secreted inside the aveoli. Called surfactant, it is produced by specialized cells and is composed of fatty proteins. It also appears to play a role in preventing lung infections.

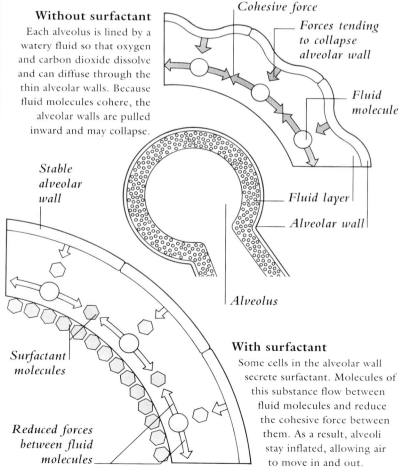

Without surfactant
Each alveolus is lined by a watery fluid so that oxygen and carbon dioxide dissolve and can diffuse through the thin alveolar walls. Because fluid molecules cohere, the alveolar walls are pulled inward and may collapse.

Cohesive force

Forces tending to collapse alveolar wall

Fluid molecule

Stable alveolar wall

Fluid layer

Alveolar wall

Alveolus

Surfactant molecules

With surfactant
Some cells in the alveolar wall secrete surfactant. Molecules of this substance flow between fluid molecules and reduce the cohesive force between them. As a result, alveoli stay inflated, allowing air to move in and out.

Reduced forces between fluid molecules

RESPIRATION *and* BREATHING

THE BODY CANNOT STORE OXYGEN, so we need to breathe day and night to move air into and out of the lungs. The rate and depth of breathing can be consciously modified, but the underlying need to breathe or not is controlled by centres in the brain stem. Here, responses to changes in the levels of oxygen and carbon dioxide control breathing of which we are usually not aware.

TWO TYPES OF RESPIRATION

External respiration refers to the exchange of oxygen and carbon dioxide within the lungs. Internal respiration occurs in body tissues when oxygen – carried in blood from the lungs in order to fuel cellular processes – is exchanged for carbon dioxide. Water and carbon dioxide are produced when cells break down nutrients such as glucose. Carbon dioxide travels in blood to the lungs and is exhaled.

Deep structure
Deep within a lung, a respiratory bronchiole (seen at top of image) brings air to the smaller alveoli, where gas exchange occurs.

SEM x 10

Oxygen in

Carbon dioxide out

Trachea

Aorta

Pulmonary arteries

Pulmonary veins

Left side of heart

Right side of heart

Alveoli

Lung

Bronchi

Body tissue cell

Blood

Vein

Artery

Glucose

Body tissue cells

Capillaries

Capillary wall

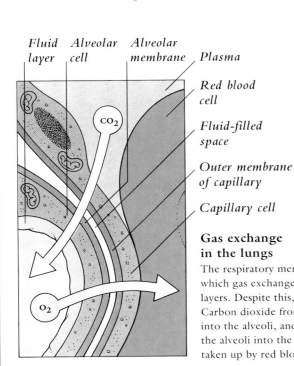

Fluid layer *Alveolar cell* *Alveolar membrane* *Plasma*

Red blood cell

Fluid-filled space

Outer membrane of capillary

Capillary cell

CO₂

O₂

Gas exchange in the lungs

The respiratory membrane, across which gas exchange occurs, has several layers. Despite this, it is extremely thin. Carbon dioxide from the blood diffuses into the alveoli, and oxygen passes from the alveoli into the capillaries to be taken up by red blood cells.

KEY

- Oxygen (O₂)
- Carbon dioxide (CO₂)
- Water (H₂O)

BREATHING

The movement of air into and out of the lungs is generated by differences in pressure inside and outside the body. The main muscle concerned is the diaphragm, assisted by internal and external muscles around the ribs. A person normally will breathe in and out about 500ml (nearly 1pt) of air 12 to 17 times a minute. The rate and volume increase automatically if the body needs more oxygen, such as during exercise.

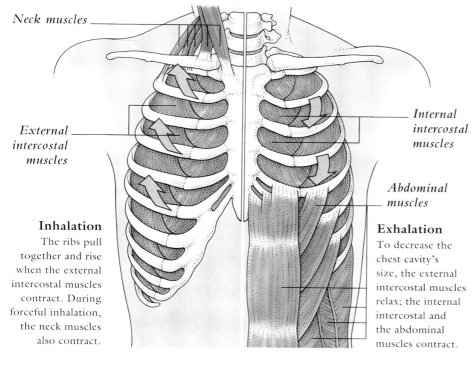

Neck muscles

External intercostal muscles

Internal intercostal muscles

Abdominal muscles

Inhalation
The ribs pull together and rise when the external intercostal muscles contract. During forceful inhalation, the neck muscles also contract.

Exhalation
To decrease the chest cavity's size, the external intercostal muscles relax; the internal intercostal and the abdominal muscles contract.

PRESSURE CHANGES

Atmospheric pressure is about 760mmHg. During an intake of breath, the contracting diaphragm increases the size of the chest cavity, and pressure within the lungs and pleural space drops. Air moves from areas of high to lower pressure and rushes into the lungs. As the diaphragm relaxes, pressure rises in the smaller chest cavity. To equalize pressure air is exhaled.

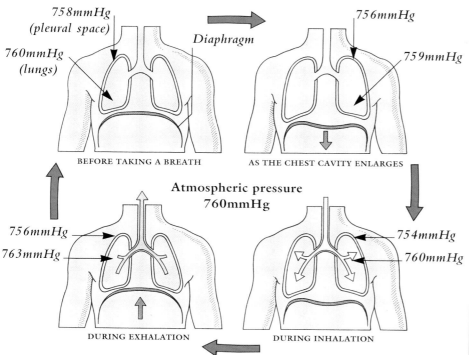

758mmHg (pleural space)

760mmHg (lungs)

Diaphragm

756mmHg

759mmHg

BEFORE TAKING A BREATH

AS THE CHEST CAVITY ENLARGES

Atmospheric pressure 760mmHg

756mmHg

763mmHg

754mmHg

760mmHg

DURING EXHALATION

DURING INHALATION

THE VOCAL CORDS

The vocal cords are paired bands of fibrous tissue at the base of the larynx. Sounds are generated when exhaled air passes through cords that have been brought together and tightened. The greater the tension in the vocal cords, the higher the pitch.

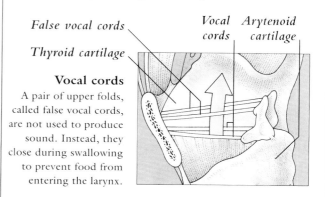

False vocal cords

Thyroid cartilage

Vocal cords

Arytenoid cartilage

Vocal cords
A pair of upper folds, called false vocal cords, are not used to produce sound. Instead, they close during swallowing to prevent food from entering the larynx.

COUGHING

Inhaled particles stimulate nerve cell receptors in the larynx, trachea, and bronchi. Nerve signals are transmitted to the brain stem, which then relays a response to trigger the coughing reflex. This expels irritants, and sometimes mucus, out of the body.

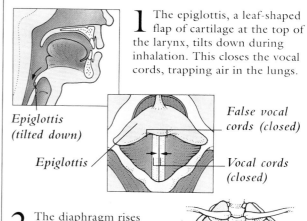

1 The epiglottis, a leaf-shaped flap of cartilage at the top of the larynx, tilts down during inhalation. This closes the vocal cords, trapping air in the lungs.

Epiglottis (tilted down)

Epiglottis

False vocal cords (closed)

Vocal cords (closed)

2 The diaphragm rises and the muscles of the abdomen contract so that the lungs are increasingly compressed. Because any decrease in the volume of a gas increases its pressure, air in the smaller space of the chest cavity is under greater pressure.

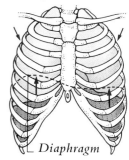

Diaphragm

3 When pressure reaches its highest point, the epiglottis tilts up and the vocal cords move apart. Air is forced up the airway and propelled out as a cough.

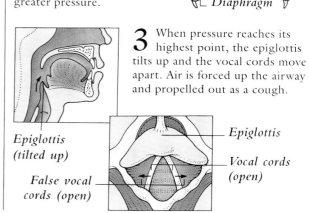

Epiglottis (tilted up)

False vocal cords (open)

Epiglottis

Vocal cords (open)

RESPIRATORY INFECTIONS

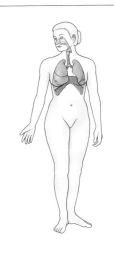

MILLIONS OF MICROORGANISMS – BACTERIA, VIRUSES, AND FUNGI – populate the air. During an intake of breath, these minute organisms can easily enter the lungs, making respiratory infections quite common. Infections affecting the upper airways, also called upper respiratory tract infections, may cause a mild illness such as the common cold or tonsillitis, or a more serious disease like sinusitis. Other respiratory infections can affect the lower air passages, causing bronchitis, or the lung tissue itself, which results in pneumonia.

UPPER AIRWAY INFECTIONS

These illnesses include infections of the nasal sinuses, pharynx, and larynx, and are caused when droplets contaminated by viruses and sometimes bacteria are inhaled. Infections often result in the inflammation and swelling of mucous membranes that line these structures. As people grow older, they become immune to most of the common viruses and have fewer infections.

Sinusitis
A bacterial infection may follow a viral infection, causing a pus-like secretion to accumulate within the nasal sinuses. Fever, headache, blocked nose, and no sense of smell are common symptoms.

Tonsillitis
Most common in young children, inflamed tonsils may cause a fever, headache, sore throat, discomfort when swallowing, and earache. The lymph nodes in the neck often swell.

Pharyngitis
Inflammation of the pharynx (throat) causes sore throat, fever, difficulty in swallowing, and sometimes swollen lymph nodes in the neck and earache.

Laryngitis
Usually caused by a virus, this infection can produce hoarseness, loss of voice, a dry cough, and sore throat.

INFLUENZA
Commonly called "flu", this serious viral infection causes fever, chills, headache, muscle aches, weakness, cough, and loss of appetite. It spreads rapidly, frequently occurring in localized outbreaks, or every few years in epidemics. Three main types of virus – A, B, and C – are recognized. Some types of virus can change their structures so that a previously acquired immunity is lost. Influenza may be life-threatening to the very young or elderly; some epidemics kill people of all ages.

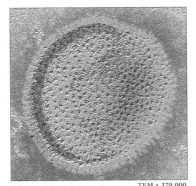

TEM x 379,000

Influenza virus

THE COMMON COLD
Colds are easily transmitted from person to person by virus-containing droplets that are released into the atmosphere when an infected person coughs or sneezes. About 200 different types of virus cause colds. Antibiotics do not have any effect and only symptoms can be treated. It is the body's immune system that must defeat the infectious organisms.

1 After being carried by infected droplets, virus particles enter the body and invade the cells that line the throat and nose. These virus particles then replicate to produce new particles, which continue to multiply rapidly.

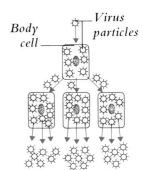

Body cell

Virus particles

Infected nasal lining

2 The blood supply brings lymphocytes (white blood cells) to the infected mucosa. The blood vessels within the nasal mucosa swell and cause the secretion of excess fluid, resulting in a "runny nose".

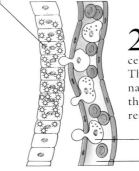

Lymphocyte

Blood vessel

3 Some types of lymphocyte make virus-specific proteins (antibodies) that immobilize the virus particles, while other types secrete chemical substances that can destroy infected cells.

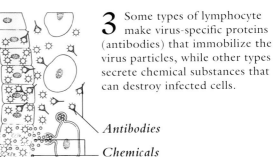

Antibodies

Chemicals

Phagocyte

4 Phagocytes, a type of white blood cell, can engulf and destroy dead viruses, immobilized virus particles, and damaged cells. Symptoms of the cold soon subside.

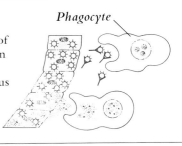

ACUTE BRONCHITIS

This form of bronchitis – which means inflammation of the bronchi – develops suddenly. It can occur as a complication of an upper respiratory tract infection, such as a common cold, or can accompany measles or influenza. Usually caused by a virus, this mild disease produces symptoms such as a cough that produces sputum, a low fever, and sometimes a slight wheeze.

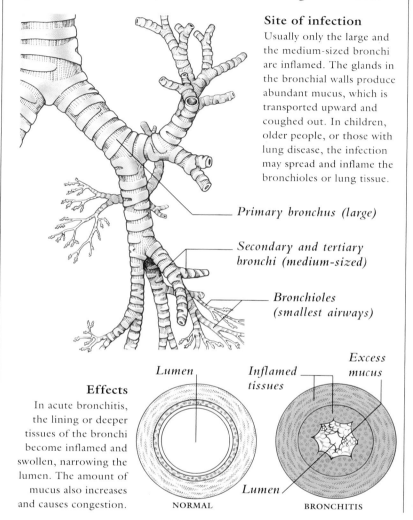

Site of infection
Usually only the large and the medium-sized bronchi are inflamed. The glands in the bronchial walls produce abundant mucus, which is transported upward and coughed out. In children, older people, or those with lung disease, the infection may spread and inflame the bronchioles or lung tissue.

Primary bronchus (large)

Secondary and tertiary bronchi (medium-sized)

Bronchioles (smallest airways)

Effects
In acute bronchitis, the lining or deeper tissues of the bronchi become inflamed and swollen, narrowing the lumen. The amount of mucus also increases and causes congestion.

Lumen

Inflamed tissues

Excess mucus

Lumen

NORMAL

BRONCHITIS

PNEUMONIA

In pneumonia, the smallest bronchioles and alveolar tissue become inflamed. There are two main types. Lobar pneumonia affects one lobe of the lung, while bronchopneumonia affects patches of tissue in one or both lungs. Usually a result of a viral or a bacterial infection, pneumonia may also be caused by fungi, yeasts, or protozoa. Symptoms include fever, loss of appetite, sweating, and joint and muscle pain. Chest pain, coughing, and breathlessness soon develop.

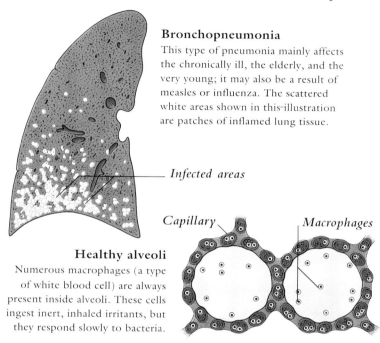

Bronchopneumonia
This type of pneumonia mainly affects the chronically ill, the elderly, and the very young; it may also be a result of measles or influenza. The scattered white areas shown in this illustration are patches of inflamed lung tissue.

Infected areas

Capillary

Macrophages

Healthy alveoli
Numerous macrophages (a type of white blood cell) are always present inside alveoli. These cells ingest inert, inhaled irritants, but they respond slowly to bacteria.

Fluid

Neutrophils

Infected alveoli
The infective process triggers changes in the capillary walls, allowing neutrophils (a type of white blood cell) in to fight the invading organisms. Fluid also flows in and accumulates.

PLEURAL EFFUSION

Pleural inflammation may result from infections, particularly pneumonia or tuberculosis. It may cause excess fluid to build up in the space between the two membrane layers of the pleura. This effusion, if extensive, can cause breathlessness. Fluid may need to be removed via a hollow needle or drain inserted through the chest wall.

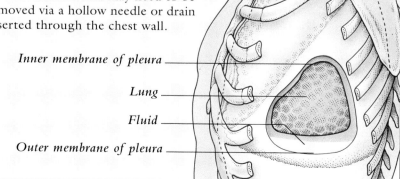

Inner membrane of pleura

Lung

Fluid

Outer membrane of pleura

LEGIONNAIRE'S DISEASE

This rare bacterial condition was described in 1976 after an outbreak of severe pneumonia among war veterans at an American Legion convention. It affects men more often than women. The symptoms include a high fever, chills, muscle aches, confusion, a severe headache, abdominal pain, and diarrhoea. Patients are usually treated in hospital, and intravenous antibiotics such as erythromycin are prescribed.

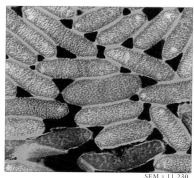

The cause
The bacterium *Legionella pneumophila* is found in small numbers in almost all water supplies. It thrives, however, in water-cooled air conditioning systems, and in plumbing systems where water stagnates.

SEM x 11,230

143

LUNG DISORDERS

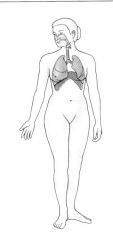

DISORDERS THAT CAUSE BREATHING PROBLEMS may be present from birth or may develop over many years. Others may occur suddenly without warning or after a traumatic injury. Inhaled substances such as mineral dust, gases, fumes, or chemicals can contribute to some disorders, while others have no known cause. Among the main groups of lung disorders are those marked by inflammation caused by infections or by allergies or other autoimmune disorders; those due to cancers and other growths; and inherited disorders.

PULMONARY HYPERTENSION

Elevated blood pressure in the pulmonary arteries leading to the lungs may be the result of a lung disorder, such as emphysema, or of blood clots from the legs that are carried to the lungs. Left-sided heart failure, which causes blood to collect in the lungs, also raises pulmonary arterial pressure.

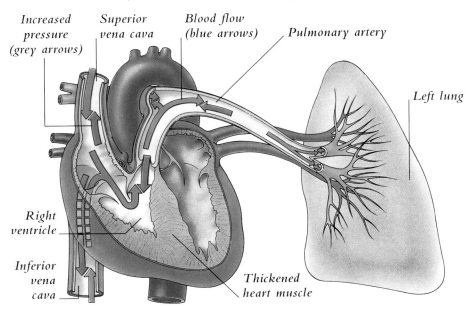

Increased pressure (grey arrows) — *Superior vena cava* — *Blood flow (blue arrows)* — *Pulmonary artery* — *Left lung* — *Right ventricle* — *Inferior vena cava* — *Thickened heart muscle*

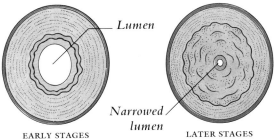

Lumen — *Narrowed lumen*

EARLY STAGES — LATER STAGES

Early and late stages

As the condition develops, the walls of the pulmonary artery thicken with muscle and fibrous tissue. This narrows the lumen, impedes blood flow, and raises pressure in the arteries. Blood volume pumped from the heart becomes progressively reduced.

PNEUMOTHORAX

A pneumothorax occurs when one of the pleural membranes ruptures, allowing air to enter the pleural space and causing the lung to collapse. A spontaneous pneumothorax can sometimes occur, while others are the result of an injury; chest pain and breathlessness are common symptoms. If air is not reabsorbed, it may compress the lung and has to be drained by a needle or tube inserted into the pleural space.

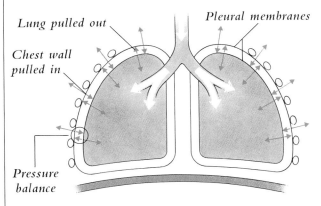

Lung pulled out — *Pleural membranes* — *Chest wall pulled in* — *Pressure balance*

Normal lungs

During normal breathing, the lungs inflate and are pulled out while the chest wall is pulled in. Within the pleural space a delicate balance is maintained between these opposing pressures.

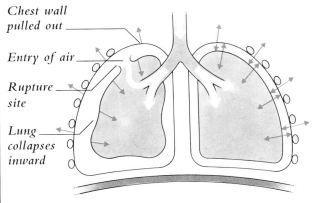

Chest wall pulled out — *Entry of air* — *Rupture site* — *Lung collapses inward*

Pneumothorax

If air enters the pleural space, it changes the pressure balance. The pressure change causes a sudden, inward collapse of the lungs.

SARCOIDOSIS

Thought to be due to an extreme immune response, sarcoidosis features multiple areas of inflammation interspersed with fibrous and grain-like tissue. The circular nodules, called granulomas (shown right), are often found in the lungs, lymph nodes, and eyes. Symptoms include breathlessness, fatigue, joint pain, and sometimes a skin rash.

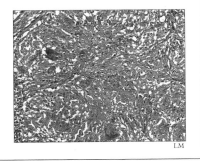

LM

FIBROSING ALVEOLITIS

Fibrosing alveolitis, which is also called idiopathic pulmonary fibrosis (IPF), is an autoimmune disorder of unknown cause. In some cases, it occurs with other immune disorders such as rheumatoid arthritis. The disease causes fibrosis (scarring) and thickening of the alveoli, the lung's air sacs, and results in severe breathlessness. Corticosteroid drugs may be given.

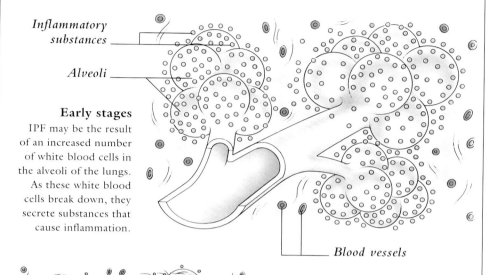

Inflammatory substances

Alveoli

Early stages
IPF may be the result of an increased number of white blood cells in the alveoli of the lungs. As these white blood cells break down, they secrete substances that cause inflammation.

Blood vessels

Growth of fibrous tissue
The inflammatory substances stimulate fibroblasts to produce an overgrowth of fibrous tissue. Thick cuboidal cells replace the usual thin cells that line the bronchi, restricting the passage of oxygen.

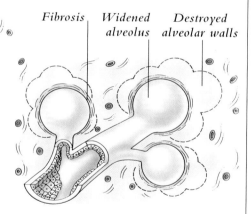

Fibrosis Widened alveolus Destroyed alveolar walls

Cuboidal cells Fibrous tissue Fibroblast

Late stages
Formation of scar tissue (fibrosis) occurs, which gradually destroys the alveolar walls. The remaining alveoli widen, reducing the surface area for gas exchange. Scar tissue may contract, restricting lung expansion.

BRONCHOSCOPY
To diagnose and sometimes to treat a lung disorder, bronchoscopy may be performed. A bronchoscope may be a rigid tube or a flexible fibreoptic tube, which can reach farther into small air passages. After a light sedative and a local anaesthetic have been given, the tube is inserted into the patient's throat and down into the bronchi. Special attachments can be passed through the tube to remove tissue samples or to perform surgery.

Flexible bronchoscope

Larynx

Trachea

Bronchi

DUST DISEASES

Asbestosis, silicosis, and pneumoconiosis are diseases caused by inhalation of dust particles. These inhaled particles irritate and inflame the lung tissue, which causes irreversible scarring. Those most at risk are people whose work exposes them to these dusts for several years. Some moulds that develop in hay, grain, or straw may cause farmer's lung, an allergic reaction that results in alveolar inflammation.

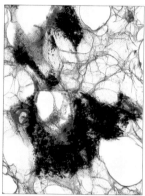

LM x 25

Coal-miner's pneumoconiosis
If coal dust is inhaled over a period of 10 to 15 years, it can lead to pneumoconiosis, or "black lung disease". The dust particles deposited in lung tissue (left) produce inflammatory nodules. Scar tissue formation – a process called fibrosis – around these nodules destroys lung tissue.

SILICOSIS

Silicosis is the world's most common occupational disease. It is a form of fibrosis in the lungs caused by silica dust, usually in the form of quartz. Quarry workers, stone masons, coal miners, and others are at risk. Symptoms such as breathlessness may not develop for many years. The disease may result in lung cancer, especially if an affected person smokes.

1 Inhaled silica particles are deposited in the lungs and ingested by scavenging white blood cells called macrophages.

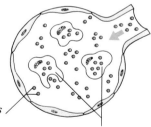

Silica particles

Macrophages

Burst cell Chemicals

2 Macrophages burst and die, releasing the silica and chemicals. The latter attract fibroblasts, which produce fibrous tissue. Silica is consumed by more macrophages and the process is repeated.

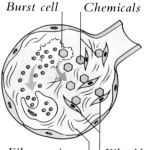

Fibrous tissue Fibroblasts

Dense nodule of scar tissue

3 More fibrous tissue develops, leading to dense nodules of scar tissue. Build-up of this tissue severely restricts functioning of the lungs.

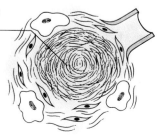

CHRONIC LUNG DISEASES

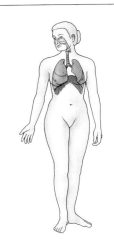

COMMON IN SMOKERS AND IN URBAN OR INDUSTRIALIZED AREAS, chronic diseases of the lung that obstruct the airways and reduce airflow have increased in every part of the world. Once more common in men, the disorders increasingly affect women, partly due to greater numbers who smoke. Known risk factors include repeated respiratory infections during childhood as well as a family member with a similar disease. In the past 20 years, the number of childhood asthma cases has doubled, but the reasons for this sudden increase are not yet clearly understood.

CHRONIC BRONCHITIS

Although recurring acute bronchitis caused by a virus or a bacterium may cause chronic inflammation of the bronchi, the most common cause is smoking and chemical irritants. At first the resulting cough is troublesome mostly in the damp, cold months, but eventually symptoms persist all year. Symptoms such as hoarseness and breathlessness also occur.

HOW BRONCHITIS DEVELOPS

If bronchi are irritated by smoking or prolonged exposure to pollutants, they begin to produce too much mucus. This results in a progressively worsening cough in order to clear the airways.

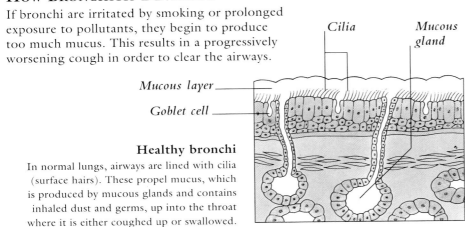

Healthy bronchi

In normal lungs, airways are lined with cilia (surface hairs). These propel mucus, which is produced by mucous glands and contains inhaled dust and germs, up into the throat where it is either coughed up or swallowed.

1 Inhaled irritants cause mucous glands to enlarge, and goblet cells to increase in number so that more mucus is produced. Damaged cilia cannot propel mucus along.

2 Mucus retained in the airway becomes a breeding ground for bacteria so that inflammation is likely to recur. Cilia are slowly destroyed; more mucus collects.

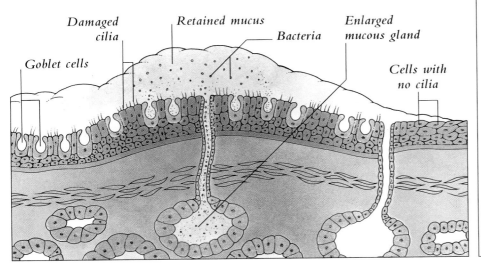

EMPHYSEMA

The lungs are filled with millions of tiny air sacs called alveoli. In emphysema, they become overstretched and rupture. Most people who are severely affected are heavy, long-term smokers, but a rare inherited enzyme deficiency is a known risk factor. At present the disorder is incurable, but stopping smoking slows its progression.

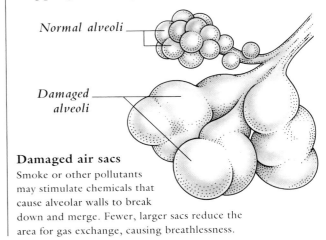

Damaged air sacs

Smoke or other pollutants may stimulate chemicals that cause alveolar walls to break down and merge. Fewer, larger sacs reduce the area for gas exchange, causing breathlessness.

DEATHS FROM SMOKING

A comparison of death rates in non-smokers and smokers caused by chronic bronchitis and emphysema is shown in the graph below.

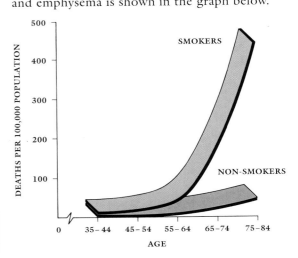

ASTHMA

Asthma attacks are recurrent episodes of breathlessness, which vary in intensity, caused by constricted airways. Asthma is diagnosed by lung function tests, and by skin and blood tests to identify substances that trigger these attacks. Allergic asthma often develops in childhood and may be accompanied by eczema. In some forms of the disease, there is no specific trigger and no known cause.

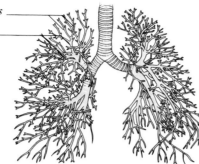

Bronchioles

Tertiary bronchi

Airways affected in asthma
The smaller bronchi and the bronchioles (the smallest airways) become constricted, inflamed, and congested with mucus. As a result, breathing becomes difficult.

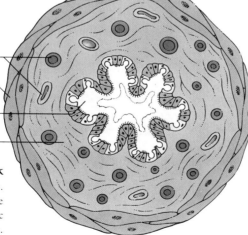

Blood vessels

Mucus

Relaxed smooth muscle

Normal airway
In a normal bronchiole, the smooth muscle in the bronchial walls is relaxed, creating a wide lumen, or space, in the centre of the air passage. This allows air to flow easily and steadily so that the body's oxygen requirements are met.

Inflammatory substances widen the blood vessels

Smooth muscle contracts

Increased mucus

Inflammation and swelling

During an asthma attack
Contracted muscle walls narrow airways. Increased mucus and inflammation due to chemicals released during an allergic response cause further narrowing.

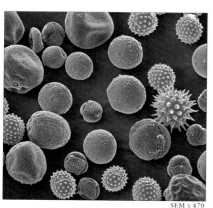

THE ROLE OF ALLERGENS
Allergens are substances that trigger an allergic response. Common allergens that may spark off or intensify asthma attacks include grass pollen, animal fur, dust, and certain foods and drugs. Other factors are anxiety or stress, vigorous exercise in cold weather, and respiratory infections.

A specific allergen
In some people, exposure to certain grass pollens triggers asthma attacks. A number of different pollen grains are shown on the left.

SEM x 470

TREATING ASTHMA

The frequency and severity of attacks may be reduced by avoiding specific allergens. Obstruction of airways may be relieved by inhaled steroids to suppress inflammation and by bronchodilator drugs, which relax bronchiole walls. These drugs are available as portable aerosol inhalers, which provide a measured dose, nebulizers to disperse the drug as a fine mist, tablets, or injections.

MAST-CELL STABILIZERS
Mast cells play a critical role in the allergic response. Antigen/antibody complexes attach to these cells and stimulate them to produce histamine. Mast-cell stabilizers help to inhibit histamine production by the mast cells, which helps to reduce inflammation of the airways.

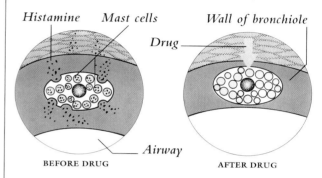

Histamine   Mast cells   Wall of bronchiole

Drug

Airway

BEFORE DRUG   **AFTER DRUG**

BRONCHODILATORS AND STEROIDS
Bronchodilator drugs work by affecting the nerve signals that control the contraction and relaxation of bronchiole muscles. They do not reduce inflammation of the mucous lining. Corticosteroid drugs, usually inhaled, widen bronchioles by reducing inflammation.

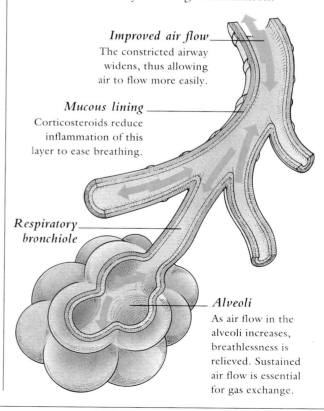

Improved air flow
The constricted airway widens, thus allowing air to flow more easily.

Mucous lining
Corticosteroids reduce inflammation of this layer to ease breathing.

Respiratory bronchiole

Alveoli
As air flow in the alveoli increases, breathlessness is relieved. Sustained air flow is essential for gas exchange.

147

LUNG CANCER

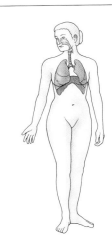

THE MOST COMMON CAUSE OF LUNG CANCER – responsible for almost 90 per cent of all cases in the UK – is tobacco smoking. In the past, lung cancer was far more common in men than women since more men than women smoked in the first half of this century; however, its incidence in women is rapidly rising and seems likely to overtake breast cancer as the most common cancer in women. Other causes of lung cancer include coal dust, asbestos, and radon gas. Lung cancer is more common in industrial areas than in rural areas.

CAUSES OF LUNG CANCER

Many inhaled irritants trigger the growth of abnormal cells in the lungs. Cigarette smoke, however, contains thousands of known carcinogenic (cancer-causing) substances, and is the main cause of lung cancer. Diagnostic tests may include a chest X-ray, biopsy, and bronchoscopy (examining the bronchi through a viewing tube).

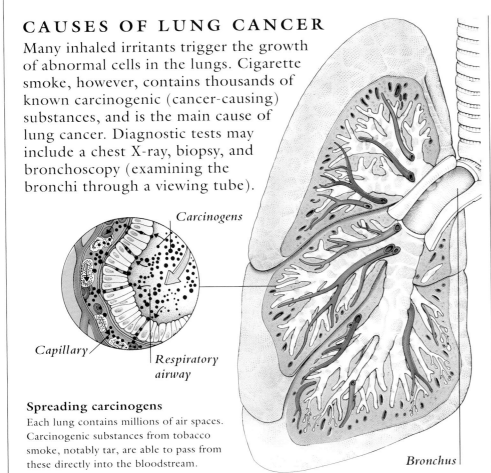

Carcinogens

Capillary

Respiratory airway

Bronchus

Spreading carcinogens

Each lung contains millions of air spaces. Carcinogenic substances from tobacco smoke, notably tar, are able to pass from these directly into the bloodstream.

GROWTH OF LUNG CANCER

In about 95 per cent of cases of lung cancer, the tumour begins growing in the bronchi where it may enlarge or bleed and obstruct breathing. Some cells of a bronchial tumour may break away and infiltrate other parts of the lung, or spread from the original site, called the primary tumour, to other organs. If cancerous tissue develops at a new site, it is known as a metastasis.

Tumour in an alveolus

A tiny tumour fills a single alveolus. A few of the cancer cells (shown in red) have broken away and begun to spread.

SEM x 230

HOW SMOKING DAMAGES THE LUNGS

Tobacco smoke is a complex mixture of over 3000 different substances, and burning cigarette tar is strongly carcinogenic. Some risk factors known to predispose toward the development of lung cancer are the number of cigarettes smoked per day, their tar content, the number of years that a person has smoked, and the depth of inhalation.

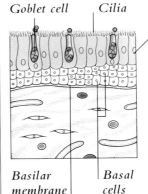

Goblet cell   *Cilia*   *Columnar cell*

Basilar membrane   *Basal cells*

1 Columnar cells topped by cilia (tiny hairs) line healthy bronchi. Under this layer are basal cells, which constantly divide to replace damaged columnar cells. Mucus produced by goblet cells lubricate the bronchi.

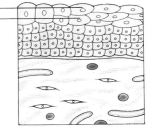

Squamous cells

2 Over a number of years, columnar cells damaged by smoking flatten and turn into squamous cells, which gradually lose their cilia.

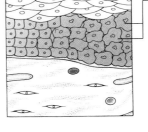

Basal cells become cancerous

3 In order to replace the squamous cells that are damaged, basal cells start to multiply at an increased rate; some of these new basal cells develop into cancerous cells.

Multiplying cancer cells break through

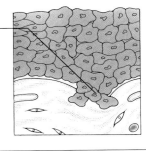

4 The cancer cells start to replace healthy cells. If these cells break through the basement membrane, they can metastasize, establishing new sites of cancer.

SYMPTOMS

A persistent cough is usually the earliest symptom of lung cancer. Because most people who develop lung cancer are smokers, this is often dismissed as simply a "smoker's cough". Other symptoms of lung cancer include coughing up blood, wheezing, weight loss, persistent hoarseness of voice, and chest pain.

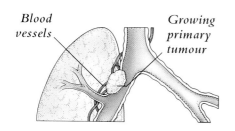

Blood vessels   *Growing primary tumour*

Symptoms from tumour growth

A tumour that grows may obstruct a bronchus, causing shortness of breath and chest pain. Sometimes a tumour presses on the oesophagus, making swallowing difficult.

Symptoms of spreading cancer

Lung cancer that metastasizes (spreads) to other body parts causes a variety of symptoms. Metastases in bones may cause pain and fractures; in the brain they may cause paralysis and confusion; in the liver they may cause loss of weight and nausea.

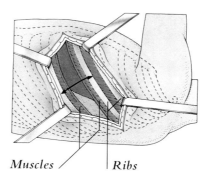

Brain metastasis

Primary tumour

Lymph node metastasis

Bone metastasis

Adrenal gland metastasis

Liver metastasis

DRUG TREATMENT

If treated with specific medications, a few types of lung cancer respond to the extent that symptoms become less severe or disappear. Because the drugs also damage normal cells, they are given at intervals of 3 to 4 weeks to allow healthy tissue to recover between treatments. Sickness, diarrhoea, or hair loss may be side-effects.

Cytotoxic antibiotics

For cells to multiply, DNA must replicate to make chromosomes in the new cell. Cytotoxic antibiotics prevent DNA replication, and thus halt the development of cancer cells.

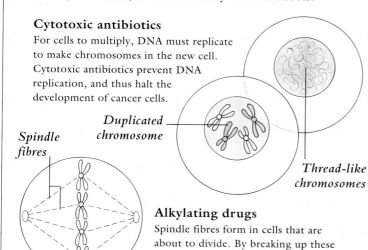

Spindle fibres   *Duplicated chromosome*   *Thread-like chromosomes*

Alkylating drugs

Spindle fibres form in cells that are about to divide. By breaking up these fibres, alkylating drugs interfere with rapidly reproducing cancer cells.

OPERATION

LOBECTOMY

If diagnostic tests confirm the presence of lung cancer, a lobectomy, or removal of a lobe of the lung, may be performed. The operation is only appropriate in certain circumstances. The tumour must be small and confined to a localized region; breakaway cancer cells must not have spread to other parts of the body; and the patient must be in reasonably good health. Suitable only for carefully selected patients, lobectomy may offer relief of symptoms as well as the possibility of a cure.

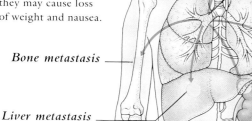

1 After administration of a general anaesthetic, the surgeon makes a skin incision around the side of the chest. The muscles between the ribs are cut and the ribs are then separated in order to expose the affected lung, which is covered by its pleura.

Muscles   *Ribs*

2 The diseased lobe is moved to one side so that the surgeon can look at the blood vessels and lymph nodes more easily. Samples of tissue are taken from the lymph nodes. These specimens are then examined microscopically to find out if the cancer has spread to the nodes.

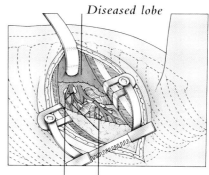

Diseased lobe

Lymph nodes   *Blood vessels*

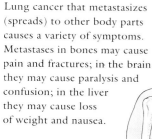

Diseased lobe

Stump of bronchus

Cut arteries

Cut vein

Healthy lung tissue

3 The arteries, veins, and the main bronchus that supply the affected lobe are first tied off and then cut. The remaining bronchial stump is permanently closed off with sutures so that air does not leak into the chest cavity, and the diseased lobe is cut away and removed.

4 Two chest drains are inserted into the chest cavity before it is closed. The drains, which remove excess blood and fluid from the area around the lungs, are left in place for 3 to 5 days and then removed.

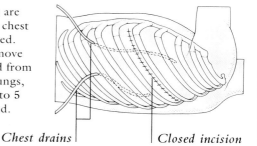

Chest drains   *Closed incision*

CHAPTER 9

The DIGESTIVE SYSTEM

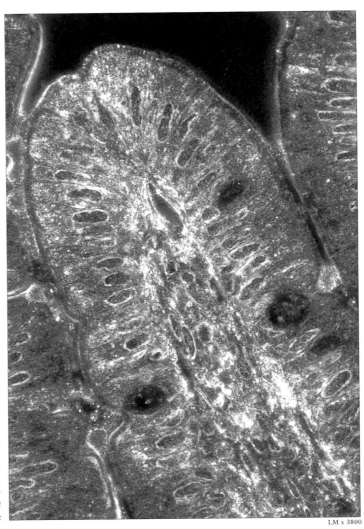

A cross-section of a villus in the small intestine

LM x 3800

INTRODUCTION

More than any other system in the human body, the digestive organs make us aware when they are in action and working well, or when they are upset and need attention. Hunger and the need to empty the bowels are just two of the messages we cannot ignore for long. Many common disorders, including gastritis, peptic ulcers, inflammatory bowel disease, and irritable bowel disease, often have a psychological component. It is thus unsurprising that digestive problems occur so frequently, or that treatment may entail psychological as well as physical intervention.

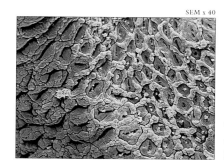

SEM x 40

The junction of the small and large intestines

Understanding of these disorders has become much more advanced over the last two decades. For instance, the recognition of the importance of a fibre-rich diet has made constipation far less troublesome. Another important advance is the identification of the bacteria that causes peptic ulcers, which has made it possible to use drugs to cure them. Lastly, the wide range of diagnostic tests available to gastroenterologists has been totally transformed. Today, endoscopy – the examination of the internal organs by means of viewing tubes – is the primary method of inspecting areas like the oesophagus, stomach, intestines, and bile ducts. This technique has made it possible to recognize cancers at an early stage, and to monitor their treatment.

Endoscopic examination of the bile ducts

THE DIGESTIVE SYSTEM

The ORGANS of DIGESTION

THE TASK OF THE DIGESTIVE SYSTEM is the physical and chemical breakdown of food. All the energy the body needs and the raw materials for growth and repair of body structures come from ingested food and drink. After ingestion, food and fluids are processed by the digestive organs into small nutrient molecules that can be absorbed from the intestines, and circulated around the body. Food that cannot be digested becomes waste material, or faeces, which is eliminated from the body by defaecation. Digestion is coordinated by the hypothalamus, hormones, and nerves.

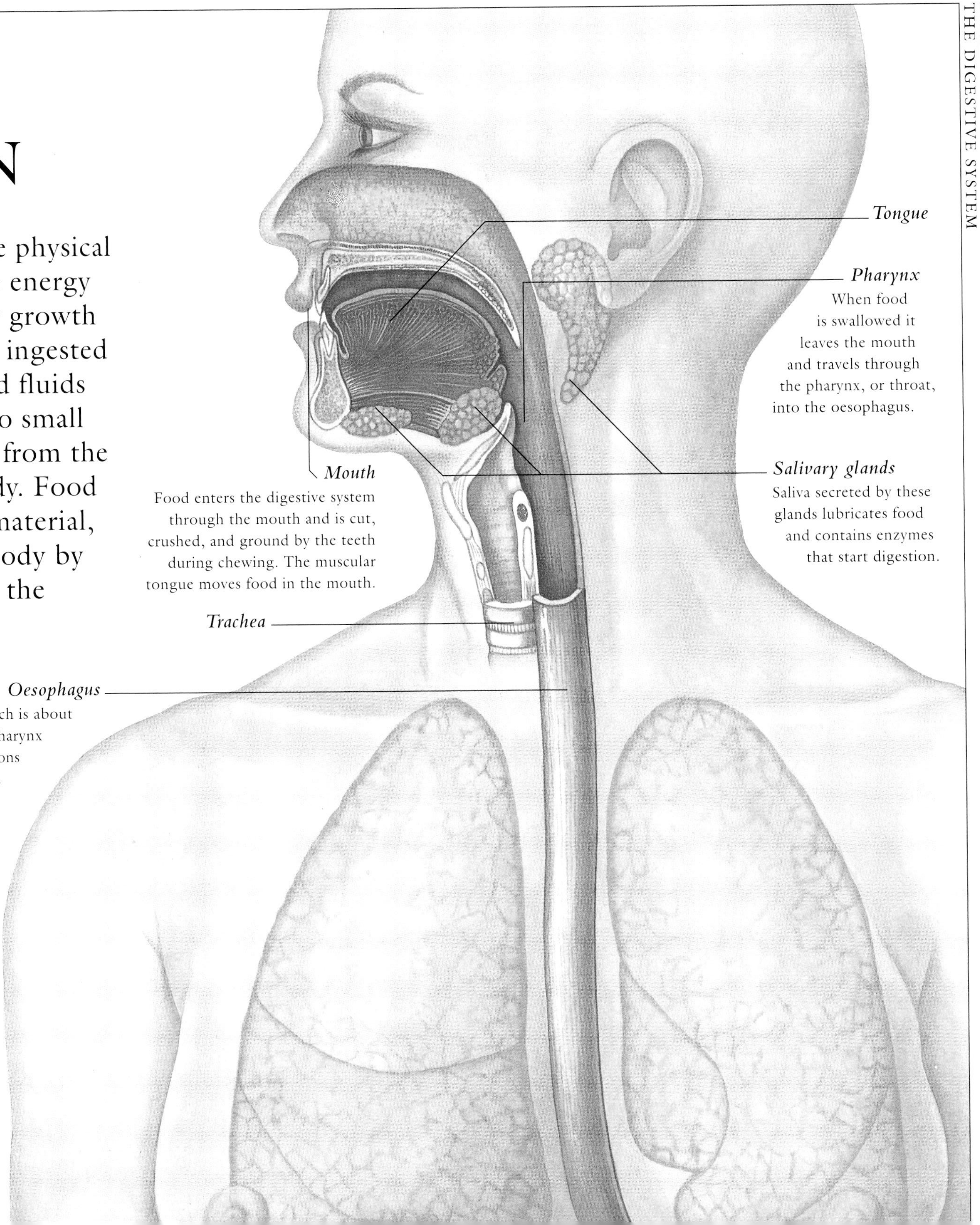

DIGESTIVE STRUCTURES

The mouth, pharynx, oesophagus, stomach, small intestine, large intestine, and anus make up the digestive tract, which is basically a food processing pipeway about 9m (30ft) long. The associated digestive structures include three pairs of salivary glands, the pancreas, the liver, and the gallbladder with their associated ducts. Each of these organs plays an important part in digestion. The appendix – a short, blind-ended tube attached to the first part of the large intestine – has no known function.

Tongue

Pharynx
When food is swallowed it leaves the mouth and travels through the pharynx, or throat, into the oesophagus.

Salivary glands
Saliva secreted by these glands lubricates food and contains enzymes that start digestion.

Mouth
Food enters the digestive system through the mouth and is cut, crushed, and ground by the teeth during chewing. The muscular tongue moves food in the mouth.

Trachea

Oesophagus
This thick-walled muscular tube, which is about 25cm (10in) long, connects the pharynx with the stomach. Waves of contractions called peristalsis propel food along.

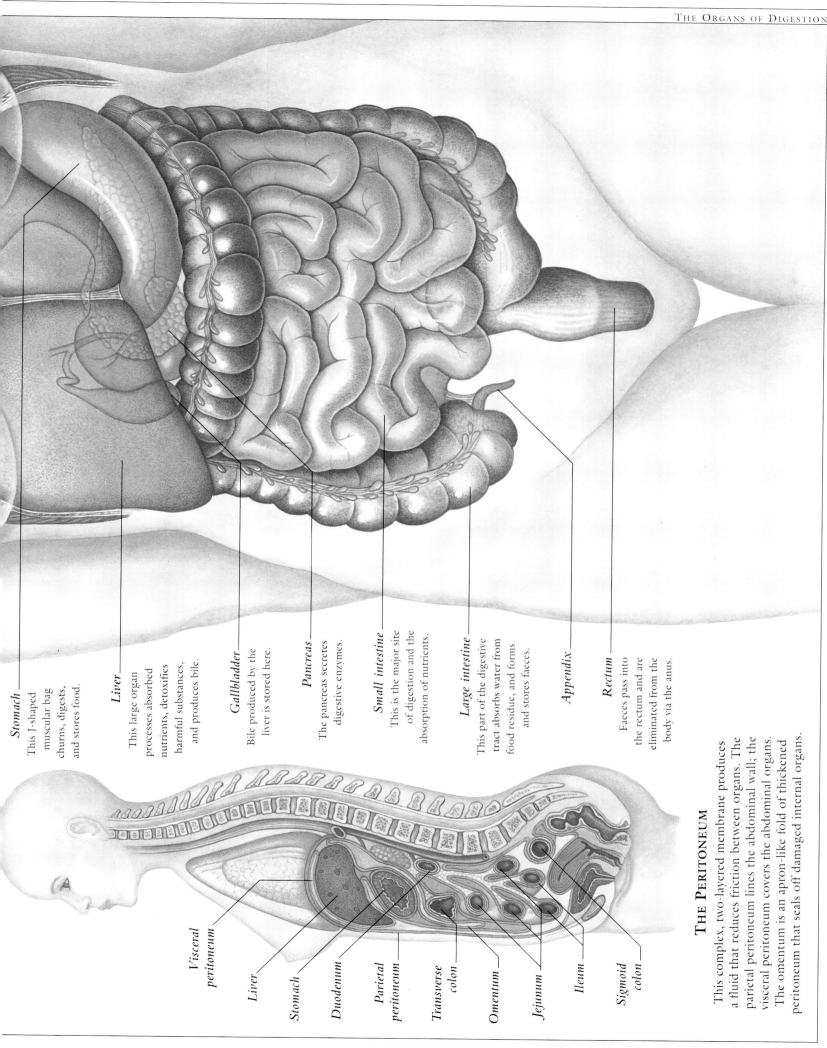

Stomach

This J-shaped muscular bag churns, digests, and stores food.

Liver

This large organ processes absorbed nutrients, detoxifies harmful substances, and produces bile.

Gallbladder

Bile produced by the liver is stored here.

Pancreas

The pancreas secretes digestive enzymes.

Small intestine

This is the major site of digestion and the absorption of nutrients.

Large intestine

This part of the digestive tract absorbs water from food residue, and forms and stores faeces.

Appendix

Rectum

Faeces pass into the rectum and are eliminated from the body via the anus.

THE PERITONEUM

This complex, two-layered membrane produces a fluid that reduces friction between organs. The parietal peritoneum lines the abdominal wall; the visceral peritoneum covers the abdominal organs. The omentum is an apron-like fold of thickened peritoneum that seals off damaged internal organs.

Visceral peritoneum

Liver

Stomach

Duodenum

Parietal peritoneum

Transverse colon

Omentum

Jejunum

Ileum

Sigmoid colon

The DIGESTIVE PROCESS

THE DIGESTIVE TRACT IS A MUSCULAR TUBE that extends from the mouth, through the stomach and intestines, to the anus. Its function is to break down food into substances that can be absorbed into the bloodstream for distribution to body cells, and to eliminate waste products. The salivary glands, pancreas, and biliary system connect to the digestive tract; all produce substances essential to healthy digestion.

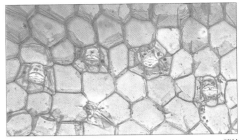

Dietary fibre (cellulose)

SEM

1 IN THE MOUTH AND OESOPHAGUS

Food is chewed by the teeth and mixed with saliva. The enzyme amylase, present in saliva, begins the breakdown of starch into sugar. Each lump of soft food, called a bolus, is swallowed and propelled by contractions down the oesophagus to the stomach.

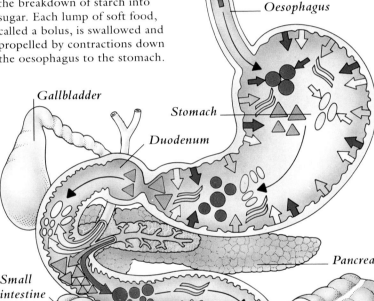
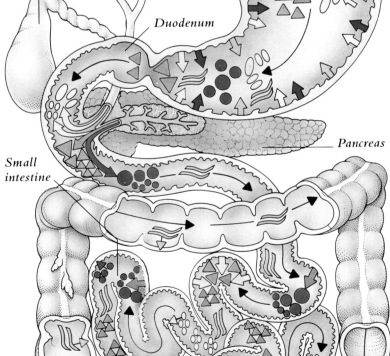

Oesophagus

Gallbladder

Stomach

Duodenum

Pancreas

Small intestine

Large intestine

THE BREAKDOWN OF FOOD

Certain nutrients, such as salts and minerals, can be absorbed directly into the circulation. Proteins, fats, and carbohydrates, however, must be broken down into smaller molecules before they can be absorbed. Food is broken down both by mechanical action and by the chemical action of digestive enzymes. Fats are split into glycerol and fatty acids; carbohydrates into monosaccharide sugars; and proteins into shorter chains and subsequently into individual amino acids.

2 IN THE STOMACH

Pepsin is an enzyme produced when inactive pepsinogen is modified by gastric acid. It breaks down proteins into smaller units called polypeptides and peptides. **Lipase** is a stomach enzyme that breaks down fats into glycerol and fatty acids. **Hydrochloric acid** is produced by the stomach lining. Its acidity is needed for the action of pepsin, and can kill bacteria.

3 IN THE DUODENUM

Lipase, a pancreatic enzyme, breaks down fats into glycerol and fatty acids. **Amylase,** another enzyme produced by the pancreas, breaks down starch into maltose, which is a disaccharide sugar. **Trypsin** and **chymotrypsin** are powerful pancreatic enzymes that split proteins into polypeptides and peptides.

4 IN THE SMALL INTESTINE

Maltase, sucrase, and **lactase** are enzymes secreted by special glands in the intestinal wall. They convert disaccharide sugars into monosaccharide sugars. **Peptidase,** another enzyme secreted by glands in the intestinal wall, splits large peptides into smaller peptides and then into individual amino acids.

5 IN THE LARGE INTESTINE

Undigested food enters the large intestine, where water and salt are absorbed by the intestinal lining. The residue, together with waste pigments, dead cells, and bacteria, is pressed into faeces and stored for excretion.

KEY

➡	*Salivary amylase*
➡	*Pancreatic amylase*
⇨	*Maltase, sucrase, and lactase*
➡	*Pepsin*
➡	*Trypsin and chymotrypsin*
➡	*Peptidase*
⇨	*Lipase*
⇨	*Bile salts*
➡	*Hydrochloric acid*
▶	*Starch*
▶	*Disaccharides (maltose, sucrose, and lactose)*
▷▷	*Monosaccharides (glucose, fructose, and galactose)*
●	*Proteins*
●	*Peptides*
⦿	*Amino acids*
⬭	*Fats*
⬯	*Fatty acids*
⦿⦿	*Glycerol*
≈≈	*Water*

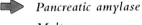

COMPONENTS OF FOOD

Food contains carbohydrates, fats, and proteins as well as vitamins, minerals, water, and fibre. Starchy and sugary foods are rich in carbohydrates, which, along with fats, are the body's main source of energy. Fats and protein are used for cell growth and repair.

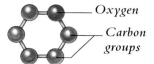

Oxygen

Carbon groups

Monosaccharides

These single sugar units have a hexagonal structure. They form the building blocks of the more complex carbohydrates.

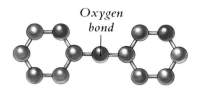

Oxygen bond

Disaccharides

Disaccharide molecules are formed from two single saccharide units chemically bonded together. Sucrose, maltose, and lactose are the main disaccharides.

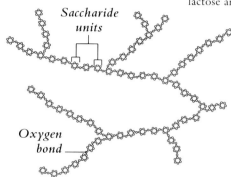

Saccharide units

Oxygen bond

Polysaccharides

Polysaccharides consist of long chains of saccharide units. Starch and glycogen, both storage carbohydrates, are examples. Cellulose is another polysaccharide, and is also the main component of fruit and vegetable fibre.

Fats

Most dietary fats consist of three fatty acids linked by oxygen bonds to a glycerol molecule. Depending upon the type and number of oxygen bonds, fatty acids are either saturated (solid at room temperature) or unsaturated.

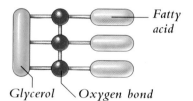

Fatty acid

Glycerol   Oxygen bond

Proteins

Proteins are complex molecules with long chains of amino acids. These acids link in various ways to form many different proteins.

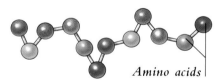

Amino acids

THE ROLE OF FIBRE

Fibre, the indigestible parts of plant foods, adds bulk to faeces and speeds their passage through the bowel. By delaying the absorption of sugar, fibre helps control its level in the blood. Fibre also binds with cholesterol and bile acids, which are derived from cholesterol, and may reduce the amount of cholesterol in blood.

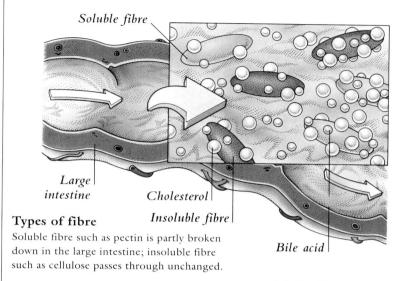

Soluble fibre

Large intestine

Cholesterol

Insoluble fibre

Bile acid

Types of fibre

Soluble fibre such as pectin is partly broken down in the large intestine; insoluble fibre such as cellulose passes through unchanged.

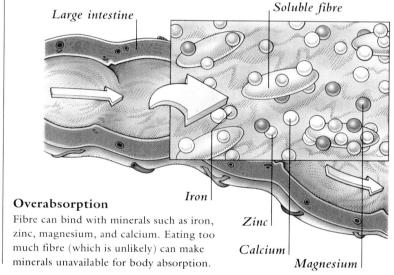

Large intestine

Soluble fibre

Iron

Zinc

Calcium

Magnesium

Overabsorption

Fibre can bind with minerals such as iron, zinc, magnesium, and calcium. Eating too much fibre (which is unlikely) can make minerals unavailable for body absorption.

HOW FOOD PROVIDES ENERGY

The breakdown products of food provide the fuel needed for the building and repair of body cells. Energy is released inside body cells by a complex chain of chemical reactions, which include the Krebs cycle. The energy released is then stored as chemical energy in the form of phosphate bonds. Splitting of these phosphate bonds releases the energy that is needed to power cell activities.

2 Energy is released when adenosine triphosphate (ATP), which is the body's main energy-carrying chemical, converts to adenosine diphosphate (ADP). ADP continuously converts back into ATP, using the energy that has been released from both glucose and fatty acids.

1 Glucose and fatty acids are the main fuels used by the Krebs cycle and linked reactions to produce energy. Amino acids may be used if these chemicals are lacking.

ATP split, forming ADP and releasing energy

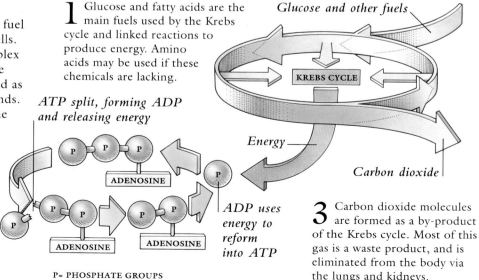

Glucose and other fuels

KREBS CYCLE

Energy

Carbon dioxide

ADP uses energy to reform into ATP

ENERGY

ADENOSINE

P= PHOSPHATE GROUPS

3 Carbon dioxide molecules are formed as a by-product of the Krebs cycle. Most of this gas is a waste product, and is eliminated from the body via the lungs and kidneys.

The MOUTH, PHARYNX, *and* OESOPHAGUS

THE PROCESS OF DIGESTION starts as soon as food enters the mouth. Food is chewed, lubricated by saliva, and mixed and pressed by the tongue. In about one minute, the food is processed into a soft, moist, round lump called a bolus. Each bolus is swallowed through the pharynx and passed into the oesophagus, a muscular tube that is able to squeeze food down to the stomach in approximately 1 to 2 seconds.

SWALLOWING

Swallowing begins as a voluntary process when food passes from the mouth into the pharynx. Automatic reflexes take over to control the subsequent stages of swallowing (see right): the muscles of the pharynx contract and move food along, and then squeeze the food so that it moves into the top of the oesophagus.

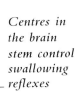

Centres in the brain stem control swallowing reflexes

Pharynx

Bolus about to enter the oesophagus

Oesophagus

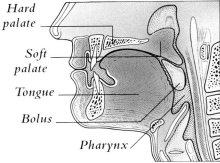

Hard palate

Soft palate

Tongue

Bolus

Pharynx

The oral stage

To initiate swallowing, the tongue rises and pushes food to the back of the mouth. The soft palate then closes onto the back of the tongue. At the same time, the floor of the mouth rises and the bolus is pushed into the pharynx.

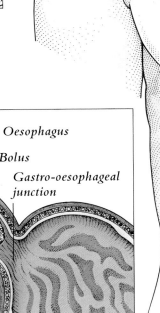

PERISTALSIS

Food is propelled along the oesophagus and into the stomach by waves of involuntary muscular contractions. The muscles in front of the bolus relax, while the muscles behind contract to squeeze the food through. This pattern of rhythmic movement is known as peristalsis; it also occurs in the stomach and the intestines.

Oesophagus

Bolus

Gastro-oesophageal junction

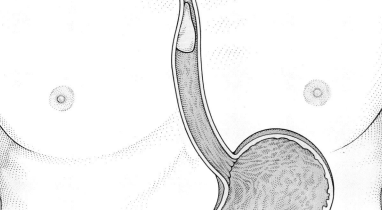

THE SALIVARY GLANDS

Saliva is produced by three pairs of salivary glands: the parotid, submandibular, and sublingual. There are also numerous small accessory glands in the mucous membrane lining the mouth and tongue. Saliva carried by ducts from the glands contains amylase, a digestive enzyme; it also makes chewing and swallowing easier.

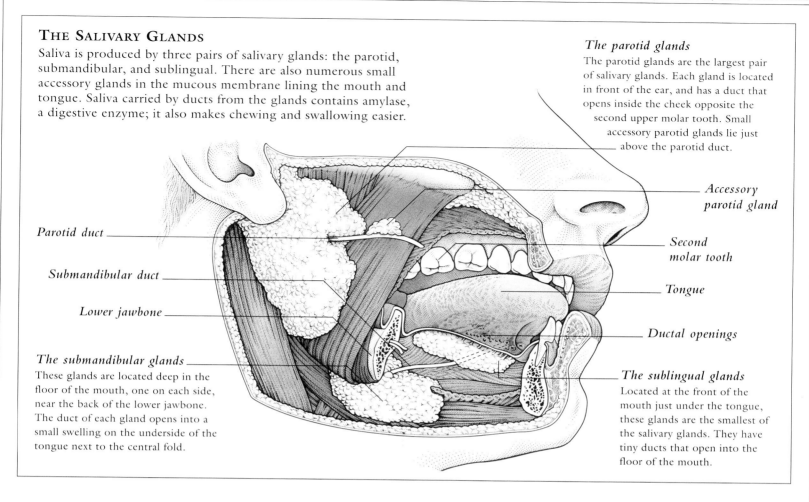

The parotid glands
The parotid glands are the largest pair of salivary glands. Each gland is located in front of the ear, and has a duct that opens inside the cheek opposite the second upper molar tooth. Small accessory parotid glands lie just above the parotid duct.

Parotid duct

Submandibular duct

Lower jawbone

The submandibular glands
These glands are located deep in the floor of the mouth, one on each side, near the back of the lower jawbone. The duct of each gland opens into a small swelling on the underside of the tongue next to the central fold.

Accessory parotid gland

Second molar tooth

Tongue

Ductal openings

The sublingual glands
Located at the front of the mouth just under the tongue, these glands are the smallest of the salivary glands. They have tiny ducts that open into the floor of the mouth.

THE ROLE OF THE TEETH

The teeth are made of hard bone-like material and are set in shock-absorbent gums. The incisors are chisel-shaped with sharp edges for cutting, while the pointed canines are designed for tearing. The premolars, with their two ridges, and the flatter molars, which are the largest and strongest teeth, crush and grind food.

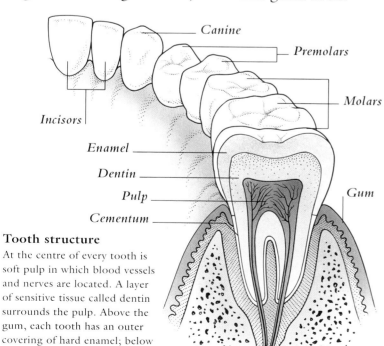

Canine

Premolars

Molars

Incisors

Enamel

Dentin

Pulp

Cementum

Gum

Tooth structure
At the centre of every tooth is soft pulp in which blood vessels and nerves are located. A layer of sensitive tissue called dentin surrounds the pulp. Above the gum, each tooth has an outer covering of hard enamel; below the gum, bone-like cementum forms the tooth's outer layer.

BREATHING AND SWALLOWING

The pharynx is a channel for air as well as food. It leads into both the larynx (voice box) for breathing and the oesophagus for swallowing. Control from the brain normally prevents food from entering the larynx during swallowing. If food goes down the wrong way, irritation of the airway triggers the coughing reflex to expel inhaled particles and prevent choking.

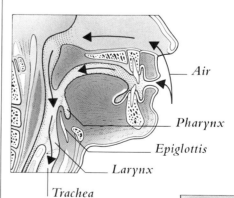

Air

Pharynx

Epiglottis

Larynx

Trachea

Breathing
During breathing, the vocal cords at the entrance to the larynx are relaxed and open, creating a space between them called the glottis. Air passes from the pharynx through the glottis into the trachea during inhalation, and passes from the trachea into the pharynx during exhalation.

Swallowing
During swallowing, the flap of cartilage known as the epiglottis tilts and the larynx rises up. The vocal cords are pressed together, which closes the glottis and seals off the entrance to the larynx. As soon as food has entered the oesophagus, the glottis reopens.

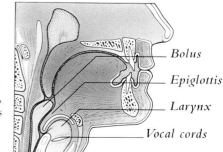

Bolus

Epiglottis

Larynx

Vocal cords

The STOMACH and SMALL INTESTINE

THE STOMACH IS A HOLLOW, ELASTIC SAC where food is churned and mixed thoroughly with juices secreted by the stomach lining. This process begins moments after food enters the stomach from the oesophagus. Processed food is released gradually into the small intestine, a coiled tube about 5m (16ft) long; here, enzymes complete the chemical breakdown of food. The products of digestion are absorbed through the intestinal lining into the bloodstream for circulation.

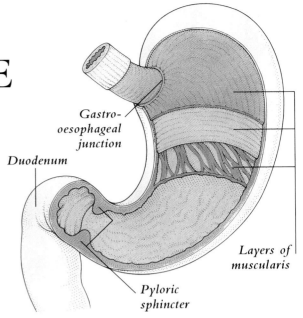

Gastro-oesophageal junction

Duodenum

Layers of muscularis

Pyloric sphincter

STRUCTURE OF THE STOMACH

The stomach is J-shaped and forms the widest part of the digestive tube. At the gastro-oesophageal junction food enters the stomach; when it reaches a muscular ring known as the pyloric sphincter, it passes into the duodenum. The stomach wall is composed of four main layers: the serosa, muscularis, submucosa, and mucosa.

Mucosa
The mucosa, which contains gastric glands, lines the stomach. The surface of the mucosa is heavily folded and covered with numerous gastric pits.

Gastric pits
Three to seven gastric glands open into the bottom of each of these small indentations.

Gastric glands
Gastric glands produce about 3L (5pt) of gastric juice each day. Deep in the glands are specialized cells that secrete acid and enzymes, all of which play an essential part in the digestive process.

Muscular layers of mucosa
Two layers of muscle are located underneath the glands of the mucosa.

Submucosa
This layer of loose tissue connects the mucosa and muscularis.

Oblique layer of muscularis

Circular layer of muscularis

Longitudinal layer of muscularis

Subserous layer
This layer of loose tissue connects the serosa and muscularis.

Serosa
The outer surface of the stomach is coated with this clear membrane.

Lymph nodule

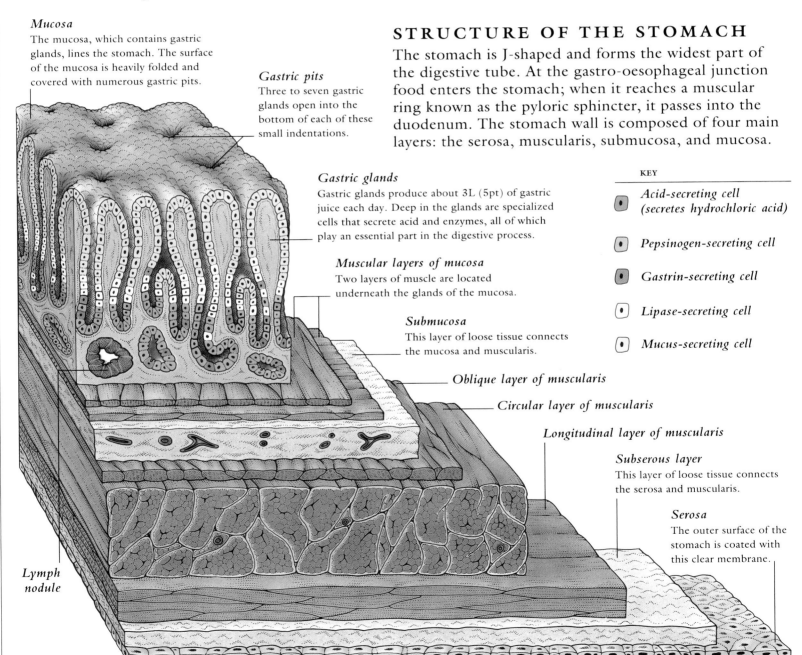

KEY

Acid-secreting cell (secretes hydrochloric acid)

Pepsinogen-secreting cell

Gastrin-secreting cell

Lipase-secreting cell

Mucus-secreting cell

SMALL INTESTINE

The duodenum, jejunum, and ileum make up the small intestine. Short and C-shaped, the duodenum receives secretions from the liver and pancreas. The jejunum and ileum are both long and coiled, but the jejunum is thicker, redder, and slightly shorter than the ileum. In the small intestine, food is broken down by pancreatic juice, bile, and intestinal secretions so that nutrients can be absorbed and utilized.

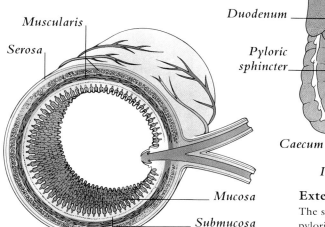

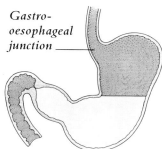

Muscularis

Serosa

Mucosa

Submucosa

Duodenum

Pyloric sphincter

Caecum

Ileum　　*Jejunum*

Extent
The small intestine starts at the pyloric sphincter and ends at the pouch-like caecum, which is the beginning of the large intestine.

Intestinal cross-section
The intestinal wall has four layers. The outermost, protective coat is known as the serosa. Next is the muscularis, which contains outer longitudinal and inner circular muscle fibres. Adjoining this is the submucosa, a loose layer carrying vessels and nerves. The innermost layer is known as the mucosa.

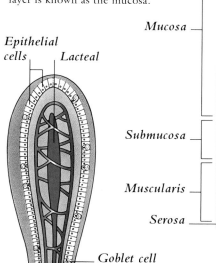

Epithelial cells　　*Lacteal*

Goblet cell

Vein

Artery

Lymph vessel

Structure of a villus
The central core of each villus contains a lacteal, or lymph vessel, and a network of minute blood vessels. Goblet cells scattered throughout the epithelium secrete mucus.

Epithelial cells　　*Villi*

Mucosa

Submucosa

Muscularis

Serosa

Intestinal villi
The mucosa has millions of projections called villi; each is covered by an epithelium, or cell layer, that absorbs nutrients. The epithelial cells have projections called microvilli. The villi and microvilli increase the surface area of the small intestine for efficient absorption.

MOVEMENT OF FOOD

Swallowing triggers relaxation of muscles at the gastro-oesophageal junction, which enables food to enter the stomach. Waves of muscular contractions, called peristalsis, move food through the stomach, and then squirt small amounts into the duodenum. Contractions of the small intestine propel food toward the large intestine.

1 The muscular action of the stomach wall mixes food with gastric juice and churns it to form a thick, creamy substance called chyme.

Gastro-oesophageal junction

2 Peristaltic waves are most marked in the lower half of the stomach. These move the stomach contents toward the still-closed pyloric sphincter.

Pyloric sphincter

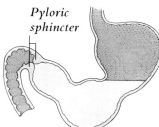

3 The valve-like pyloric sphincter, stimulated by chyme, opens to let only small quantities of food pass into the duodenum at a time.

Duodenum

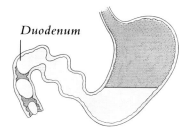

INTESTINAL MOVEMENT
The small intestine moves by peristalsis, pendular movements, and segmentation. Peristalsis consists of contraction waves that propel food. Pendular movements are the lengthening and shortening motions of short intestinal sections. Segmentation involves ring-like, evenly spaced contractions.

CONTRACTION 1

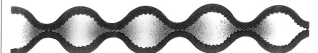

CONTRACTION 2

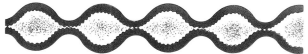

CONTRACTION 3

Segmentation
This series of concentric contractions, mixing chyme up to 12 times a minute, is the small intestine's main movement.

The LIVER, PANCREAS, *and* GALLBLADDER

THE LIVER, PANCREAS, AND GALLBLADDER are closely connected with the digestive tract but not actually part of it. The liver is the largest and one of the most important internal organs. It is like a chemical processing factory and has many functions, including production of a digestive liquid called bile. The pancreas produces a powerful digestive juice, and the gallbladder stores and concentrates bile. These organs secrete their digestive substances into the duodenum, which is the first part of the small intestine.

LIVER FUNCTIONS

Cholesterol and bile are produced by the liver from the breakdown products of dietary fat and old red blood cells. The liver produces proteins, and stores glycogen, iron, and some vitamins. It also removes toxic substances (poisons and waste products) from the blood, and converts them into safer substances.

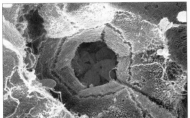

Cells of liver lobule
SEM x 1050

LIVER STRUCTURE

The wedge-shaped liver is divided by a ligament into two lobes, with the left lobe smaller than the right. It is composed of thousands of distinctive hexagon-shaped lobules made up of billions of cells. Tiny tubes known as bile ducts form a network throughout the liver.

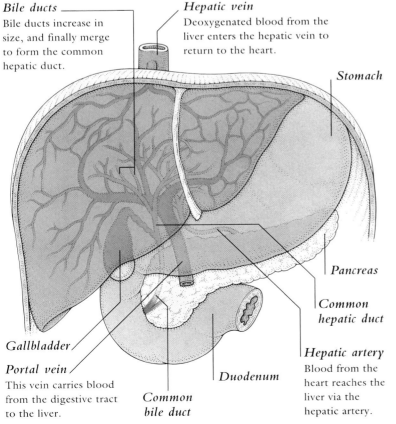

Bile ducts
Bile ducts increase in size, and finally merge to form the common hepatic duct.

Hepatic vein
Deoxygenated blood from the liver enters the hepatic vein to return to the heart.

Stomach

Pancreas

Common hepatic duct

Gallbladder

Portal vein
This vein carries blood from the digestive tract to the liver.

Duodenum

Common bile duct

Hepatic artery
Blood from the heart reaches the liver via the hepatic artery.

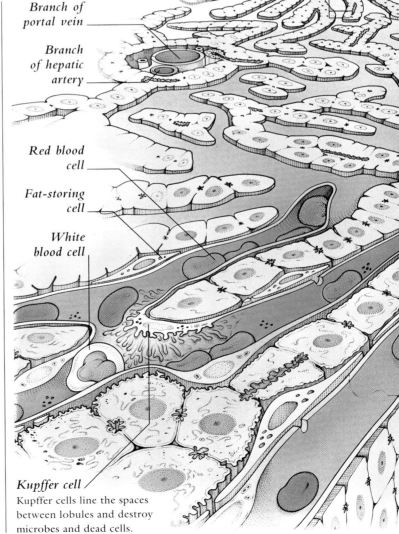

Canaliculi

Branch of portal vein

Branch of hepatic artery

Red blood cell

Fat-storing cell

White blood cell

Kupffer cell
Kupffer cells line the spaces between lobules and destroy microbes and dead cells.

160

PANCREAS: ROLE IN DIGESTION

The pancreas secretes a juice in response to food in the upper digestive tract. Rich in enzymes that break down fats, nucleic acids, proteins, and carbohydrates, this juice also contains sodium bicarbonate to neutralize stomach acid. The enzymes are secreted into ducts that converge to form the pancreatic duct. This duct transports the enzymes to the duodenum.

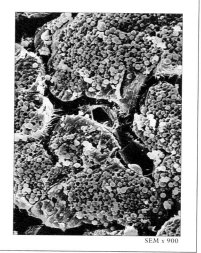

SEM x 900

Acinar cells of the pancreas

Grape-like clusters of cells in the pancreas, known as acini, contain globules of pancreatic enzymes.

THE BILIARY SYSTEM

The right and left hepatic ducts from the liver, the bile ducts, and the gallbladder form the biliary system. Bile is a waste product produced by the liver's chemical processes, but it also plays a part in the digestion of fats. The common bile duct joins the pancreatic duct at the ampulla of Vater, the entry into the duodenum.

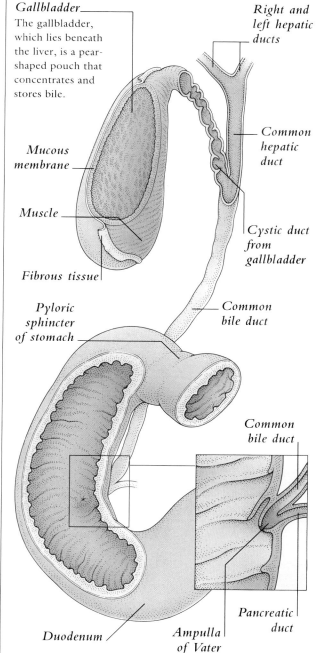

Gallbladder
The gallbladder, which lies beneath the liver, is a pear-shaped pouch that concentrates and stores bile.

Right and left hepatic ducts

Mucous membrane

Common hepatic duct

Muscle

Fibrous tissue

Cystic duct from gallbladder

Pyloric sphincter of stomach

Common bile duct

Common bile duct

Duodenum

Ampulla of Vater

Pancreatic duct

Branch of hepatic vein
(central vein of lobule)

Lobule
Thousands of hexagonal units, known as lobules, make up the liver. Each lobule is about 1mm in diameter. Within each lobule is a central vein from which rows of hepatocytes radiate.

Hepatocytes
The liver's chemical activities take place within millions of these cells, which are packed with organelles and enzymes, as well as storage particles. Hepatocytes manufacture bile and secrete it into tiny channels called canaliculi, which drain into bile ducts.

Bile duct

Branch of hepatic artery

Branch of portal vein

Lymphatic vessel

Sinusoid
Blood flows from small branches of the hepatic artery and portal vein via sinusoids into the central vein.

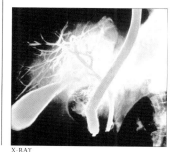

X-RAY

Site of stored bile

The sac-like gallbladder, shown in orange, squeezes stored bile into the cystic duct when food is eaten. This duct then joins the common bile duct. To create the image, dye was introduced through the tube shown in green.

The COLON, RECTUM, *and* ANUS

THE FINAL PART OF THE DIGESTIVE TRACT is made up of the colon, the rectum, and the anus. A short pouch called the caecum links the small intestine to the colon. The caecum, colon, and rectum form the large intestine. About 1.5m (5ft) long, the colon changes digestive waste products into a form that the body excretes as faeces via the rectum and anus. By the time digested food reaches the colon, the nutrients that are essential for bodily functions have been absorbed.

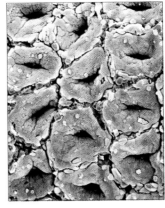

SEM x 120

Colonic glands
This microscopic image shows the openings to several of the tubular glands lining the colon. They absorb water from faeces.

DIGESTIVE TRANSIT TIMES

After the first, voluntary stage of swallowing, the passage of food through different parts of the digestive system is governed by reflex actions. Below is an illustration showing the approximate time food takes to pass through each part. The time that food spends in the stomach and the colon depends on its type and on the individual person. People with longer transit times may be more prone to disorders such as cancer of the colon.

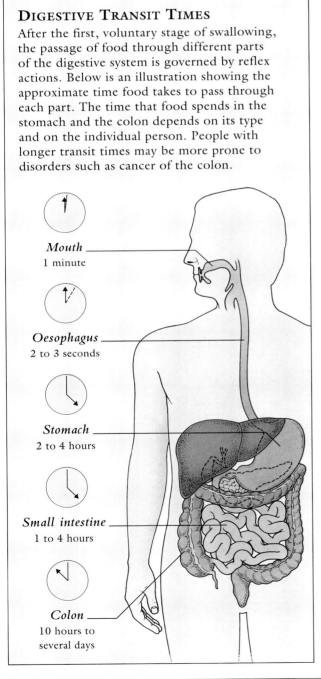

Mouth
1 minute

Oesophagus
2 to 3 seconds

Stomach
2 to 4 hours

Small intestine
1 to 4 hours

Colon
10 hours to several days

ACTIVITY IN THE COLON

The main function of the colon is to convert liquid from the small intestine, called chyme, into faeces. Billions of bacteria within the colon produce the vitamins K and B, as well as the gases hydrogen, carbon dioxide, hydrogen sulphide, and methane. The lining of the colon secretes mucus to lubricate the inside of the intestine to ease the passage of faeces. Mucus contains antibodies that protect against disease.

Absorption of water from faeces
Sodium, chloride, and water are absorbed through the lining of the colon into blood and lymph so that the faeces become drier. Both bicarbonate and potassium are secreted by the colon to replace sodium and chloride.

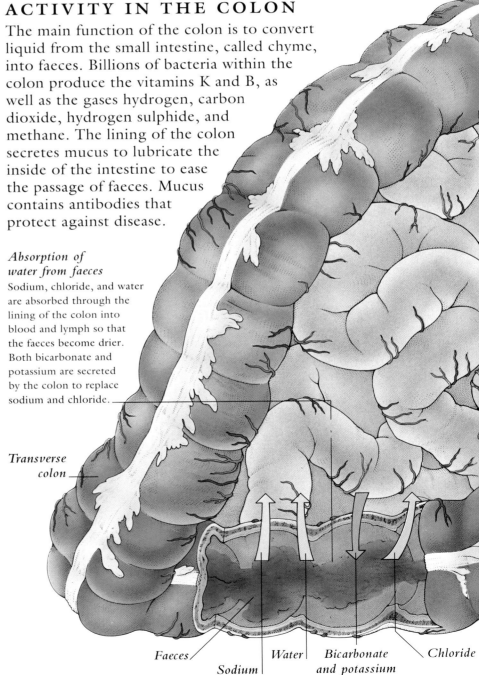

Transverse colon

Faeces

Sodium

Water

Bicarbonate and potassium

Chloride

COLONIC MOVEMENT

Muscular movement in the wall of the colon mixes and propels faeces along the colon toward the rectum. The movement of faeces within the colon varies in rate, intensity, and nature. Types of movement are known as segmentation, peristaltic contractions, and mass movements. Faecal material passes more slowly through the colon than through the small intestine, permitting the reabsorption of approximately 1.4L (2.5pt) of water every day.

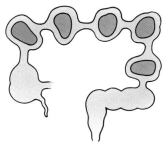

Segmentation
Segmentation describes a series of ring-like contractions that occur at regular intervals; these churn and mix faeces but do not propel them.

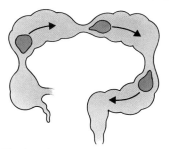

Peristaltic contractions
Waves of peristaltic contractions propel faeces toward the rectum. Muscles behind food contract, while the muscles in front relax.

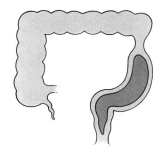

Mass movements
Mass movements are strong peristaltic waves that propel faeces relatively long distances about two or three times a day.

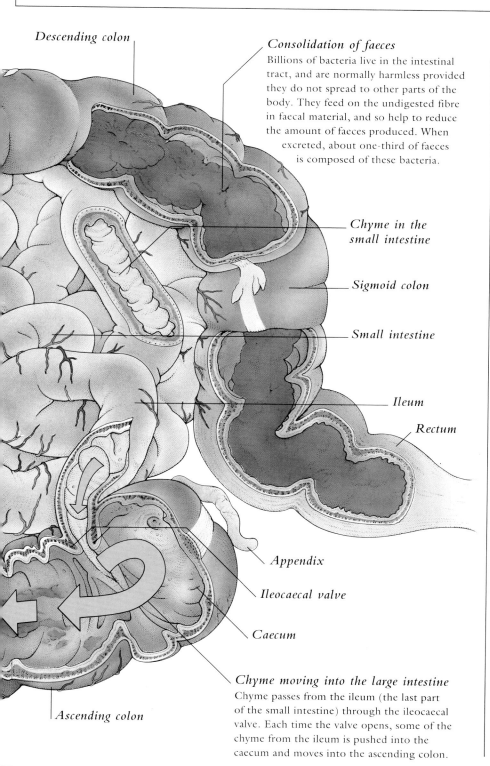

Descending colon

Consolidation of faeces
Billions of bacteria live in the intestinal tract, and are normally harmless provided they do not spread to other parts of the body. They feed on the undigested fibre in faecal material, and so help to reduce the amount of faeces produced. When excreted, about one-third of faeces is composed of these bacteria.

Chyme in the small intestine

Sigmoid colon

Small intestine

Ileum

Rectum

Appendix

Ileocaecal valve

Caecum

Chyme moving into the large intestine
Chyme passes from the ileum (the last part of the small intestine) through the ileocaecal valve. Each time the valve opens, some of the chyme from the ileum is pushed into the caecum and moves into the ascending colon.

Ascending colon

THE RECTUM AND ANUS

The rectum is about 12cm (5in) long, and it is normally empty except just before and during defaecation. Below the rectum lies the anal canal, which is about 4cm (1.5in) long and lined with vertical ridges called anal columns. In the walls of the anal canal are two strong, flat sheets of muscles called the internal and external sphincters, which act like valves and relax during defaecation.

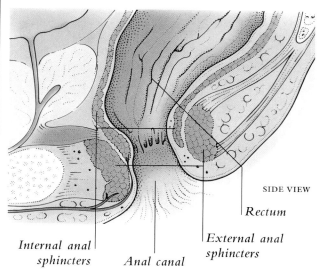

SIDE VIEW

Rectum

Internal anal sphincters

Anal canal

External anal sphincters

DEFAECATION

Peristaltic waves in the colon push faeces into the rectum, which triggers the defaecation reflex. Contractions push the faeces along, and the anal sphincters relax to allow faeces to pass out of the body. The defaecation reflex may be aided by voluntary contraction of the abdominal muscles, or overridden by conscious control.

Faeces

Anal canal

FRONT VIEW

STOMACH *and* DUODENAL DISORDERS

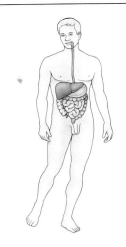

ULCERS OF THE STOMACH AND DUODENUM, also called peptic ulcers, are among the most common conditions treated by gastroenterologists. Other important conditions include hiatal hernia, inflammation (gastritis and duodenitis), and cancer of the stomach. Doctors often investigate such disorders by endoscopy, in which a flexible, fibreoptic viewing tube is passed down through the mouth.

HERNIAS

Hiatal hernia is the protrusion of part of the stomach into the chest through a weakness in muscles of the diaphragm. It occurs most frequently in overweight, middle-aged, or elderly people, especially women. In a diaphragmatic hernia, abdominal organs protrude through an abnormal opening in the diaphragm.

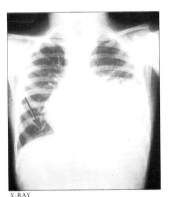

X-RAY

Diaphragmatic hernia

This type may be diagnosed shortly after birth by X-ray. The opaque region above the level of the diaphragm (arrow) in the X-ray at left indicates abdominal organs protruding up into one side of the chest. The disorder can be life-threatening and requires urgent treatment by surgery.

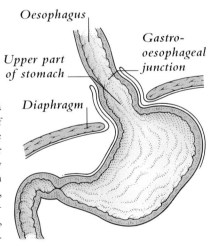

Oesophagus

Upper part of stomach

Gastro-oesophageal junction

Diaphragm

Sliding hiatal hernia

This is the most common type of hiatal hernia. It occurs when the lower oesophagus and the upper stomach slide into the chest cavity through an opening, or hiatus, in the diaphragm. As a result of this, pressure conditions at the gastro-oesophageal junction are disturbed, causing acid reflux and heartburn.

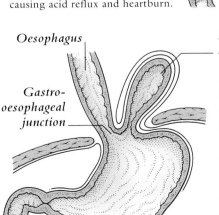

Oesophagus

Gastro-oesophageal junction

Pouch of stomach

Paraoesophageal hiatal hernia

About 10 per cent of all hiatal hernias are of this type. Part of the stomach lies adjacent to the lower oesophagus after being pushed upward through the diaphragm. Because the gastro-oesophageal junction is not disturbed, acid reflux does not occur.

STOMACH CANCER

The incidence of stomach cancer has declined during the past 50 years, but it still accounts for over 10 per cent of UK cancer deaths. It appears most commonly in men aged 50 to 70, and the symptoms, if present, are more or less identical with those of a peptic ulcer. Gastrectomy offers a hope of cure if the cancer has not yet spread beyond the stomach to other organs.

Total gastrectomy

Rarely, the entire stomach is removed, and the oesophagus is then joined to the jejunum. The cut end of the duodenum is closed. People who have undergone a total gastrectomy may become anaemic if not given injections of vitamin B$_{12}$.

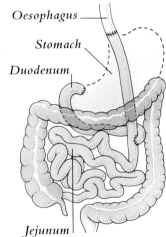

Oesophagus

Stomach

Duodenum

Jejunum

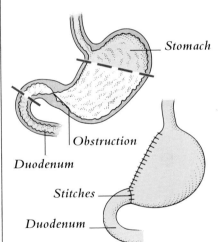

Stomach

Obstruction

Duodenum

Stitches

Duodenum

Partial gastrectomy

Even if a complete cure is not possible, partial gastrectomy (surgical removal of part of the stomach) may help if a cancer is obstructing the upper or, as shown here, the lower stomach.

GASTRITIS

The possible causes of gastritis, or inflammation of the stomach lining, include irritation caused by alcohol, non-steroidal anti-inflammatory drugs (NSAIDs), and/or smoking tobacco. Recent research has focused on the role of infection with the bacterium *Helicobacter pylori* (shown at right) as another possible cause. Gastritis may appear suddenly or develop slowly over time. Symptoms may include nausea, upper abdominal pain, and indigestion.

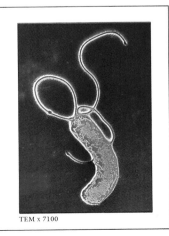

TEM x 7100

PEPTIC ULCER

About 10 per cent of people in developed countries may have experienced peptic ulceration at some stage. The precise cause remains unclear, but the bacterium *Helicobacter pylori* may cause inflammation and ulceration by increasing stomach acid. Other contributory factors include alcohol, smoking tobacco, NSAIDs, stress, family history, and diet. The main symptom of a peptic ulcer is upper abdominal pain. The problem can occur at any age.

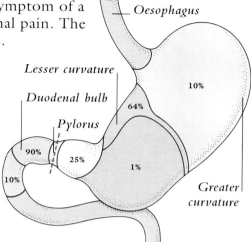

Oesophagus

Lesser curvature

Duodenal bulb

Pylorus

10%

64%

90%

25%

10%

1%

Greater curvature

Sites of peptic ulcers

Peptic ulcers are found mainly in the duodenum, the most common site being the first part, sometimes called the bulb. In the stomach, the most common site of ulceration is the lesser curvature. The illustration shows the distribution of peptic ulcers in the US population.

DEVELOPMENT OF A PEPTIC ULCER

A layer of mucus secreted by the mucosal cells normally protects the lining of the stomach and duodenum from attack by hydrochloric acid, pepsin (a digestive enzyme), and other substances that are potentially harmful.

1 Damage occurs when the protective mucus barrier breaks down and stomach juice comes into contact with cells of the lining. In the early stages, the mucosa is only partly destroyed, producing a shallow area of damage known as an erosion.

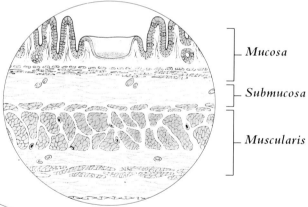

Mucosa

Submucosa

Muscularis

2 A true ulcer penetrates the entire mucosal layer, and usually also the submucosa and muscularis layers. Peptic ulcers tend to be round or oval. They are chronic, with destruction of tissue and healing occurring at the same time.

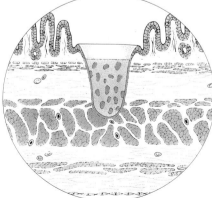

3 A peptic ulcer may burrow through the entire thickness of the wall. This can result in erosion into a large artery, causing a haemorrhage, or perforation of the wall and inflammation of the abdominal lining (peritonitis). Another complication is narrowing of the outlet from the stomach by scar tissue.

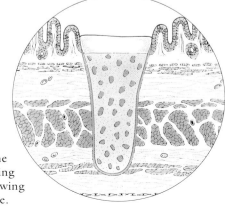

DRUG TREATMENT

Various drugs can help treat a peptic ulcer. Antacids neutralize stomach acid, while mucosal protectors provide a protective coat. H_2 blockers and proton pump inhibitors block production of acid by cells in the stomach lining. Newer treatments are designed to eliminate *Helicobacter pylori* by using combinations of bismuth and various antibacterial agents.

Action of antacids

Antacids, such as magnesium trisilicate and calcium carbonate, are basically alkaline substances that neutralize stomach acid. They help relieve the pain of ulceration and promote healing.

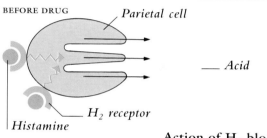

Parietal cells of stomach lining

Mucus

Neutralized acid

Drug

BEFORE DRUG

Parietal cell

Acid

H_2 receptor

Histamine

AFTER DRUG

Acid

H_2 blocker

Histamine

Action of H_2 blockers

Normally, histamine (H_2) stimulates the secretion of acid by occupying specific H_2 receptors on the surface of parietal cells in stomach mucosa. H_2 blockers occupy these receptors, inhibiting the action of histamine and reducing acid secretion.

SURGICAL TREATMENT

In spite of improved drug therapy for peptic ulcers, some people are in need of surgery for persistent ulceration, perforation, bleeding, obstruction, or scarring. A partial gastrectomy can involve either removing the acid-secreting part of the stomach or, in the case of a stomach ulcer, the ulcer itself.

Vagotomy

Vagotomy reduces stomach acid secretion by preventing nerve signals from reaching the stomach lining. In truncal vagotomy, the whole vagus nerve is cut. In selective types of vagotomy, only certain nerve branches are cut (as shown here).

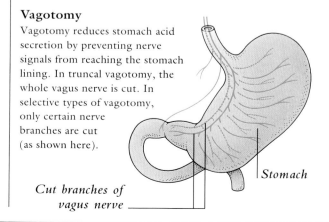

Cut branches of vagus nerve

Stomach

LIVER DISORDERS

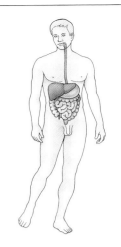

A COMMON CAUSE OF LIVER DISEASE in developed countries is the excessive consumption of alcohol. Other causes are viral infection of the liver and drug reactions. Long-term damage from any of these causes can lead to cirrhosis. Cancer can arise in the liver, but more often spreads from another part of the body, such as the lungs or breast. In a rare condition known as biliary atresia, the bile ducts are abnormal at birth. Unless this is treated within a few weeks, the affected infant becomes jaundiced and may develop serious liver damage.

ALCOHOLIC LIVER DISEASE

Persistent alcohol abuse leads to liver damage, which can be irreversible. In the early stages alcoholic liver disease may produce no symptoms, but blood tests can reveal abnormal liver function. Some people may be genetically more susceptible to the disease. Alcohol is broken down by stomach enzymes; because women have fewer enzymes than men, they are at greater risk.

PROGRESSION OF THE DISEASE

Alcohol damage to the liver initially causes an abnormal accumulation of fat in liver cells (fatty liver). Sometimes damage causes inflammation, or alcoholic hepatitis. If people who have either fatty liver or alcoholic hepatitis continue to abuse alcohol, cirrhosis and liver failure can develop.

How damage occurs
Some alcohol is excreted in the urine or breath unchanged, but most is converted by enzymes in the liver into acetaldehyde. Both alcohol and acetaldehyde are poisonous to liver cells.

Alcohol   *Liver cell*

Fat-laden cells   *Acetaldehyde*   *Water*

H   H
| |
H—C—C—OH
| |
H   H
ALCOHOL

▼

OXIDATION IN
LIVER CELLS

▼

H
|
H—C—C=O
| |
H   H
ACETALDEHYDE

+

H   H
\ /
O
WATER

Fatty liver
The liver cells become infiltrated with globules of fat, which results in enlargement of the liver.

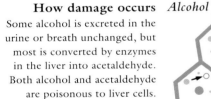

Alcoholic hepatitis
As a result of the production of acetaldehyde, liver cells become acutely inflamed and damaged so that liver function is impaired.

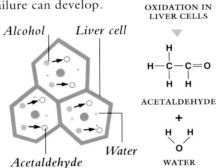

Damaged tissue

Scar tissue

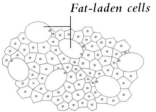

Cirrhosis
In cirrhosis, bands of scar tissue separate nodules of overgrown cells. At this stage damage is irreversible. Cirrhosis may also be due to other causes, such as chronic viral hepatitis.

PORTAL HYPERTENSION

Cirrhotic scar tissue can obstruct blood flow in the liver, leading to a rise in pressure in the portal vein. Increased pressure causes enlargement of veins in the lower oesophagus and upper stomach. The enlarged veins may burst, causing a haemorrhage. As liver function worsens, toxins may impair mental function.

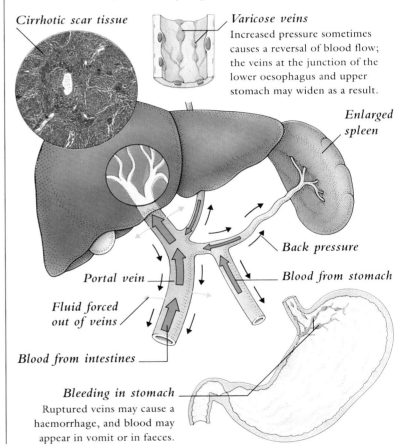

Cirrhotic scar tissue

Varicose veins
Increased pressure sometimes causes a reversal of blood flow; the veins at the junction of the lower oesophagus and upper stomach may widen as a result.

Enlarged spleen

Back pressure

Blood from stomach

Portal vein

Fluid forced out of veins

Blood from intestines

Bleeding in stomach
Ruptured veins may cause a haemorrhage, and blood may appear in vomit or in faeces.

SIGNS OF LIVER DISEASE

An important sign of liver disease is jaundice, which causes the eyes and skin to appear yellow (seen at right). Other signs of liver disease are nausea, loss of appetite, weight loss, abdominal swelling and pain, abnormal blood clotting, dilation of capillaries in the skin, and, in men, enlargement of the breasts.

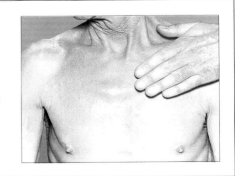

HEPATITIS

Hepatitis, or liver inflammation, is commonly caused by a viral infection, particularly with hepatitis A, B, or C viruses. Viral hepatitis is usually an acute, short-lived illness. Chronic inflammation, however, can lead to cirrhosis; it also increases the risk of liver cancer. Hepatitis A and B can be prevented by immunization. Some other causes of hepatitis include adverse drug reactions, poisoning by toxic chemicals – including drugs and alcohol – and certain bacterial infections.

Hepatitis B virus

A protein coat with surface antigens (proteins) surrounds the DNA core of this virus. This infection is transmitted through contaminated blood or drug needles, sexual intercourse, or from an infected mother to her baby at birth.

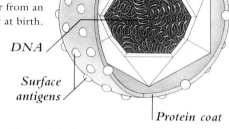

DNA

Surface antigens

Protein coat

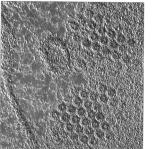

TEM x 139,000

Hepatitis A virus

Hepatitis A virus particles (red circles) are small, 20-sided structures containing RNA. Hepatitis A is usually contracted by ingesting contaminated food or water.

LIVER ABSCESS

An abscess, or a collection of pus, in the liver can be caused by infection with bacteria or amoebae. Bacteria may have spread from an infected site in another part of the body, for example the appendix. Amoebic liver abscess is common in tropical countries and may be preceded by diarrhoea. Liver abscesses can cause fever, nausea, weight loss, liver enlargement, and chest pain.

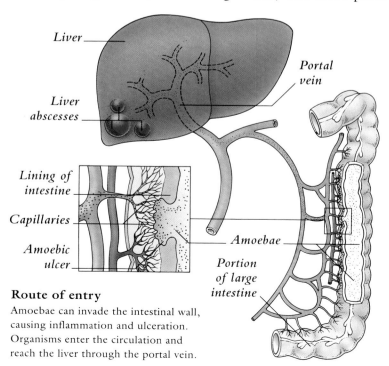

Liver

Liver abscesses

Portal vein

Lining of intestine

Capillaries

Amoebic ulcer

Amoebae

Portion of large intestine

Route of entry

Amoebae can invade the intestinal wall, causing inflammation and ulceration. Organisms enter the circulation and reach the liver through the portal vein.

OPERATION

LIVER TRANSPLANT

The replacement of a diseased liver with a healthy one from a donor may benefit people who have a disabling or life-threatening liver disease such as advanced chronic hepatitis, congenital biliary atresia, or primary biliary cirrhosis (an autoimmune disorder). Patients should be free from major infection, and not have a heart or lung disease. Immunosuppressant drugs to prevent organ rejection must be taken for the rest of the patient's life.

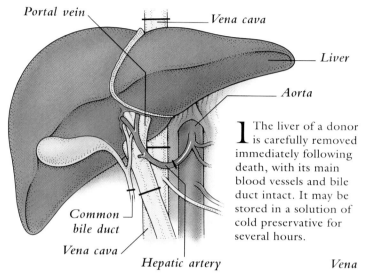

Portal vein

Vena cava

Liver

Aorta

Common bile duct

Vena cava

Hepatic artery

1 The liver of a donor is carefully removed immediately following death, with its main blood vessels and bile duct intact. It may be stored in a solution of cold preservative for several hours.

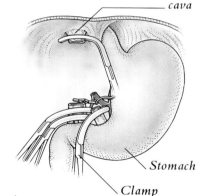

Vena cava

Stomach

Clamp

2 The recipient's abdomen is opened, and the vena cava – the major vein in the abdomen – is clamped above and below the liver. During the operation, venous blood is diverted via a bypass. The hepatic artery, the bile duct, and the portal vein are all cut so that the entire diseased liver can be removed.

3 The new liver is stitched to the vena cava and to other blood vessels, and the cut ends of the bile duct are joined. A T-shaped tube is temporarily inserted into the reconstructed bile duct to allow drainage while tissue healing occurs.

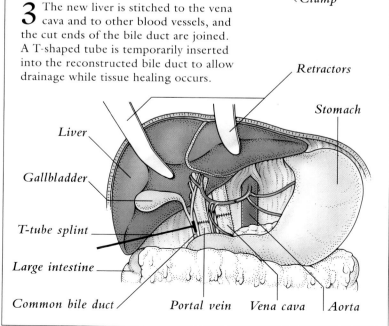

Retractors

Stomach

Liver

Gallbladder

T-tube splint

Large intestine

Common bile duct

Portal vein

Vena cava

Aorta

GALLBLADDER *and* PANCREATIC DISORDERS

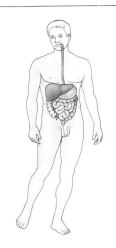

MOST DISORDERS OF THE GALLBLADDER are due to the presence of gallstones. However, people with gallstones do not necessarily experience any symptoms. Inflammation of the pancreas may be due to gallstones, alcohol abuse, or viral infections. Other pancreatic disorders are cancer and pseudocysts. Malfunction of the pancreas can cause diabetes mellitus and impair absorption of nutrients.

CANCER OF THE PANCREAS

Pancreatic cancer occurs most commonly in elderly people. The main symptom of this type of cancer is a dull pain in the upper abdomen penetrating to the back. Other symptoms include loss of appetite and weight, and jaundice. The cancer may spread from the head of the pancreas directly into the duodenum, and through the bloodstream to the liver and lungs.

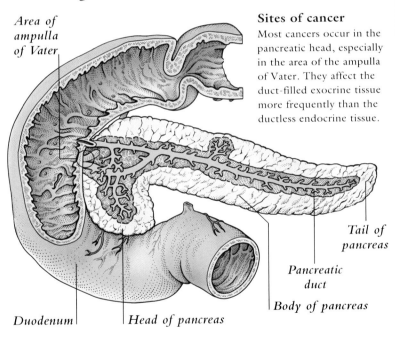

Area of ampulla of Vater

Sites of cancer
Most cancers occur in the pancreatic head, especially in the area of the ampulla of Vater. They affect the duct-filled exocrine tissue more frequently than the ductless endocrine tissue.

Tail of pancreas

Pancreatic duct

Body of pancreas

Duodenum *Head of pancreas*

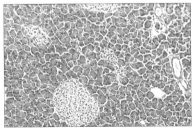
LM

Healthy tissue
The duct-filled exocrine tissue is composed of cell clusters known as acini, which secrete digestive enzymes. The large pale circle is an islet of Langerhans, endocrine tissue that secretes hormones directly into the bloodstream.

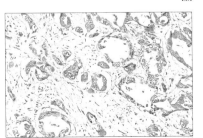
LM

Cancerous tissue
In pancreatic cancer, groups of irregularly shaped malignant cells with enlarged nuclei replace the smaller healthy cells. The tissue lacks the organized appearance of normal pancreatic tissue.

OPERATION

DRAINING A PSEUDOCYST

A pancreatic pseudocyst is a fluid-filled sac that usually develops between the pancreas and the stomach. These sacs are often a result of inflammation of the pancreas, called pancreatitis. Symptoms include nausea, fever, and swelling in the upper abdomen. Many cysts disappear without treatment, but others require surgery.

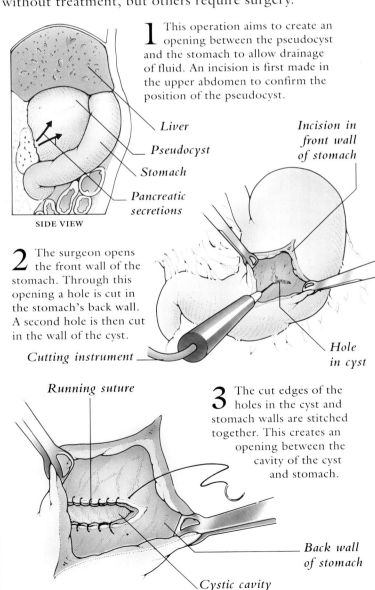

1 This operation aims to create an opening between the pseudocyst and the stomach to allow drainage of fluid. An incision is first made in the upper abdomen to confirm the position of the pseudocyst.

Liver

Pseudocyst

Stomach

Pancreatic secretions

SIDE VIEW

Incision in front wall of stomach

2 The surgeon opens the front wall of the stomach. Through this opening a hole is cut in the stomach's back wall. A second hole is then cut in the wall of the cyst.

Cutting instrument

Hole in cyst

Running suture

3 The cut edges of the holes in the cyst and stomach walls are stitched together. This creates an opening between the cavity of the cyst and stomach.

Back wall of stomach

Cystic cavity

GALLSTONES

Most gallstones, which are made of bile pigment and cholesterol, result from an imbalance in the chemical composition of bile. These gallstones are particularly common among overweight, middle-aged women. Gallstones can travel from the gallbladder into the cystic duct, but may then fall back into the cavity of the gallbladder, pass through the common bile duct into the duodenum, or become impacted in ducts.

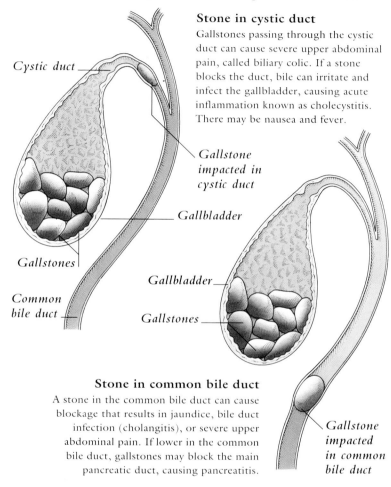

Stone in cystic duct

Gallstones passing through the cystic duct can cause severe upper abdominal pain, called biliary colic. If a stone blocks the duct, bile can irritate and infect the gallbladder, causing acute inflammation known as cholecystitis. There may be nausea and fever.

Cystic duct

Gallstone impacted in cystic duct

Gallbladder

Gallstones

Gallbladder

Gallstones

Common bile duct

Stone in common bile duct

A stone in the common bile duct can cause blockage that results in jaundice, bile duct infection (cholangitis), or severe upper abdominal pain. If lower in the common bile duct, gallstones may block the main pancreatic duct, causing pancreatitis.

Gallstone impacted in common bile duct

LESS COMMON COMPLICATIONS

An inflamed gallbladder may become filled with pus, a condition called empyema, or it may perforate and leak. A mucocele may form if a stone blocks the cystic duct and the gallbladder becomes distended with mucus. A fistula, an abnormal passage, sometimes forms between the gallbladder and the intestine. Repeated episodes of cholecystitis can shrink or scar the entire gallbladder.

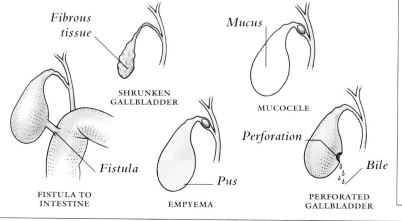

Fibrous tissue

Mucus

SHRUNKEN GALLBLADDER

MUCOCELE

Perforation

Fistula

Pus

Bile

FISTULA TO INTESTINE

EMPYEMA

PERFORATED GALLBLADDER

TREATMENT OF GALLSTONES

Gallstones require treatment if they are causing symptoms, when removal of the gallbladder (cholecystectomy) or of the stones that obstruct the common bile duct becomes necessary. Increasingly, cholecystectomies are being carried out laparoscopically rather than by an operation in which the abdomen is opened. Where symptoms are mild, small or medium-sized stones may be dissolved by certain drugs.

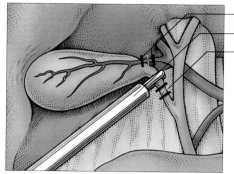

Clips

Grasping forceps

Incision

Laparoscopic cholescystectomy

An endoscope, a fibreoptic viewing instrument, is inserted through a small incision that is made near the umbilicus. The gallbladder is severed from its connections and removed.

OPERATION

REMOVING A GALLSTONE

Gallstones can be removed from the lower end of the common bile duct by a flexible endoscope, which is a fibreoptic viewing instrument. The tube is passed into the mouth, down the oesophagus, through the stomach, and finally into the duodenum. Fine wire instruments are passed down the endoscope through the ampulla of Vater into the common bile duct.

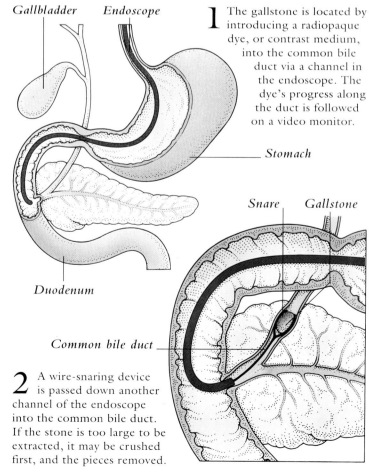

Gallbladder

Endoscope

1 The gallstone is located by introducing a radiopaque dye, or contrast medium, into the common bile duct via a channel in the endoscope. The dye's progress along the duct is followed on a video monitor.

Stomach

Duodenum

Snare

Gallstone

Common bile duct

2 A wire-snaring device is passed down another channel of the endoscope into the common bile duct. If the stone is too large to be extracted, it may be crushed first, and the pieces removed.

INTESTINAL, RECTAL, *and* ANAL DISORDERS

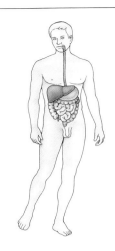

INTESTINAL INFECTIONS OCCUR WORLDWIDE and are the commonest disorders of the digestive tract. In developing regions of the world, many children die from these disorders; in industrialized countries, where cancer and chronic intestinal inflammation are more serious conditions, they usually cause minor problems. Diarrhoea, constipation, fever, chills, pain, and rectal bleeding are symptoms.

INFLAMMATORY BOWEL DISEASE

The term inflammatory bowel disease includes ulcerative colitis and Crohn's disease; both result in chronic intestinal inflammation. They may be caused by the immune system attacking the body's own tissues; a genetic predisposition is probable. Symptoms include fever, bleeding, abdominal pain, and diarrhoea. Diagnosis is usually made by means of barium X-ray, colonoscopy, and microscopy of bowel tissue specimens. Treatment may include anti-inflammatory drugs.

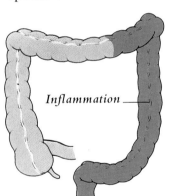

Inflammation

Ulcerative colitis

Ulcerative colitis affects all or part of the colon. It causes diarrhoea as well as the appearance of blood, and sometimes pus, in the faeces. Those affected are at increased risk of intestinal cancer and should have regular check-ups.

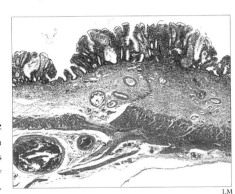
LM

Inflamed membrane

This sample of tissue from a colon affected by ulcerative colitis shows the typical pattern of irregularity and inflammation of the mucosa.

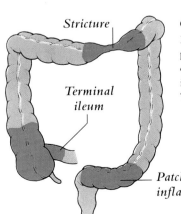

Stricture

Terminal ileum

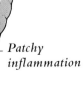
Patchy inflammation

Crohn's disease

In Crohn's disease, narrowing, or stricture, and patches of inflammation may occur anywhere in the digestive tract. The area where the large and small intestine meet (the terminal ileum) is often affected. The disease can cause malabsorption of food.

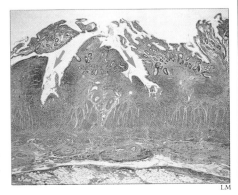
LM

Inflamed wall

Inflammation of the intestinal wall with ulceration that extends into the submucous layer (arrows) is a typical effect of Crohn's disease.

DIVERTICULAR DISEASE

Diverticular disease most often affects the lower colon in elderly people. The disease includes diverticulosis (the appearance of pouches, or diverticula, in the intestinal wall) and diverticulitis (inflammation of these pouches). Many affected people have no symptoms, but some have abdominal pain and swelling, diarrhoea, constipation, gas, and rectal bleeding. Low-fibre diets and constipation are contributing factors.

Hard, dry faeces

Wall of colon

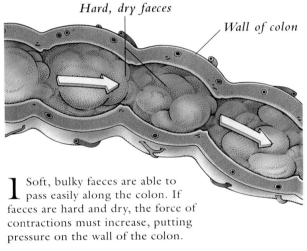

1 Soft, bulky faeces are able to pass easily along the colon. If faeces are hard and dry, the force of contractions must increase, putting pressure on the wall of the colon.

Hard, dry faeces

Diverticula push through weak parts of muscle walls

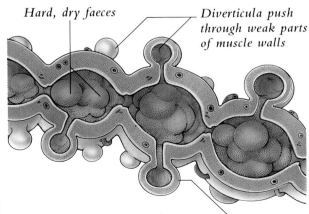

Pouches can become inflamed

2 Eventually, the increased pressure pushes intestinal lining through points of weakness in the muscle of the intestinal wall. The pouches that form easily trap bacteria and may become inflamed, causing pain and swelling.

IRRITABLE BOWEL SYNDROME

Irritable bowel syndrome may affect as much as 40 per cent of the population, but relatively few seek medical help. The chronic condition results from a disturbance of muscular movement within the large intestine. Symptoms can be aggravated by anxiety and include diarrhoea, constipation, abdominal pain, bloating, and intestinal gas. Treatment may include a change of diet, relaxation, and antispasmodic drugs.

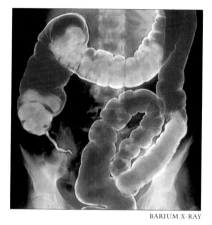

BARIUM X-RAY

Making a diagnosis
Before the diagnosis of irritable bowel syndrome can be made, a doctor needs to rule out other conditions. A barium X-ray helps to distinguish the disorder from diverticular disease, inflammatory bowel disease, and cancer of the large intestine. The colon shown at left appears normal.

CANCER OF THE COLON

Cancer of the colon is one of the commonest cancers in industrialized countries. Risk factors include family history of the condition, inflammatory bowel disease, intestinal polyps, and ageing. Symptoms are blood in the faeces, a change in bowel habits, and pain in the abdomen. People over the age of 50 should be tested for faecal blood; if positive, colonoscopy follows.

Colonoscopy
A colonoscope (flexible viewing tube) is passed through the anus into the colon to help establish the cause of intestinal symptoms, to locate tumours and inflamed areas, and to obtain intestinal tissue samples for examination.

Colonoscope

Colon

Rectum

Polyp in colon
Polyps are abnormal growths projecting from a mucous membrane, such as the lining of the colon shown at left. They may cause rectal bleeding or anaemia, or undergo malignant change. They can be removed during colonoscopy.

ENDOSCOPIC VIEW

OPERATION

PARTIAL COLECTOMY

Cancer of the colon can be treated by removing the growth as well as a border of normal intestine above and below it and any affected lymph nodes. The rest of the healthy colon is then rejoined. This procedure is sometimes preceded by the creation of a temporary colostomy, in which a small opening in the abdominal wall is made to permit faeces to pass out of the body.

1 Cancer of the colon often begins as a polyp in the mucous glands of the lining of the intestine. The cancer may invade the intestinal wall or may spread to nearby lymph nodes, and then to more distant organs.

Invading tumour

Midline incision

Intestinal wall

Descending colon

Ascending colon

Tumour

2 An incision is made in the abdominal wall to provide access to the abdominal cavity. The colon is inspected, and the tumour position is confirmed.

Incision   *Clamp*   *Tumour*

Transverse colon tied off

Blood vessels

Mesentery

3 The colon is then clamped both above and below the diseased area, and the section of colon with the tumour is cut out. Surrounding lymph and blood vessels and the intestinal membrane, called mesentery, are tied and cut.

Clamps   *Incision in sigmoid colon*

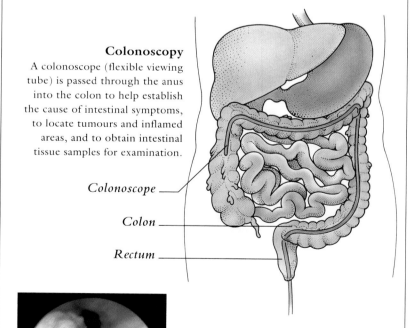

Mesentery

Ascending colon

Cut ends rejoined

4 The healthy cut ends of the colon are sutured together. In some cases, the surgeon uses a special type of surgical stapling instrument to connect the colon directly to the rectum.

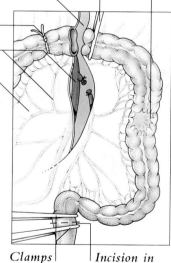

INTESTINAL INFECTIONS

The most common intestinal infection is viral gastroenteritis, but infection can also be caused by bacteria and protozoa. Most forms are transmitted via contaminated water or food. Common symptoms include vomiting, diarrhoea, and abdominal pain. Viral gastroenteritis usually clears up in a few days, and the only treatment needed is replacement of lost fluid. Other infections are treated with antimicrobial drugs.

Giardia

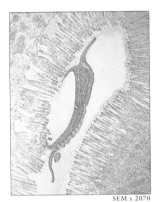

SEM x 2070

Giardia lamblia is a protozoan that is shaped like a pear. It attaches to the upper small intestine. Infection is a risk to people travelling to areas of the world where the water supplies are contaminated.

Salmonella

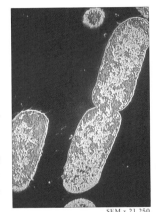

SEM x 21,250

Salmonella typhimurium (seen at right) causes outbreaks of gastroenteritis that may be triggered by infected eggs or poultry. Other species of salmonella are able to enter the bloodstream, causing chills, fever, or abscesses.

APPENDICITIS

Inflammation of the appendix is common, especially in children. It causes acute pain and tenderness in the lower right part of the abdomen. Other symptoms include mild fever, nausea, vomiting, and loss of appetite. Surgical removal of the appendix, appendicectomy, is the usual treatment. Left untreated, an inflamed appendix can rupture, causing peritonitis (inflammation of the abdominal lining) and abscesses.

Inflamed appendix

A short, closed-ended tube, the appendix projects from a cul-de-sac called the caecum. Appendicitis can be triggered by blockage of the appendix or by ulceration of its lining.

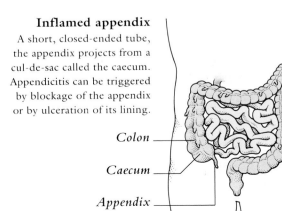

Colon

Caecum

Appendix

INTESTINAL OBSTRUCTION

An obstruction in the intestine can be a surgical emergency. It can cause abdominal pain and distension, the absence of the faecal excretion, dehydration, and sometimes vomiting. Obstruction can be confirmed by taking abdominal X-rays. Treatment usually includes administration of intravenous fluids and the suctioning of fluid from the stomach.

Volvulus

Volvulus, or intestinal twisting, can cause obstruction. It can occur intermittently, causing attacks of severe abdominal pain, distention, and vomiting. Surgery is needed to unravel and secure the twisted section. Untreated volvulus can block intestinal blood supply, causing gangrene.

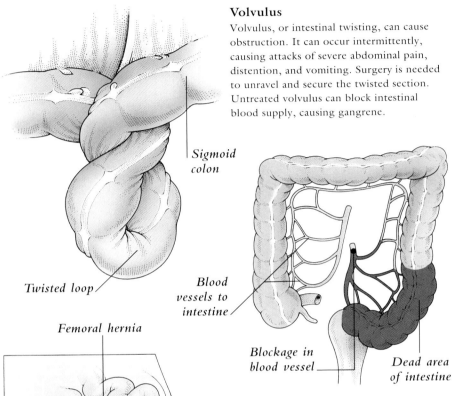

Sigmoid colon

Twisted loop

Blood vessels to intestine

Femoral hernia

Blockage in blood vessel

Dead area of intestine

Mesenteric infarction

The blockage of a blood vessel in the intestinal membrane – the mesentery – deprives a segment of intestine of its blood supply. This condition, called mesenteric infarction, is rare but serious. The affected segment becomes gangrenous and dies unless prompt treatment is received.

Hernia

A hernia is an abnormal intestinal protrusion through a weakness in the abdominal wall. In the type shown, the intestine passes through the narrow femoral canal and can become trapped, causing obstruction and severe pain.

BLOCKAGE IN CHILDREN

Intestinal obstruction in young children can be the result of intussusception, symptoms of which include severe abdominal pain and faeces that resemble redcurrant jelly. It is unblocked by a barium enema or surgery.

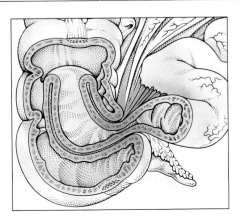

Intussusception

This condition occurs when part of the intestine telescopes in on itself, forming a tube within a tube.

RECTAL AND ANAL DISORDERS

Common symptoms of disorders affecting the rectum and anus are bleeding, pain, constipation, discharge, itching, and the presence of a lump. Rectal and anal infections, including sexually transmitted ones, occur more often among people who have anal intercourse. Anal cancer is less common than rectal cancer and can follow infection by anal wart virus.

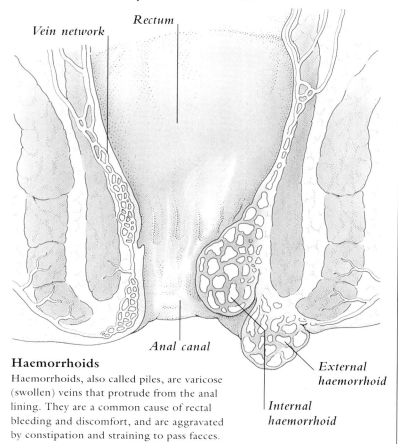

Vein network

Rectum

Anal canal

External haemorrhoid

Internal haemorrhoid

Haemorrhoids
Haemorrhoids, also called piles, are varicose (swollen) veins that protrude from the anal lining. They are a common cause of rectal bleeding and discomfort, and are aggravated by constipation and straining to pass faeces.

RECTAL CANCER
Rectal cancer accounts for one-quarter to one-third of cancers of the large intestine, and is more common in people between the ages of 50 and 70. Usually a rectal examination and tissue biopsy help to confirm the diagnosis. Treatment is surgery to remove the cancer.

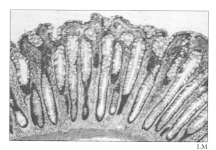

Normal rectal cells
This section of normal rectal tissue shows the organized structure of the mucous membrane lining. Parallel columns of gland cells lie perpendicular to the surface.

LM

Cancerous rectal cells
The normal arrangement of glandular tissue in the rectal lining has been completely disrupted by cancer cells so that the specimen has a disorganized appearance.

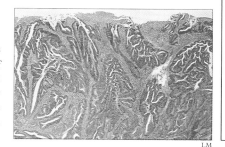

LM

OPERATION

ANTERIOR RESECTION OF RECTUM
Cancer of the upper rectum may be treated by anterior resection. This operation removes the tumour together with some normal bowel on either side. The remaining rectum is then joined to the colon. Cancer of the lower rectum requires the removal of the diseased area and the anus, and the creation of a colostomy.

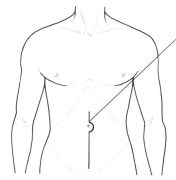

Incision

1 The patient is prepared for surgery with antibiotics, and a catheter is inserted into the bladder. After the patient has been given an anaesthetic, a vertical incision is made in the abdominal wall to gain access to the diseased rectum.

Catheter in bladder

Rectum

Tumour

2 After locating the cancer by feel, the surgeon establishes the extent of the tissue that needs to be removed. The rest of the exposed abdominal cavity is also examined to make sure the cancer has not spread.

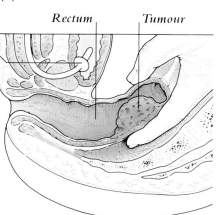

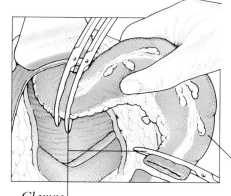

3 Clamps are placed on either side of the cancer. The isolated part of the intestine is then cut away from the surrounding structures and carefully removed.

Diseased rectum

Clamps

Staple gun

4 A staple gun is used to rejoin the cut ends of healthy intestine. The gun is inserted into the rectum through the anus and delivers a ring of tiny metal staples that hold the edges firmly together. Alternatively, the ends are sutured together.

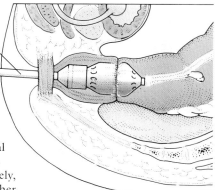

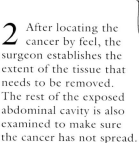

CHAPTER TEN

C H A P T E R   1 0

The URINARY SYSTEM

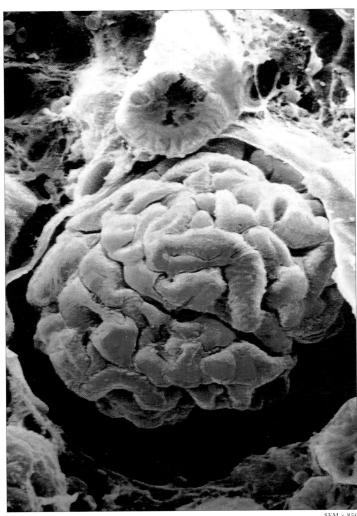

A glomerulus – one
of the tiny filtering
units in the kidney

SEM x 850

INTRODUCTION

Water is an essential constituent of all living things, and it accounts for around 60 per cent of an adult's body weight. Different tissues contain different quantities of water: fat holds little moisture, while blood, skeletal muscle, and skin have the highest concentrations. Water helps distribute heat around the body, it transports nutrients and hormones both within and between body cells, and it is also the vital medium in which chemical reactions occur. Working in conjunction with the kidneys, water helps to dilute toxic substances and absorb waste products. To stay in good health, an adult needs to drink about 2L (nearly half a gallon) of fluid a day. This replaces water lost in exhaled air and sweat, and passed in faeces. It also enables the kidneys to produce sufficient urine to keep the body's inner chemistry in balance. Under the influence of a range of hormones, the kidneys regulate the volume, acidity, and salinity of the urine. After being formed in the kidneys, urine is stored in the bladder, which is normally emptied three or four times a day. Malfunctioning of the kidneys, if left without treatment, may lead to chronic kidney failure. Symptoms such as an increase in frequency of urination, discomfort or pain felt during urination, or any odour or discoloration of the urine, suggest a urinary tract disorder, and should be investigated promptly.

A kidney

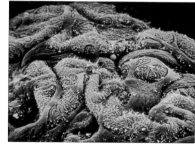

SEM x 920

Cells on the surface of a glomerulus

THE URINARY SYSTEM

ANATOMY *of the* URINARY SYSTEM

THE URINARY SYSTEM REGULATES THE VOLUME AND COMPOSITION of fluids in the body and removes waste products and excess fluid. Waste products are filtered from the blood by the kidneys for excretion in the urine, which descends through the ureters to the hollow urinary bladder. Urine is stored here until a convenient time, when the muscles at the bladder outlet relax, allowing it to be expelled from the body through the urethra.

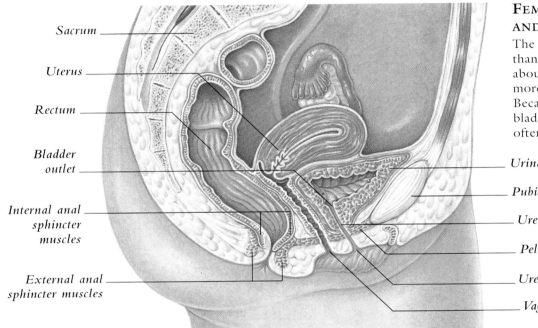

Sacrum

Uterus

Rectum

Bladder
outlet

Internal anal
sphincter
muscles

External anal
sphincter muscles

FEMALE BLADDER AND URETHRA

The bladder is lower in a woman's pelvis than it is in a man's, and the urethra is about one-fifth as long, which leads to more frequent urinary tract infections. Because the uterus rests just above the bladder, its enlargement in pregnancy often causes frequent urination.

Urinary bladder

Pubic symphysis

Urethra

Pelvic floor

Urethral outlet

Vagina

MALE BLADDER AND URETHRA

A man's urethra is about 20cm (8in) long, and is made up of three sections named for their location: the spongy urethra, the membranous urethra, and the prostatic urethra. Its role is to transport urine and semen out of the body. The prostate gland encircles the urethra at the base of the bladder; as men grow older, its enlargement may compress the urethra, causing problems with urination.

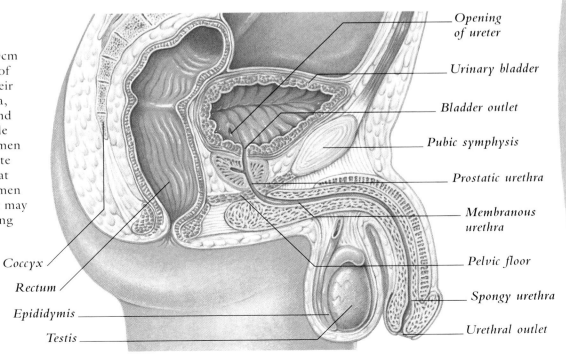

Coccyx

Rectum

Epididymis

Testis

Opening
of ureter

Urinary bladder

Bladder outlet

Pubic symphysis

Prostatic urethra

Membranous
urethra

Pelvic floor

Spongy urethra

Urethral outlet

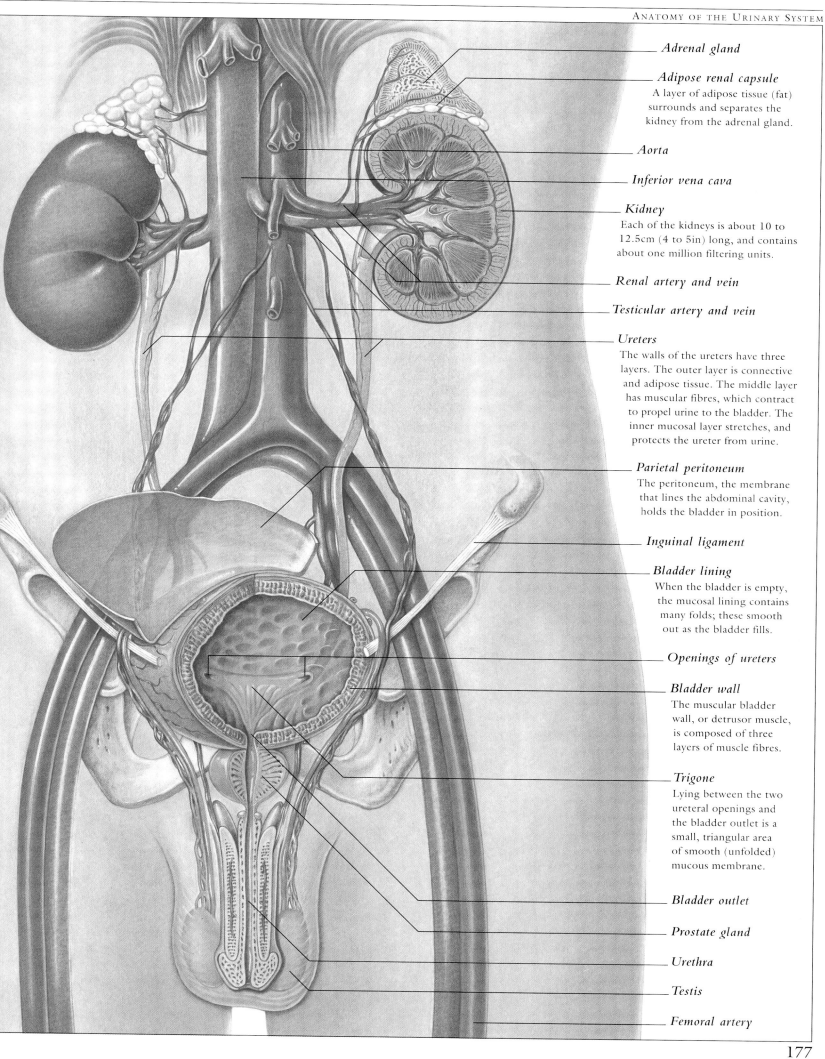

Adrenal gland

Adipose renal capsule
A layer of adipose tissue (fat)
surrounds and separates the
kidney from the adrenal gland.

Aorta

Inferior vena cava

Kidney
Each of the kidneys is about 10 to
12.5cm (4 to 5in) long, and contains
about one million filtering units.

Renal artery and vein

Testicular artery and vein

Ureters
The walls of the ureters have three
layers. The outer layer is connective
and adipose tissue. The middle layer
has muscular fibres, which contract
to propel urine to the bladder. The
inner mucosal layer stretches, and
protects the ureter from urine.

Parietal peritoneum
The peritoneum, the membrane
that lines the abdominal cavity,
holds the bladder in position.

Inguinal ligament

Bladder lining
When the bladder is empty,
the mucosal lining contains
many folds; these smooth
out as the bladder fills.

Openings of ureters

Bladder wall
The muscular bladder
wall, or detrusor muscle,
is composed of three
layers of muscle fibres.

Trigone
Lying between the two
ureteral openings and
the bladder outlet is a
small, triangular area
of smooth (unfolded)
mucous membrane.

Bladder outlet

Prostate gland

Urethra

Testis

Femoral artery

KIDNEY STRUCTURE *and* FUNCTION

THE KIDNEYS ARE PAIRED, REDDISH-BROWN ORGANS in the back of the abdominal cavity on either side of the spinal column. Their main functions are to regulate the amount of water in the body and to maintain body fluids at a constant concentration and acidity level. They achieve these life-sustaining functions by filtering blood and excreting waste products and excess water as urine.

ANATOMY OF A KIDNEY

Each kidney has an outer rim, the renal cortex; this rim surrounds an inner region, the renal medulla, which is composed of many conical segments known as renal pyramids. Kidney tissue consists of numerous urine-making units, known as nephrons, and urine-collecting tubules. Urine drains from these small tubules into wider tubes called ducts of Bellini. These open at the tips of the renal pyramids into calyces (cavities).

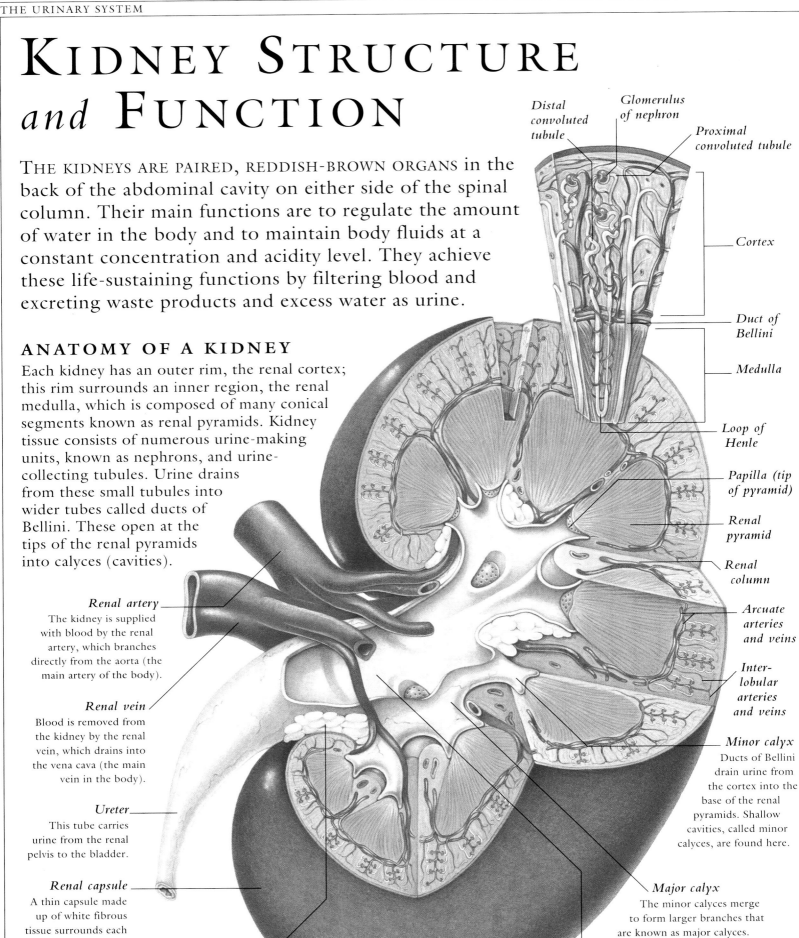

Distal convoluted tubule

Glomerulus of nephron

Proximal convoluted tubule

Cortex

Duct of Bellini

Medulla

Loop of Henle

Papilla (tip of pyramid)

Renal pyramid

Renal column

Arcuate arteries and veins

Inter-lobular arteries and veins

Renal artery
The kidney is supplied with blood by the renal artery, which branches directly from the aorta (the main artery of the body).

Renal vein
Blood is removed from the kidney by the renal vein, which drains into the vena cava (the main vein in the body).

Ureter
This tube carries urine from the renal pelvis to the bladder.

Renal capsule
A thin capsule made up of white fibrous tissue surrounds each of the kidneys.

Adipose tissue
The kidney and its blood vessels are embedded in a cushion of fatty adipose connective tissue.

Minor calyx
Ducts of Bellini drain urine from the cortex into the base of the renal pyramids. Shallow cavities, called minor calyces, are found here.

Major calyx
The minor calyces merge to form larger branches that are known as major calyces.

Renal pelvis
The renal pelvis is a funnel-shaped tube that divides into two or three branches called major calyces.

STRUCTURE OF THE NEPHRON

The kidney contains more than one million nephrons. Each nephron contains a glomerulus (a rounded tuft of tiny capillary blood vessels) and a long, thin renal tubule. One end of the renal tubule is a cup-shaped membrane, Bowman's capsule, which envelops the glomerulus. The other end joins a straight urine-collecting tubule. The glomeruli are located mainly in the renal cortex, and the tubules in the medulla.

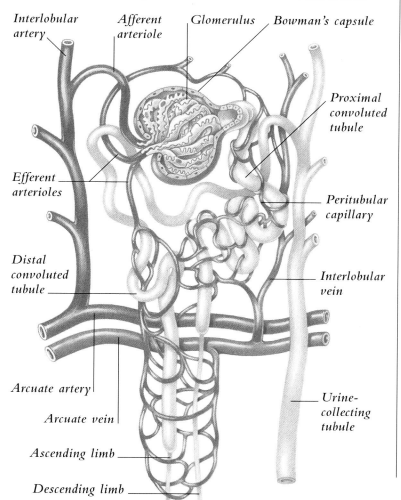

Interlobular artery

Afferent arteriole

Glomerulus

Bowman's capsule

Proximal convoluted tubule

Efferent arterioles

Peritubular capillary

Distal convoluted tubule

Interlobular vein

Arcuate artery

Arcuate vein

Ascending limb

Descending limb

Loop of Henle

Urine-collecting tubule

SEM x 270

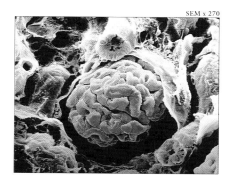

Site of blood filtration
Located beneath Bowman's capsule is the glomerulus, a mass of capillaries shown here in red. The filtrate produced by the glomerulus is collected by Bowman's capsule and distributed to a network of tubules, two of which are shown in blue.

GLOMERULAR FILTRATION

Blood passing through the glomerular capillaries is filtered under pressure into Bowman's capsule. This filtrate, or filtered fluid, contains water, potassium, bicarbonate, sodium, glucose, and amino acids, as well as the waste products urea and uric acid. Larger particles, such as blood cells, stay in the capillaries.

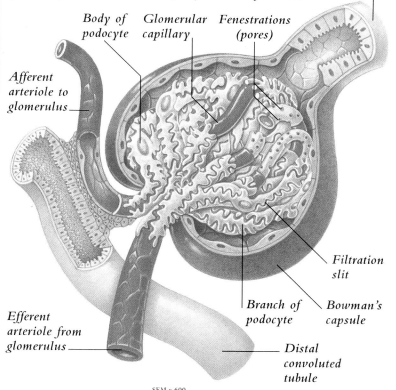

Proximal convoluted tubule

Body of podocyte

Glomerular capillary

Fenestrations (pores)

Afferent arteriole to glomerulus

Filtration slit

Branch of podocyte

Bowman's capsule

Efferent arteriole from glomerulus

Distal convoluted tubule

SEM x 600

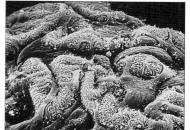

Podocytes

Podocytes are specialized branching cells that rest on the glomerular surface. These cells aid filtration by restricting the size of molecules that pass through capillary membranes. Filtration slits are located between the branches of the podocytes.

URINE FORMATION

Water and other substances are reabsorbed from the filtrate as it passes along the coiled renal tubules. Surplus acids and, in only one area, potassium, are secreted. The kidneys can vary the amount of a substance that is reabsorbed or secreted, and thus alter both the volume and composition of urine.

KEY

▢ Glucose	⇨ Water
⬭ Sodium	△ Acid
◯ Potassium	⊙ Blood cells
▯ Bicarbonate	⊛ Protein
◊ Urea	

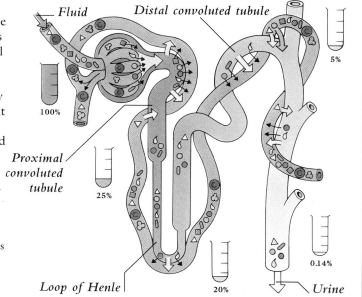

Fluid

Distal convoluted tubule

Proximal convoluted tubule

Loop of Henle

100%

25%

5%

20%

0.14%

Urine

URINARY TRACT DISORDERS

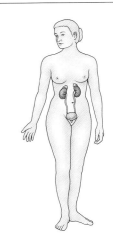

THE URINARY TRACT IS VERY SUSCEPTIBLE TO INFECTION, especially in women, and is also prone to chronic, debilitating disorders. Kidney failure, once an important cause of death in early adult life, is now remediable by dialysis and transplantation, but other common urinary symptoms such as incontinence remain troublesome despite substantial advances in their management.

SITES OF DISORDERS

Although each of the urinary organs is affected by its own characteristic diseases, a disorder of any single organ can also affect other parts of the system. For example, stones that form in the kidney may damage the ureters, and obstruction to the outflow of urine may damage the kidneys as a result of back pressure.

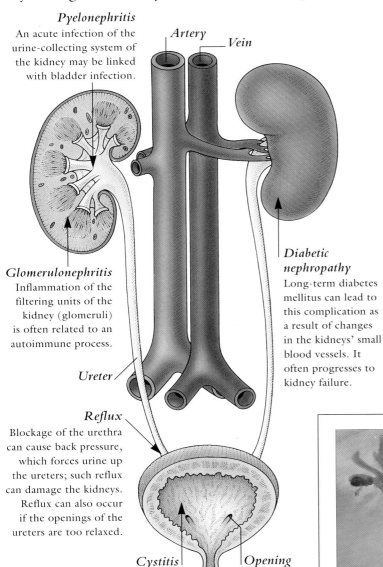

Pyelonephritis
An acute infection of the urine-collecting system of the kidney may be linked with bladder infection.

Artery

Vein

Glomerulonephritis
Inflammation of the filtering units of the kidney (glomeruli) is often related to an autoimmune process.

Diabetic nephropathy
Long-term diabetes mellitus can lead to this complication as a result of changes in the kidneys' small blood vessels. It often progresses to kidney failure.

Ureter

Reflux
Blockage of the urethra can cause back pressure, which forces urine up the ureters; such reflux can damage the kidneys. Reflux can also occur if the openings of the ureters are too relaxed.

Cystitis
An inflammation inside the bladder caused by infection, cystitis affects both sexes but is more common in women.

Opening of ureter

Urethra

INCONTINENCE

Urinary incontinence is the tendency to involuntary leakage of urine. It occurs more in women than in men, mainly because women often have a weakness in the pelvic floor muscles if they have had children. Incontinence is especially common in elderly people, often as a result of dementia. Damage to the brain or spinal cord is another possble cause of incontinence.

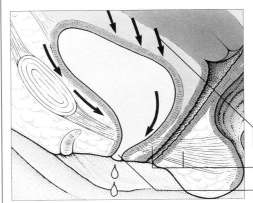

Stress incontinence
Weak pelvic floor muscles may allow small amounts of urine to escape during exertion, such as running, or less strenuous activities, such as coughing.

Pressure

Pelvic floor muscles

Urethra

Bladder contractions

Urge incontinence
An urgent desire to urinate is sometimes triggered by a sudden change of body position. Once urination starts, the bladder contracts involuntarily until empty.

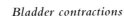

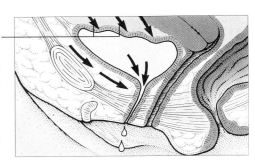

KIDNEY STONES
Concentrated substances in the urine may precipitate to form kidney stones. These may occur in the urine-collecting part of the kidneys, or in the ureters or bladder, and can be very painful.

Imaging a kidney stone
After a dye is injected, an X-ray (pyelogram) can reveal stones, such as the one shown here in orange.

X-RAY

KIDNEY FAILURE

Serious kidney disease may so severely damage the organ that it is no longer capable of carrying out its function of removing waste products from the blood. The failure of a single kidney does not endanger life, but diseases often affect both organs. If both of the kidneys fail, dialysis or transplantation of a healthy organ is often required.

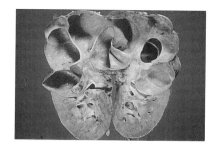

POLYCYSTIC KIDNEY

The presence of multiple cysts (left) in the kidney may occur as a genetic abnormality that may cause death in the first year of life. Adult polycystic disease can also be due to a hereditary cause. Congenital small cysts gradually enlarge, which causes high blood pressure and loss of kidney function. About half of sufferers eventually require dialysis.

DIALYSIS

Dialysis involves filtering blood by passing it through a semi-permeable membrane immersed in a special solution, known as dialysate. Smaller molecules, such as urea and other waste products, pass through the membrane into the dialysate for disposal, but larger molecules such as proteins are retained. The most common type of procedure is haemodialysis.

Haemodialysis

Blood from an artery passes through a coiled membrane tube and back into a vein. The tube is immersed in a tank filled with dialysate. Waste products filter out into the dialysate.

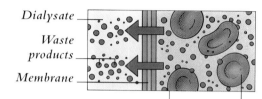

Dialysate · *Waste products* · *Membrane* · *Blood cell*

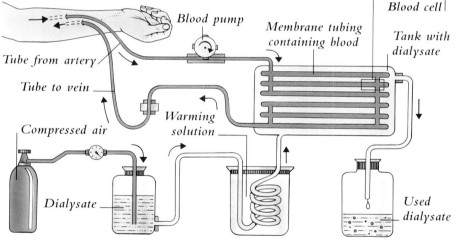

Blood pump · *Membrane tubing containing blood* · *Tank with dialysate* · *Tube from artery* · *Tube to vein* · *Compressed air* · *Warming solution* · *Dialysate* · *Used dialysate*

Peritoneal dialysis

In this procedure, 2L (3.5pt) of dialysate are run into the peritoneal cavity and changed around every 4 hours. Waste products pass from the capillaries lining the peritoneal cavity through the membrane of the peritoneum into the dialysate.

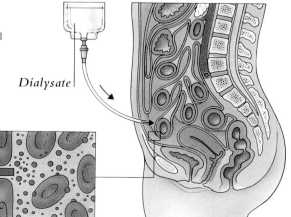

Dialysate

Dialysate · *Peritoneal membrane* · *Capillary wall*

KIDNEY TRANSPLANT

The definitive treatment for failure of both the kidneys is a kidney transplant. This most successful of all organ transplant procedures is often performed using a kidney donated by a close relative. Alternatively, a computer can arrange a tissue match, most often with someone who has suffered accidental death.

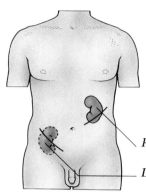

Incision sites
One or both diseased kidneys are removed via an incision made under the ribs. The donated kidney is inserted low in the pelvis through an incision in the groin.

Removed kidney · *Donated kidney*

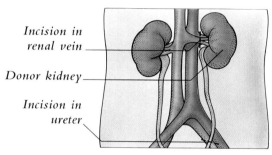

Incision in renal vein · *Donor kidney* · *Incision in ureter*

1 The donor's renal artery and vein are cut. The left kidney, located higher in the body, is usually removed because its longer ureter allows better repositioning of the kidney in the recipient.

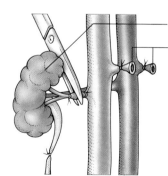

Diseased kidney · *Cut blood vessels*

2 The diseased kidney(s) may be removed since a diseased kidney can cause hypertension. The ureters and the renal blood vessels are tied and cut.

3 The donated kidney is positioned in the pelvis. The cut end of the longer ureter is pushed through a stab incision into the bladder and is stitched in position. The clamps are removed, and the incision in the lower abdomen is closed.

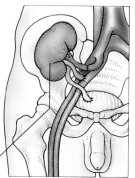

Donated kidney

CHAPTER ELEVEN

C H A P T E R   11

The REPRODUCTIVE SYSTEM

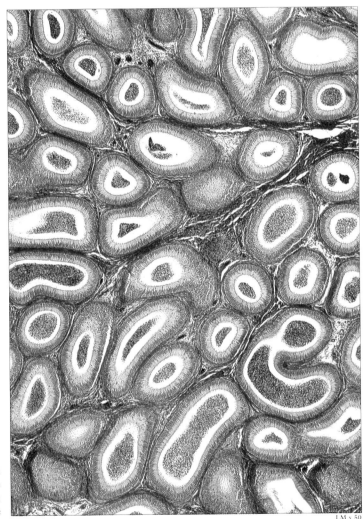

The epididymis (seen in cross-section), the convoluted duct in which sperm mature

LM x 50

INTRODUCTION

In biological terms, the primary function of the human body is to replicate itself, and the sexual and parenting instincts are among the strongest of our basic drives. During the present century, sexual behaviour in western society has been transformed by the availability of reliable contraception. This has enabled many couples to delay childbearing until relatively late in their lives, when fertility has already begun to decline, and a whole new science of assisted reproduction has evolved to help them become parents. Other research has looked at the hormones controlling the development of sperm and eggs, and the process of conception. This has led to improvements in the treatment of many disorders of the reproductive system. But cancers of the male and female reproductive systems (mostly those of the prostate, breast, ovary, and uterus) still account for a large proportion of cancer deaths. Today, researchers are seeking ways of detecting these disorders at an earlier stage, and better treatments for them. The social upheavals of the twentieth century have had a marked effect on the incidence of sexually transmitted diseases (STDs). These spread rapidly during World War II, but declined later as antibiotics were developed. Some STDs, such as herpes and acquired immune deficiency syndrome (AIDS), are incurable.

Cross-section of an ovary, showing a maturing egg

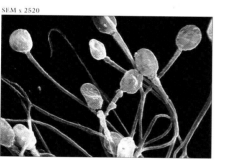

SEM x 2520

A group of sperm

THE REPRODUCTIVE SYSTEM

The MALE REPRODUCTIVE ORGANS

THE TESTES, A PAIR OF ROUNDED GLANDS that lie in a pouch called the scrotum, produce sperm and male sex hormones. From each testis, sperm pass into a long coiled tube, the epididymis, where they mature and are stored until they are ejaculated or reabsorbed by the body. During sexual arousal, spongy tissue in the penis fills with blood and the organ becomes erect. Before ejaculation, sperm are propelled along a long duct called the vas deferens. Fluid secreted by the two seminal vesicles and the prostate gland is added to the sperm to produce semen, which is ejaculated through the urethra.

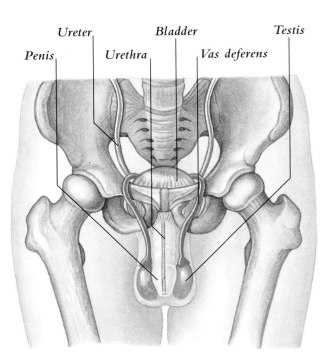

Penis　**Ureter**　**Urethra**　**Bladder**　**Vas deferens**　**Testis**

LOCATION OF THE ORGANS

Unlike the reproductive glands of the female, those of the male, the testes, do not lie within the pelvis. Instead, they are located externally in the scrotum. This arrangement maintains sperm at slightly below body temperature, which is necessary for them to survive. The male pelvis is narrower and deeper, and has thicker, stronger bones than the female pelvis, which is better adapted for pregnancy and childbirth.

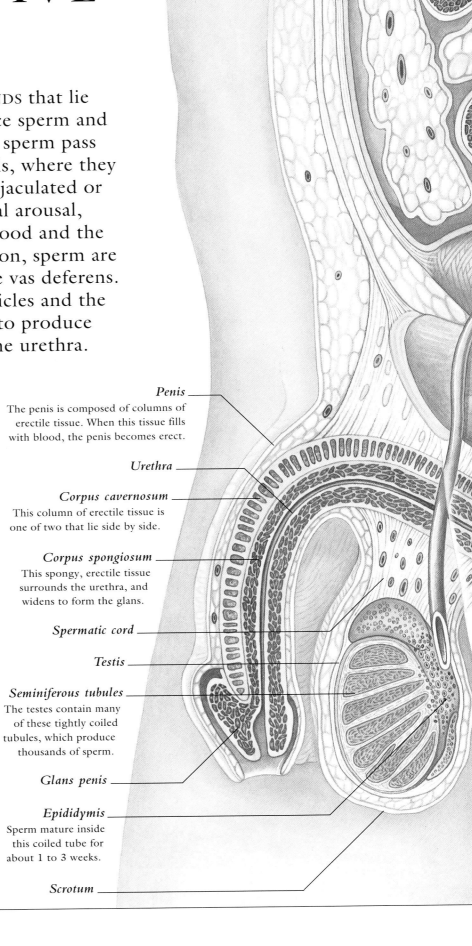

Penis
The penis is composed of columns of erectile tissue. When this tissue fills with blood, the penis becomes erect.

Urethra

Corpus cavernosum
This column of erectile tissue is one of two that lie side by side.

Corpus spongiosum
This spongy, erectile tissue surrounds the urethra, and widens to form the glans.

Spermatic cord

Testis

Seminiferous tubules
The testes contain many of these tightly coiled tubules, which produce thousands of sperm.

Glans penis

Epididymis
Sperm mature inside this coiled tube for about 1 to 3 weeks.

Scrotum

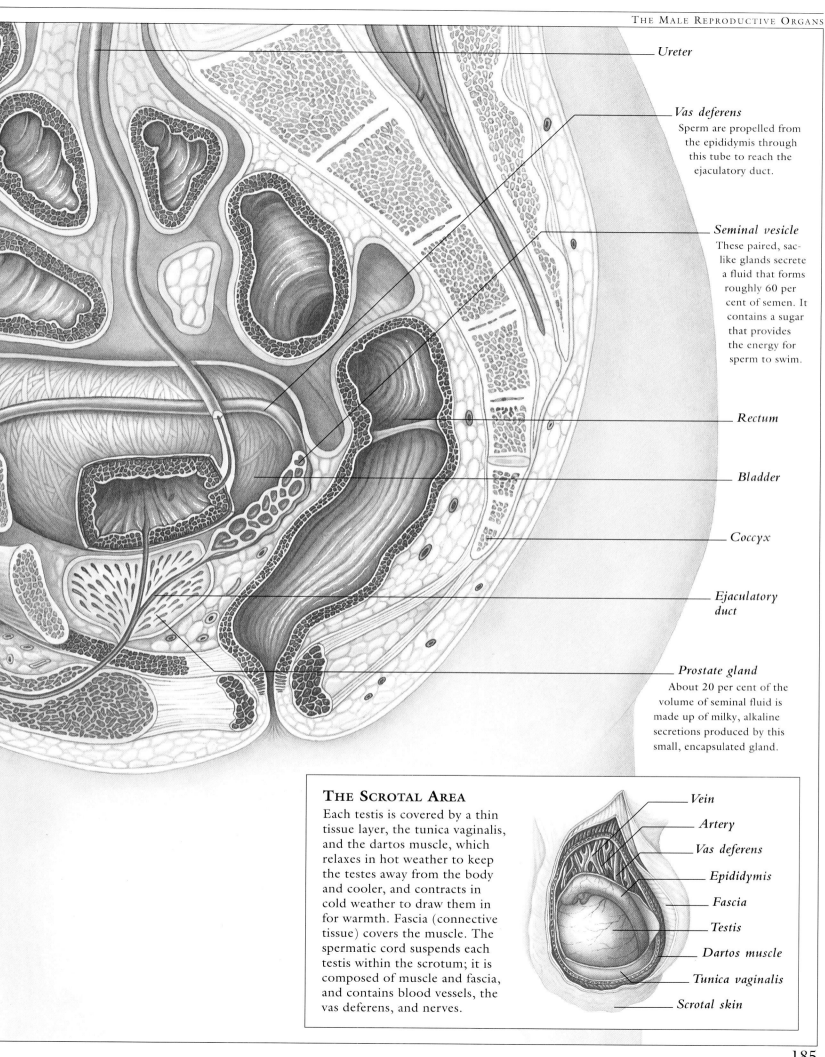

Ureter

Vas deferens
Sperm are propelled from the epididymis through this tube to reach the ejaculatory duct.

Seminal vesicle
These paired, sac-like glands secrete a fluid that forms roughly 60 per cent of semen. It contains a sugar that provides the energy for sperm to swim.

Rectum

Bladder

Coccyx

Ejaculatory duct

Prostate gland
About 20 per cent of the volume of seminal fluid is made up of milky, alkaline secretions produced by this small, encapsulated gland.

THE SCROTAL AREA

Each testis is covered by a thin tissue layer, the tunica vaginalis, and the dartos muscle, which relaxes in hot weather to keep the testes away from the body and cooler, and contracts in cold weather to draw them in for warmth. Fascia (connective tissue) covers the muscle. The spermatic cord suspends each testis within the scrotum; it is composed of muscle and fascia, and contains blood vessels, the vas deferens, and nerves.

Vein

Artery

Vas deferens

Epididymis

Fascia

Testis

Dartos muscle

Tunica vaginalis

Scrotal skin

The FEMALE REPRODUCTIVE ORGANS

THE ESSENTIAL SEX GLANDS IN WOMEN are the two ovaries. From puberty, these paired glands release the female sex cells, the ova; they also manufacture the sex hormones, notably oestrogen, that influence the development of female sexual characteristics, such as the general body shape, enlargement of the breasts, and menstrual cycles. Each month an ovum is released and travels down one of the two fallopian tubes to the uterus, a hollow structure in the centre of the pelvis; if the egg is not fertilized, menstruation occurs.

LOCATION OF ORGANS

Female reproductive organs are located within the pelvic cavity, a broad, empty space between the encircling pelvic bones. Because the uterus has to enlarge during pregnancy as the fetus grows, this space is much wider and shallower in a woman than in a man.

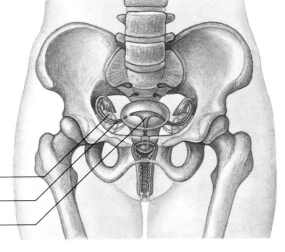

Ovary

Fallopian tube

Uterus

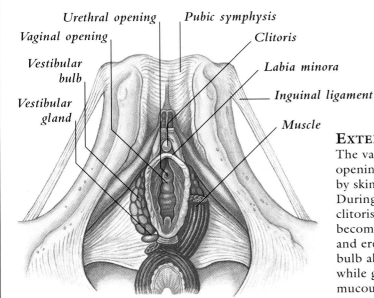

Urethral opening

Vaginal opening

Vestibular bulb

Vestibular gland

Pubic symphysis

Clitoris

Labia minora

Inguinal ligament

Muscle

Colon

Ligament

Bladder

Pubic symphysis

Clitoris
Like the penis, this organ contains spongy, erectile tissue and nerve endings.

Labia minora

Labia majora

EXTERNAL GENITALS

The vaginal and urethral openings are surrounded by skin folds called labia. During sexual arousal, the clitoris swells with blood, becoming highly sensitive and erect. The vestibular bulb also becomes erect, while glands lubricate the mucous membranes.

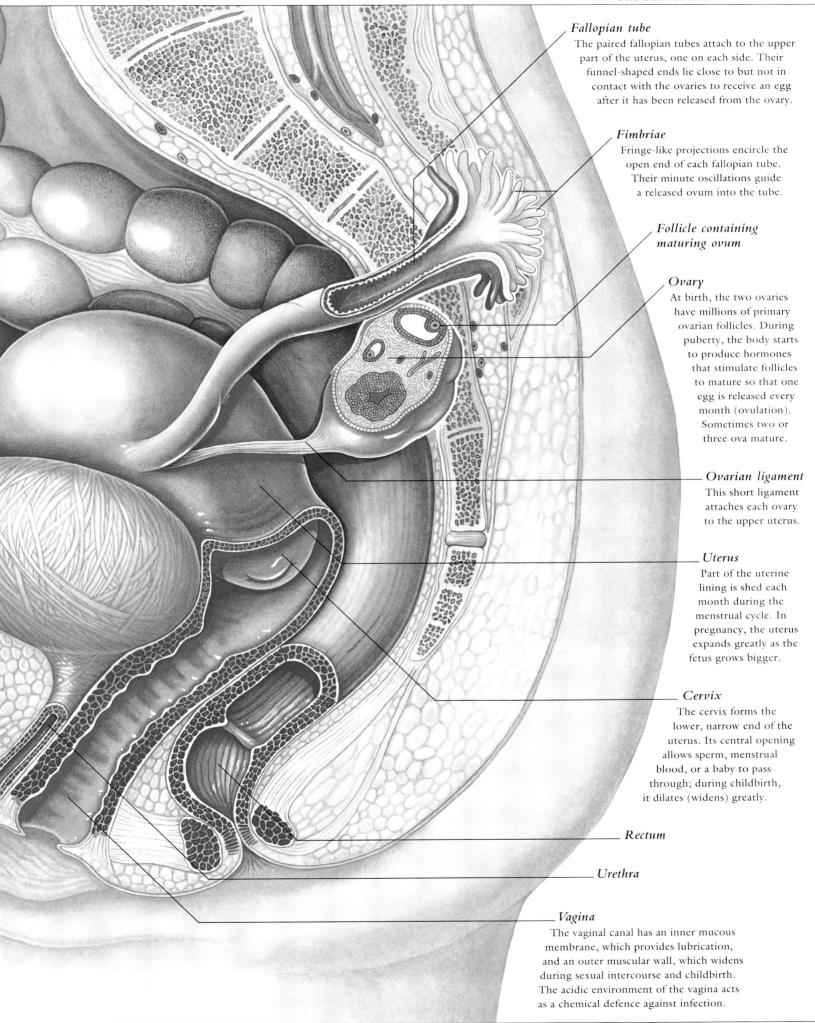

Fallopian tube
The paired fallopian tubes attach to the upper part of the uterus, one on each side. Their funnel-shaped ends lie close to but not in contact with the ovaries to receive an egg after it has been released from the ovary.

Fimbriae
Fringe-like projections encircle the open end of each fallopian tube. Their minute oscillations guide a released ovum into the tube.

Follicle containing maturing ovum

Ovary
At birth, the two ovaries have millions of primary ovarian follicles. During puberty, the body starts to produce hormones that stimulate follicles to mature so that one egg is released every month (ovulation). Sometimes two or three ova mature.

Ovarian ligament
This short ligament attaches each ovary to the upper uterus.

Uterus
Part of the uterine lining is shed each month during the menstrual cycle. In pregnancy, the uterus expands greatly as the fetus grows bigger.

Cervix
The cervix forms the lower, narrow end of the uterus. Its central opening allows sperm, menstrual blood, or a baby to pass through; during childbirth, it dilates (widens) greatly.

Rectum

Urethra

Vagina
The vaginal canal has an inner mucous membrane, which provides lubrication, and an outer muscular wall, which widens during sexual intercourse and childbirth. The acidic environment of the vagina acts as a chemical defence against infection.

BREAST DISORDERS

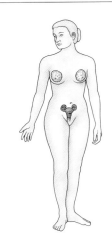

THE BREASTS ARE STRONGLY INFLUENCED by female sex hormones. Many women notice breast sensations that are related to hormonal changes of the menstrual cycle or during pregnancy. Common symptoms are pain, nipple discharge, and lumps. About 80 per cent of breast lumps are not cancerous, but tests are needed if one is found. The main tests include mammography (X-ray of the breasts), ultrasound scanning, and needle aspiration in order to remove fluid or cells from the lump for examination under a microscope.

COMMON PROBLEMS

Many women experience cyclical changes in their breasts, causing pain known as mastalgia. Symptoms commonly start about a week before menstruation and disappear within a day of the period starting, and the pain can become quite severe. Symptoms may be relieved by drug treatments; in some cases, gamolenic acid (found in evening primrose oil) or reducing the dietary intake of saturated fat has helped.

Gynaecomastia

Gynaecomastia is the abnormal development of breast tissue on one or both sides in males. It is common in puberty and may be due to hormone disorders, side-effects from either prescribed or illicit drugs, or alcohol abuse.

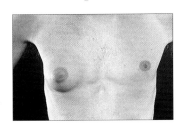

Fibroadenoma

Fibroadenomas are common non-cancerous breast lumps. Occurring most frequently in women under age 30, they are painless, fibrous growths that can be removed under local or general anaesthesia.

Cyst

Cysts are fluid-filled sacs within the breast. Usually non-cancerous, many are filled with a clear fluid, which can be drawn out through a needle and syringe during a technique called aspiration.

Fibrocystic disease

An overgrowth of fibrous tissue in the breast may cause breast pain and increased lumpiness in the last few days of each menstrual cycle.

Fatty tissue

Abscess

Breast abscess

An abscess (collected pus) may develop in the breast after bacteria enter through a crack in the nipple. This is common in women who are breastfeeding. The area of the abscess becomes red and very painful, and chills and fever may occur. Treatment includes antibiotic drugs and surgery.

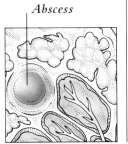

BREAST CANCER

Breast cancer is a leading cause of death in women, and about one in nine develops the disease. The risk increases with age and with the number of close female relatives affected. The outlook depends on the type of cancer and how far it has spread.

Symptoms

The main symptom of breast cancer is a lump. Other signs are a blood-stained discharge from the nipple, indrawing of the nipple, and sometimes dimpling of the skin over the breast (shown at right). In a small percentage of cases, the disease affects both breasts.

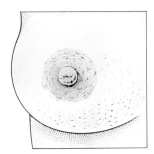

MAMMOGRAPHY

Mammography is a simple X-ray procedure used to screen women for breast cancer. Most useful for women over 50, the technique permits the detection of cancers at an early stage, sometimes even before a tumour can be felt by hand. Most breast cancers can be treated more effectively if they are detected at a very early stage.

Mammogram

On an X-ray film, a breast tumour usually appears as a dense mass with an irregular border, such as that seen at left (orange). Most tumours start in the mammary ducts. Analysis of a biopsy sample will usually confirm whether a breast lump is cancerous.

X-RAY

The procedure

The breast rests on an X-ray plate, and is compressed against the plate by a plastic cover attached to the X-ray machine. X-ray pictures are taken of each breast in turn.

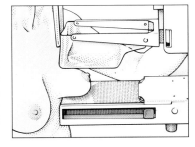

SURGICAL PROCEDURES

A range of surgical operations can be performed to remove breast lumps and to treat breast cancer. The procedure carried out depends on the size and nature of the tumour. Sometimes breast surgery known as mammoplasty is performed for cosmetic reasons to either increase or reduce the size of the breast.

LUMPECTOMY

In this procedure, the breast lump is removed with a small area of surrounding tissue. For smaller breast cancers, it offers as good a chance for survival as more extensive surgery.

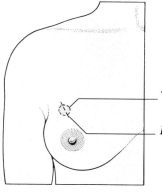
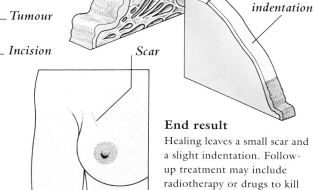

Tissue removed

Tumour

Small indentation

Tumour

Incision

Scar

The incision
A small incision is made over the lump. The tumour and some surrounding tissue is removed, along with lymph nodes on the affected side.

End result
Healing leaves a small scar and a slight indentation. Follow-up treatment may include radiotherapy or drugs to kill any remaining cancer cells.

PARTIAL MASTECTOMY

Partial mastectomy is the surgical removal of part of the breast. In some cases, the cancer and a segment of the surrounding breast tissue are removed (segmental mastectomy). In other cases, the affected quarter of the breast is removed (quadrantectomy). Sometimes the lymph nodes in the armpit are also removed.

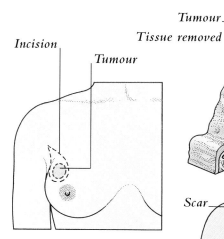

Incision

Tumour

Tumour

Tissue removed

Indentation

Scar

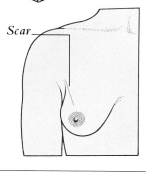

The incision
The affected section of breast tissue is removed along with the overlying skin. The lymph nodes from the armpit on the same side as the breast may be removed.

End result
Healing leaves a visible scar and a depression in the skin. The breast may be slightly smaller than before. Drugs and radiotherapy may also be part of the treatment.

SUBCUTANEOUS MASTECTOMY

In this procedure, all or most of the internal breast tissue is removed, but the nipple and overlying skin are left intact. A variable number of lymph nodes are removed from the armpit for examination under a microscope. Mastectomy operations are most often used to treat cancer, but may also be performed as a preventive measure for women at high risk.

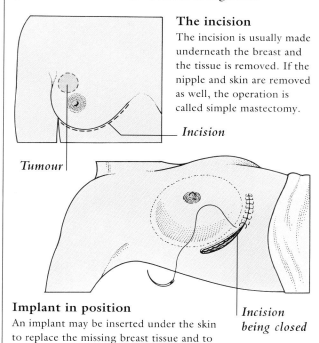

The incision
The incision is usually made underneath the breast and the tissue is removed. If the nipple and skin are removed as well, the operation is called simple mastectomy.

Incision

Tumour

Implant in position
An implant may be inserted under the skin to replace the missing breast tissue and to restore the appearance of the breast.

Incision being closed

MODIFIED RADICAL MASTECTOMY

In this procedure, the entire breast and the lymph nodes in the armpit are removed. The breast can be reconstructed at the time of mastectomy or at a later date. A radical mastectomy, in which the pectoral (chest) muscles are also removed, is now regarded as disfiguring and is rarely performed.

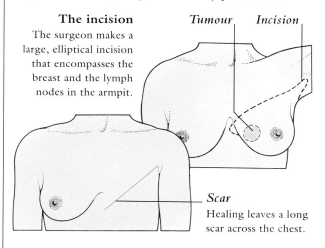

The incision
The surgeon makes a large, elliptical incision that encompasses the breast and the lymph nodes in the armpit.

Tumour

Incision

Scar
Healing leaves a long scar across the chest.

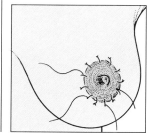

Breast reconstruction
Skin and underlying fat taken from a site near the breast or from the abdomen are used to help reconstruct the breast. An implant may be inserted and the nipple is reconstructed.

UTERUS DISORDERS

A WOMAN'S UTERUS UNDERGOES MORE CHANGES than any other organ in her body. From around age 13 up to about age 55, it sheds its lining during the monthly menstrual cycle. Normally only about the size of a woman's fist, it enlarges enormously during pregnancy. Apart from complications that follow childbirth, for example a torn cervix, disorders of the uterus include fibroids, prolapse, endometriosis, polyps, and cancer. Medications or surgery are used to alleviate most of the symptoms of these common disorders.

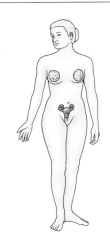

FIBROIDS

About one in five women over the age of 35 develops a fibroid, a non-cancerous uterine tumour composed of fibrous tissue and muscle. Often fibroids remain small and cause no symptoms. Larger ones, however, may cause discomfort, heavier periods, and frequent urination; these may require surgery to remove the fibroid from its covering or to remove the uterus.

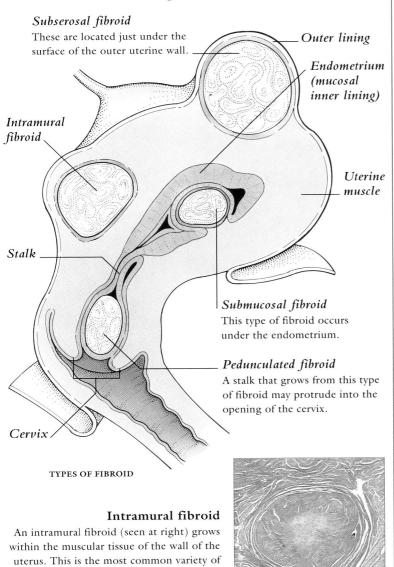

Subserosal fibroid
These are located just under the surface of the outer uterine wall.

Outer lining

Endometrium (mucosal inner lining)

Intramural fibroid

Uterine muscle

Stalk

Submucosal fibroid
This type of fibroid occurs under the endometrium.

Pedunculated fibroid
A stalk that grows from this type of fibroid may protrude into the opening of the cervix.

Cervix

TYPES OF FIBROID

Intramural fibroid

An intramural fibroid (seen at right) grows within the muscular tissue of the wall of the uterus. This is the most common variety of fibroid. As it grows, the uterus may become enlarged and deformed, causing distortion of the cavity and affecting menstruation.

LM

ENDOMETRIOSIS

In this disorder, fragments of endometrium migrate to other parts of the pelvic cavity via the fallopian tubes, and implant in other organs. The fragments can bleed during each period. Cysts may form, and pain occurs during menstruation and intercourse. Medications to suppress menstruation are prescribed, or surgery may be needed to cauterize implanted endometrium, or to remove cysts or affected tubes, ovaries, and uterus.

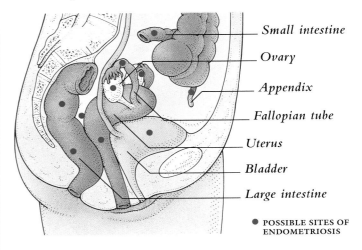

Small intestine

Ovary

Appendix

Fallopian tube

Uterus

Bladder

Large intestine

● **POSSIBLE SITES OF ENDOMETRIOSIS**

PROLAPSE OF UTERUS

Pregnancy and childbirth can stretch the ligaments that hold the uterus in place, especially in women who have had many children. Lax ligaments allow the uterus to sag; this can distort the vagina and cause problems with bowel movements and urination. An operation may be performed to tighten the lax ligaments, or a pessary, a plastic device that provides support, may be inserted.

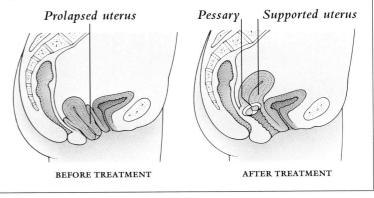

Prolapsed uterus

Pessary *Supported uterus*

BEFORE TREATMENT **AFTER TREATMENT**

CERVICAL CANCER

The neck of the uterus, called the cervix, is an important site of cancer. The cervical smear test involves scraping cells from the surface of the cervix and smearing them onto a glass slide. When examined under a microscope, this cervical smear may show abnormal changes, called dysplasia, before cancer develops or spreads. Treatment at an early stage can prevent progression.

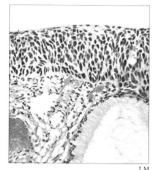

Non-invasive cancer
Severe dysplasia is indicated by the abnormally large cells confined above the basement membrane (arrow), the lowest layer of the cervical lining.

LM

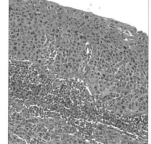

Invasive cervical cancer
Seen at right are tumour cells that have broken through the basement membrane (arrow) and spread from the cervical lining into deeper tissue.

LM

DIAGNOSIS AND TREATMENT

If a cervical smear reveals dysplasia, a colposcopy may follow. A magnifying viewing instrument with a strong light is used to examine the cervix. Small biopsy samples are taken of suspicious areas; more of the cervical tissue may be removed if necessary. Alternatively, abnormal tissue can be destroyed by either freezing (cryocautery) or laser treatment.

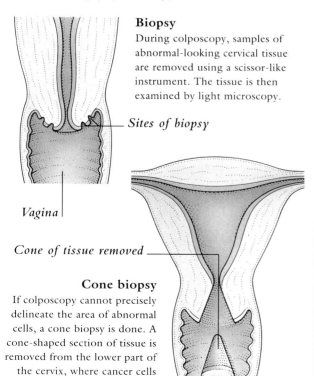

Biopsy
During colposcopy, samples of abnormal-looking cervical tissue are removed using a scissor-like instrument. The tissue is then examined by light microscopy.

Sites of biopsy

Vagina

Cone of tissue removed

Cone biopsy
If colposcopy cannot precisely delineate the area of abnormal cells, a cone biopsy is done. A cone-shaped section of tissue is removed from the lower part of the cervix, where cancer cells are most likely to develop.

HYSTERECTOMY

Hysterectomy, which means removal of the uterus, is the most common major operation performed on women in developed countries. It may be done to treat menorrhagia (heavy periods), fibroids, endometriosis, uterine prolapse, and cancer of the cervix or the body of the uterus.

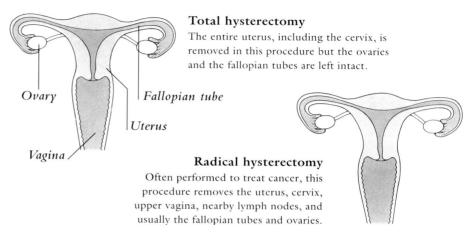

Total hysterectomy
The entire uterus, including the cervix, is removed in this procedure but the ovaries and the fallopian tubes are left intact.

Ovary

Fallopian tube

Uterus

Vagina

Radical hysterectomy
Often performed to treat cancer, this procedure removes the uterus, cervix, upper vagina, nearby lymph nodes, and usually the fallopian tubes and ovaries.

OPERATION

ABDOMINAL HYSTERECTOMY

Removal of the uterus is usually performed through an incision in the abdominal wall. A woman in good health may expect to be up and about within a week, and to have made a full recovery within 4 to 6 weeks. Vaginal incision carries more risks and is now rare.

1 An incision is made in the abdomen either horizontally parallel to the upper pubic hair line or vertically between the navel and pubic hair.

Vertical incision

Horizontal incision

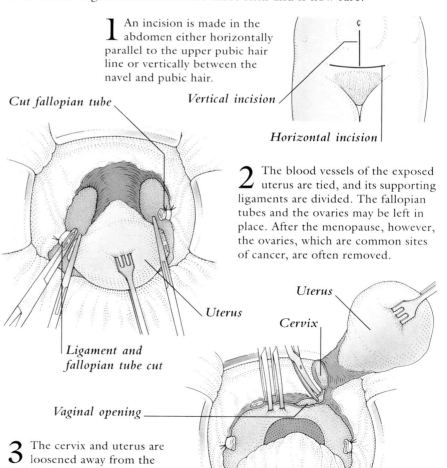

Cut fallopian tube

2 The blood vessels of the exposed uterus are tied, and its supporting ligaments are divided. The fallopian tubes and the ovaries may be left in place. After the menopause, however, the ovaries, which are common sites of cancer, are often removed.

Uterus

Uterus

Cervix

Ligament and fallopian tube cut

Vaginal opening

3 The cervix and uterus are loosened away from the bladder and are disconnected from the wall of the vagina before being removed.

OVARY, TESTIS, *and* PROSTATE DISORDERS

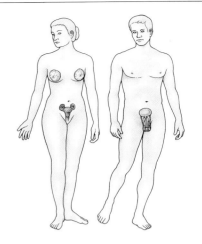

THE OVARIES, TESTES, AND PROSTATE GLAND are possible sites of cancers, non-malignant swellings, and sexually transmitted infections. Diseases of the ovaries and testes can also be responsible for disorders elsewhere in the body related to the hormones they secrete. Some of the conditions that directly affect the organs themselves are described here.

OVARIAN DISORDERS

The ovaries may rarely be affected by viral or bacterial infections. The most common disorder is the presence of one or more cysts. These fluid-filled swellings may develop at any age, and may occasionally grow to an enormous size. Most, however, cause no symptoms, and only 5 per cent are malignant.

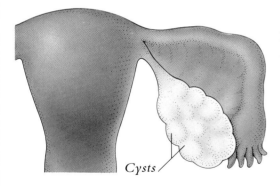

Uterus   *Cyst*   *Twisted fallopian tube and pedicle*

Twisted pedicle
The stalk, or pedicle, of a cyst may become twisted, cutting off the pedicle's blood supply and causing sudden, severe abdominal pain. Immediate surgery may be required.

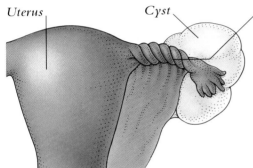

Polycystic ovaries
Many small cysts may form due to a hormone imbalance. A common cause of infertility, this syndrome is sometimes diagnosed by symptoms such as excessive body hair, irregular or absent periods, and obesity.

Cysts

LAPAROSCOPY
This technique involves the use of a flexible fibreoptic viewing tube to examine the abdominal cavity directly. It is used to determine causes of pelvic pain or infertility. Laparoscopy is also used in the diagnosis and treatment of a range of gynaecological disorders, including ovarian cysts, endometriosis, and ovarian and uterine cancer.

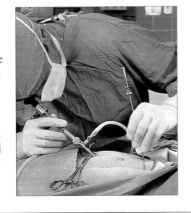

OVARIAN CANCER
Cancer of the ovary kills more women than cancers of the uterus and cervix together, essentially because it is rarely detected while still at a curable stage. It is most common in women over age 50 and those who are childless. Long-term use of the oral contraceptive pill may be protective against the disease. Anticancer drugs can prolong survival, even when a tumour is advanced.

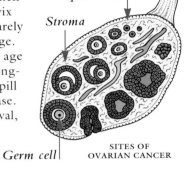

Surface epithelium
Stroma
Germ cell

SITES OF OVARIAN CANCER

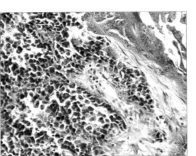

Cancerous cells
Seen in the tissue section at left are darkly stained cancerous cells invading the normal tissue of the surface epithelium. This is the most common site for ovarian cancer.

TESTICULAR DISORDERS

The most common symptom of a testicular disorder is swelling. Most swellings are painless and harmless, but should be checked. Swellings may be due to an injury or to a collection of fluid, sperm, or blood. Some are associated with a fever, possibly due to an infection of the testis. Only rarely is a swelling a sign of cancer.

Hydrocele
A straw-coloured fluid may accumulate in the space around the testis. Called a hydrocele, this type of swelling very commonly affects middle-aged men. It is usually soft and painless, and requires no treatment unless it becomes so large that it causes embarrassment or discomfort. In these cases, the fluid can be aspirated (drawn out) through a thin, hollow needle.

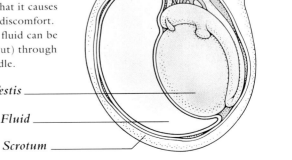

Testis

Fluid

Scrotum

TESTICULAR CANCER

Cancer of the testis is rare, but occurs most commonly in men under the age of 40, especially those who had an undescended testis in childhood. It first appears as a firm, usually painless swelling, often discovered during self-examination. In a few instances there is pain and inflammation. Ultrasound scans help to confirm the diagnosis. Surgical removal of the affected testis and anticancer drugs will cure the disease in most cases.

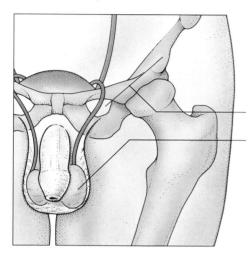

Removing the testis
A surgeon makes an incision in the groin to remove the affected testis. A synthetic implant may be inserted.

Site of incision

Testis to be removed

Testicular tumour
Seen on the right is a cross-section of an excised testis. The large white area is a tumour. Removal of one testis does not usually affect subsequent fertility.

PROSTATE DISORDERS

The prostate gland located at the base of the bladder surrounds the urethra. The gland sometimes becomes swollen and inflamed as a result of bacterial infection, possibly sexually transmitted. An enlarged prostate is common in men aged over 50, as are symptomless cancerous changes. Prostate cancer is one of the main causes of death from cancer in men.

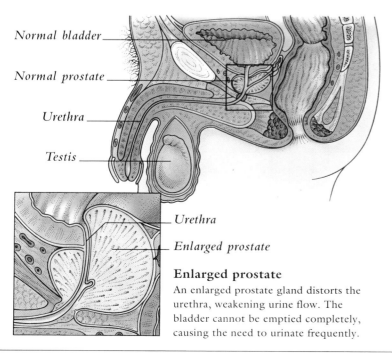

Normal bladder

Normal prostate

Urethra

Testis

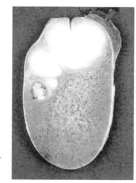

Urethra

Enlarged prostate

Enlarged prostate
An enlarged prostate gland distorts the urethra, weakening urine flow. The bladder cannot be emptied completely, causing the need to urinate frequently.

OPERATION

TRANSURETHRAL PROSTATECTOMY

Two main methods are available to treat an enlarged prostate gland. One is transurethral prostatectomy, in which only part of the gland – the part that blocks the flow of urine – is removed. The procedure requires no surgical incision and only a brief hospital stay.

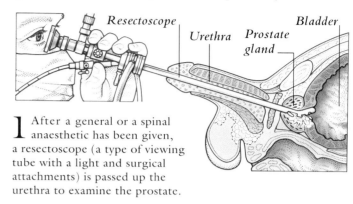

Resectoscope   *Bladder*

Urethra *Prostate gland*

1 After a general or a spinal anaesthetic has been given, a resectoscope (a type of viewing tube with a light and surgical attachments) is passed up the urethra to examine the prostate.

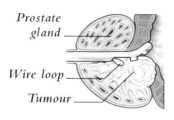 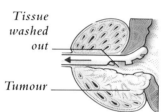

Prostate gland

Tissue washed out

Wire loop

Tumour   *Tumour*

2 A cutting instrument or a heated wire loop is used to shave away as much of the tumour as necessary to restore the normal flow of urine.

3 Fragments of prostate tissue are washed away through the resectoscope. A catheter is left in the bladder until healing is complete.

RADICAL RETROPUBIC PROSTATECTOMY

The entire prostate gland may need to be removed if it is cancerous or is greatly enlarged. There is a risk of impotence following this surgical procedure and, in some cases, infertility and incontinence occur.

1 When the patient has been fully anaesthetized, the surgeon makes a vertical incision low in the abdomen to gain access to the prostate gland.

Incision

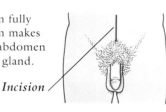

Bladder

Seminal vesicle

Prostate gland

Tumour   *Urethra*

2 The surgeon removes the diseased prostate gland and adjacent structures. A catheter is then passed up into the bladder to maintain urine flow.

3 The bladder and urethra are reconnected. The catheter creates a passage for urine flow as healing occurs, and is usually removed about one week later.

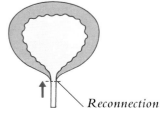

Reconnection

SEXUALLY TRANSMITTED DISEASES

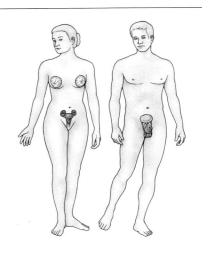

INFECTIONS SPREAD BY SEXUAL INTERCOURSE are called STDs. These are very common worldwide, especially among young adults. In developed countries, syphilis and gonorrhoea declined after World War II, increased in the 1960s and '70s, declined in the 1980s, and are rising again in some areas. Some STDs increase the risk of transmitting HIV, the AIDS virus.

PELVIC INFLAMMATORY DISEASE

Pelvic inflammatory disease, PID, means infection of the upper female reproductive tract. The disorder is usually caused by untreated gonorrhoea or chlamydial infection. The diagnosis is based on the symptoms and on tests carried out on samples of cervical or vaginal discharge taken during a physical examination. PID is usually treated with a combination of antibiotics.

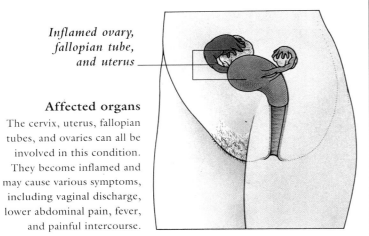

Inflamed ovary, fallopian tube, and uterus

Affected organs
The cervix, uterus, fallopian tubes, and ovaries can all be involved in this condition. They become inflamed and may cause various symptoms, including vaginal discharge, lower abdominal pain, fever, and painful intercourse.

COMPLICATIONS

Pelvic inflammatory disease is serious as it can cause severe damage and scarring in the reproductive tract. Worldwide, it is the most common cause of infertility. Other complications of PID include chronic pelvic pain and abnormal menstrual bleeding. Scarring in the fallopian tubes can block passage of a fertilized egg, increasing the risk of an ectopic pregnancy, in which the egg implants outside the uterine cavity.

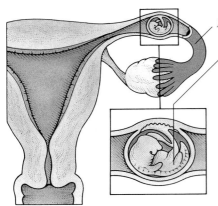

Fallopian tube

Embryo

Ectopic pregnancy
The most common site for an ectopic pregnancy is one of the fallopian tubes. The pregnancy can lead to rupture of the tube, causing vaginal blood loss and severe lower abdominal pain. Internal bleeding can be severe.

NON-GONOCOCCAL URETHRITIS

Non-gonococcal, also called non-specific, urethritis is inflammation of the urethra caused by an infection other than gonorrhoea. This infection is among the most prevalent of all STDs. The incubation period is usually 1 to 3 weeks. In women, the main symptom is vaginal discharge; effects in men are described below. Treatment consists of antibiotics such as tetracycline.

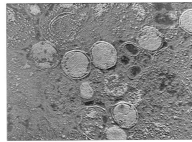

TEM x 29,100

A common cause
The most common cause of non-specific urethritis is the bacterium *Chlamydia trachomatis* (shown left). Unlike other bacteria, it lives and multiplies only inside human cells. The organism also causes various other diseases, including a tropical STD known as lymphogranuloma venereum and an eye infection.

Effects in men
As a result of inflammation of the urethra, males commonly experience discharge from the penis and pain when passing urine. Infection may spread to the epididymis, producing pain and swelling of the scrotum.

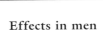

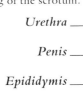

Urethra

Penis

Epididymis

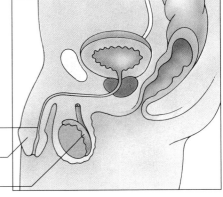

TEM x 49,850

Human papillomavirus

GENITAL WARTS
Warts that grow on the genitals are due to infection with human papillomavirus (HPV). The virus can also infect the anal region. Infection with HPV can precede the development of cancer of the anus and cervix; affected women should therefore have regular cervical smear tests. Warts can be destroyed by freezing, burning, or application of podophyllin.

GONORRHEA

Gonorrhoea, a bacterial infection, causes discharge of pus from the penis or vagina, and pain on urination. The principal sites of infection are the urethra and, in women, the cervix, from where organisms can spread to the uterus, fallopian tubes, and ovaries. The rectum can also be affected. A pregnant woman risks passing the infection to her baby at delivery. Gonorrhoea is treated by antibiotics, but in some parts of the world the organism has developed resistance to drugs.

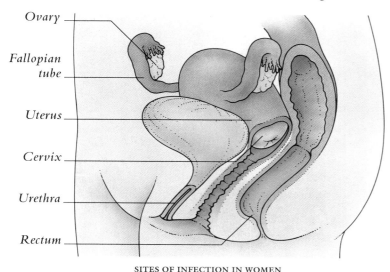

Ovary
Fallopian tube
Uterus
Cervix
Urethra
Rectum

SITES OF INFECTION IN WOMEN

SYPHILIS

Before effective treatments became available, syphilis was feared as AIDS is today. The early symptoms are ulceration of the genital region, followed by a rash, mouth ulcers, and lymph node enlargement. Later effects include brain, heart, and bone disorders. A pregnant woman can pass the infection to her baby.

Infecting organism

The organism that causes syphilis is a spiral bacterium, *Treponema pallidum*. The bacteria are seen here as wavy and extended threads inside a testicular cell. Treatment with penicillin can cure syphilis if given early, but the effects of late stages of syphilis are irreversible.

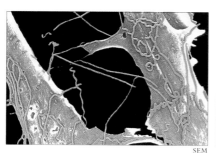

SEM

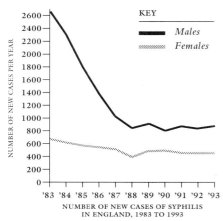

KEY
━━━ Males
░░░ Females

NUMBER OF NEW CASES PER YEAR

'83 '84 '85 '86 '87 '88 '89 '90 '91 '92 '93
NUMBER OF NEW CASES OF SYPHILIS
IN ENGLAND, 1983 TO 1993

Decrease in syphilis

The number of syphilis cases is much higher in men than in women. Numbers of new cases in men decreased significantly from 1983 to 1988; the cause is presumed to be an increase in safe sex practices in homosexual men. Female cases showed a much smaller overall decrease during the same period.

GENITAL HERPES

One of the commonest STDs is genital herpes, which is caused by an organism called herpes simplex virus. Its reported incidence has increased over recent years in some countries. Genital herpes tends to recur, with the first episode being the most severe and subsequent occurrences decreasing in severity and frequency.

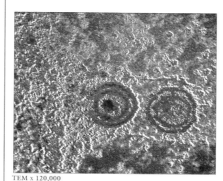

TEM x 120,000

Herpes simplex virus

Here two herpes simplex virus particles can be seen emerging from a host cell's nucleus into the surrounding cytoplasm. The herpes simplex virus also causes mouth ulcers and cold sores.

Genital ulcers

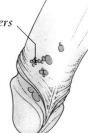

Symptoms

During an episode of genital herpes, crops of small blisters develop on the penis or around the vagina, then form shallow, painful ulcers. Genital ulcers may be accompanied by fever, headache, and sore throat in the first episode.

TREATMENT

There is no cure for genital herpes. Painkillers, such as aspirin, and warm salty baths can provide relief from symptoms. The antiviral drug acyclovir can relieve pain and speed healing in people suffering an attack, and can also reduce the frequency and severity of recurrences.

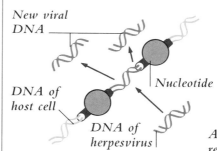

New viral DNA

DNA of host cell

Nucleotide

DNA of herpesvirus

Replication of herpesvirus

The herpesvirus can multiply only within a host cell. It makes new copies of itself by using the host's DNA (genetic material), which is composed of nucleotides.

Replication prevented

Acyclovir works by interfering with the process of viral replication. When inside herpes-infected cells, the drug is activated to resemble a nucleotide and blocks the synthesis of viral DNA.

Acyclovir blocks replication

DNA of host cell

DNA of herpesvirus

PREVENTION OF STDs

To prevent STDs, sexually active people should limit the number of their sexual partners, use a condom for penetrative sex, and avoid practices that could damage the delicate lining of the vagina or anus. People with symptoms of an STD (or those being treated) should not have sex; their partners should be checked for infection.

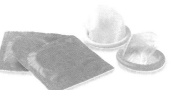

Condoms

Latex rubber condoms can provide an effective barrier against microorganisms, but they can burst and should always be used correctly.

INFERTILITY

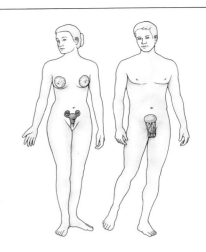

AS MANY AS ONE COUPLE IN SIX asks for medical advice about infertility. These numbers may be growing for social as well as medical reasons: many women are delaying childbearing, and after the age of 30, fertility begins to decline. However, in only about one-third of infertile couples is the cause a disorder in the woman; in one-third of cases, the cause is a disorder in the man, usually a low sperm count. Approximately half of all couples treated for infertility manage to achieve a pregnancy.

ENDOMETRIOSIS

Worldwide, one of the most common causes of infertility is blockage of the fallopian tubes, which may be the result of untreated endometriosis. Normally, fertilization takes place when a sperm and ovum meet in the fallopian tube, but a blockage prevents this. Drugs or surgery may be required.

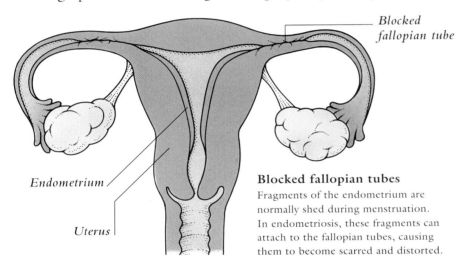

Blocked fallopian tube

Endometrium

Uterus

Blocked fallopian tubes
Fragments of the endometrium are normally shed during menstruation. In endometriosis, these fragments can attach to the fallopian tubes, causing them to become scarred and distorted.

ANTIBODIES TO SPERM

Sometimes infertility is due to the formation of antibodies to sperm by either partner. Antibodies may develop against sperm after a vasectomy, immobilizing sperm by making them stick together. Should this occur, fertility may not be restored after a technically successful reversal operation.

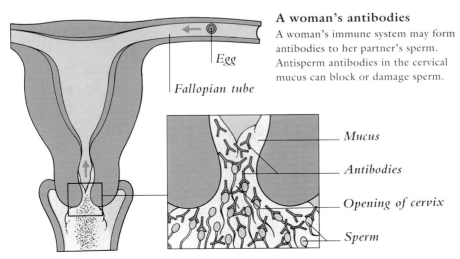

Egg

Fallopian tube

A woman's antibodies
A woman's immune system may form antibodies to her partner's sperm. Antisperm antibodies in the cervical mucus can block or damage sperm.

Mucus

Antibodies

Opening of cervix

Sperm

CAUSES OF FEMALE INFERTILITY

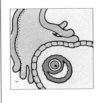

Egg release
Ovaries may fail to release mature eggs, or may release them at irregular intervals. The causes include hormone imbalance due to obesity or excessive weight loss, or to polycystic ovarian disease.

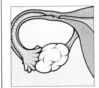

Blocked or damaged fallopian tubes
Narrowed or blocked tubes as a result of scarring from infection, endometriosis, or an ectopic pregnancy may sometimes prevent fertilization or implantation.

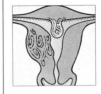

Abnormalities of the uterus
Structural abnormalities are a rare cause of infertility. The uterus may have been defective from birth, or may have been damaged by the formation of fibroids, by surgery, or by an infection.

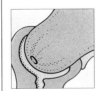

Cervical problems
A hormone imbalance may result in a thick cervical mucus, which blocks sperm as they try to travel along the woman's reproductive tract. Damage to the cervix may result in repeated miscarriages.

CAUSES OF MALE INFERTILITY

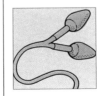

Abnormal sperm
The most common cause of male infertility is an inadequate number of sperm; sperm may also be misshapen or unable to move rapidly. These problems may be the result of hormone imbalance, drugs, or illness.

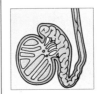

Difficult passage of sperm
Sperm must make their way through the tubal systems of the epididymis and the vas deferens before mixing with semen to be ejaculated. Blockage of these pathways may be a cause of male infertility.

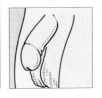

Ejaculation problems
Nerve reflexes may be damaged by spinal disorders or impaired by drugs. Following a prostate operation, ejaculate sometimes is propelled in reverse so that semen enters the bladder, resulting in infertility.

INFERTILITY TESTS

Tests are not usually considered until a couple has been trying to conceive for at least a year. Both partners are tested: the woman is examined to confirm that she is ovulating, and the man is checked to see that he is producing healthy sperm. More elaborate investigations may be needed.

SEMEN ANALYSIS

Semen is obtained after a man masturbates or it is taken from his partner's vagina after sexual intercourse. About 20 per cent of the millions of sperm produced each day are abnormal; only if a higher number are defective is infertility likely.

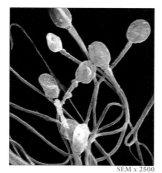

SEM x 2500

Normal sperm

The number of sperm in the semen is counted, and their appearance and mobility are assessed. Normal sperm, such as those shown at left, are of a uniform size and shape, and also swim vigorously.

Abnormal sperm

Analysis of semen may show too few sperm, or sperm that are immobile or abnormally shaped. Shown at right are sperm of varying sizes with irregularly shaped bodies.

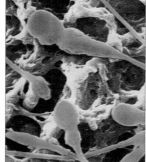

SEM x 2500

CHECKING THE FALLOPIAN TUBES

Once ovulation has been confirmed, the next step is to check whether the fallopian tubes are blocked by passing dye into the uterus. This is followed by serial X-rays or direct viewing with a laparoscope to track the dye as it flows through the tubes.

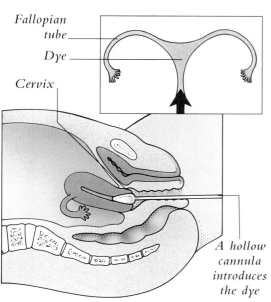

Fallopian tube

Dye

Cervix

A hollow cannula introduces the dye

INFERTILITY TREATMENT

If a woman is ovulating irregularly or not at all, her overall general health may need to be improved, especially if she is seriously underweight. She may also need treatment with fertility drugs or hormones so that her ova will mature and be released. If the man has a low sperm count or sperm of low quality, treatment of the underlying cause may help. If sperm are healthy, they can be used to fertilize the mature ova of his partner or a surrogate in an assisted conception technique. The couple may consider donor insemination.

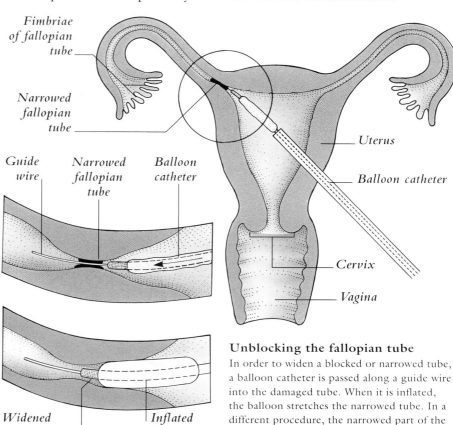

Fimbriae of fallopian tube

Narrowed fallopian tube

Guide wire

Narrowed fallopian tube

Balloon catheter

Uterus

Balloon catheter

Cervix

Vagina

Widened fallopian tube

Inflated balloon

Unblocking the fallopian tube

In order to widen a blocked or narrowed tube, a balloon catheter is passed along a guide wire into the damaged tube. When it is inflated, the balloon stretches the narrowed tube. In a different procedure, the narrowed part of the tube is removed and the wider parts rejoined.

IN VITRO FERTILIZATION (IVF)

IVF may be the best chance for a couple to conceive if the woman's fallopian tubes are blocked, or if the cause of infertility cannot be determined. Her eggs are first collected, then mixed with sperm and incubated in a hospital laboratory. After fertilization, eggs are transferred into the woman's uterus. Other assisted fertilization techniques are being developed to aid infertile couples.

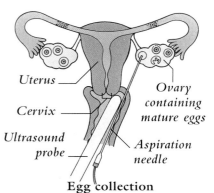

Uterus

Cervix

Ultrasound probe

Ovary containing mature eggs

Aspiration needle

Egg collection

The woman is given fertility drugs to stimulate several eggs to mature. These are collected using a laparoscope or a needle guided by an ultrasound probe.

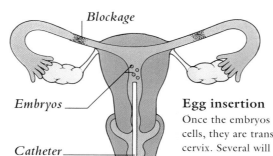

Blockage

Embryos

Catheter

Egg insertion

Once the embryos have grown to about eight cells, they are transferred into the uterus via the cervix. Several will be transferred so that the chances of a successful pregnancy are increased.

CHAPTER TWELVE

C H A P T E R   1 2

The HUMAN LIFE CYCLE

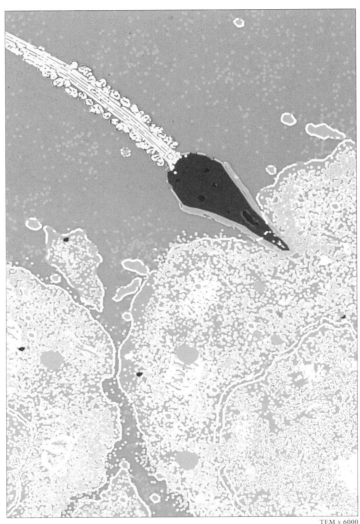

A human sperm
penetrates the outer
covering of an egg

TEM x 6000

INTRODUCTION

After an egg has been fertilized, it divides and then differentiates into three layers of cells. These embryonic layers later develop into tissues and organs. Instructions for this development are held in the nucleus of the original cell by the genes, units that together make up 23 pairs of structures called chromosomes. Deciphering the code of the genes is one of the most exciting tasks of modern biology: the human genome project has located the precise position of many thousands of genes. This has made it possible to give advice to families in which hereditary diseases are discovered. The replacement of faulty genes with healthy ones is likely to be an important issue in future decades. Alternative ways to reduce the risks of birth defects include immunizing women against rubella, and giving supplements of folic acid in the weeks before and after conception. Children born in the 1990s should live longer than those born previously. Most people who now live to age 80 or more remain in reasonably good health, though they are more susceptible to some diseases. The challenge for medicine in the coming century is to ensure that longer life is accompanied by better health for society's oldest members.

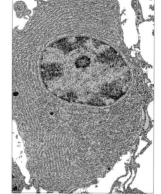

A cell nucleus – location of the chromosomes

TEM x 10,800

The ninth month of pregnancy

Chromosomes separating during sperm or egg formation

The EMBRYO

DURING ITS FIRST 8 WEEKS OF DEVELOPMENT, the unborn child is called an embryo. For the rest of the pregnancy, it is known as a fetus. The embryo develops from a cluster of cells formed by repeated division of the fertilized egg. Some of these cells form membranes to protect both the embryo and its placenta, which nourishes the embryo and removes its waste products.

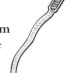

The sperm's journey
After each ejaculation, about 300 million sperm enter the cervix. Only about 300 of these will reach the fallopian tube, and only one will fertilize the female ovum.

Egg
Uterus
Sperm
Vagina
Penis

FERTILIZATION

Fertilization takes place high in the fallopian tube when the head of the sperm penetrates a mature ovum. After penetration occurs, the nuclei of the sperm and ovum, each of which contains 23 chromosomes, fuse to form the zygote. With its 46 chromosomes, the zygote starts to divide as it travels down the tube to the uterus.

Sperm fertilizing egg

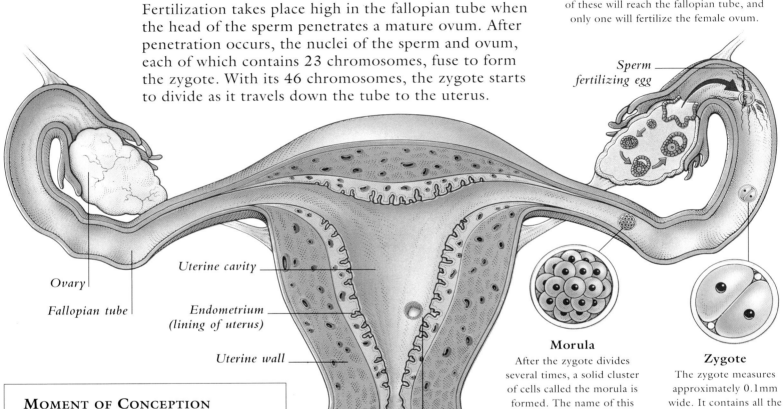

Ovary
Fallopian tube
Uterine cavity
Endometrium (lining of uterus)
Uterine wall
Cervix
Vagina

Morula
After the zygote divides several times, a solid cluster of cells called the morula is formed. The name of this stage of development is the Latin word for "mulberry".

Zygote
The zygote measures approximately 0.1mm wide. It contains all the genetic material needed for fetal development.

Blastocyst
About 6 days after fertilization, the cell mass develops a hollow cavity. Now called a blastocyst, it is ready to become embedded in the endometrial tissue.

MOMENT OF CONCEPTION
Fertilization begins when a single sperm penetrates the female ovum's outer layer, known as the corona radiata. After one sperm head penetrates the ovum, chemical changes triggered by enzymes prevent the entry of any other sperm. The sperm sheds its body and tail, while the head containing the nucleus and genetic material continues to move toward the ovum's nucleus.

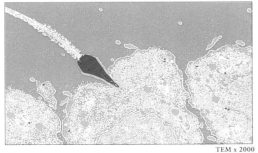

TEM x 2000

Sperm penetrating egg

Acrosome
Head
Flagellum (tail)

Structure of sperm
Each sperm is about 0.5mm long. The head contains genetic material, while the acrosome capping the head holds enzymes that stop other sperm from penetrating the ovum. The whip-like tail propels sperm.

IMPLANTATION AND EARLY DEVELOPMENT

Once the blastocyst forms, it floats freely within the uterine cavity for about 48 hours before drifting toward a site in the endometrium. Part of the uterine lining erodes and softens to facilitate the process of implantation. By about the tenth day after fertilization, the embryo is completely embedded in the uterine wall. If levels of oestrogen and progesterone are too low, the endometrium may break down, causing a miscarriage.

1 The blastocyst is covered by an outer layer called the trophoblast. After the blastocyst becomes attached, specialized trophoblast cells secrete an enzyme that softens the tissue of the endometrium; other trophoblast cells burrow more deeply, eventually forming the nourishing placenta. The inner cell cluster in the blastocyst's fluid-filled cavity develops into the embryo.

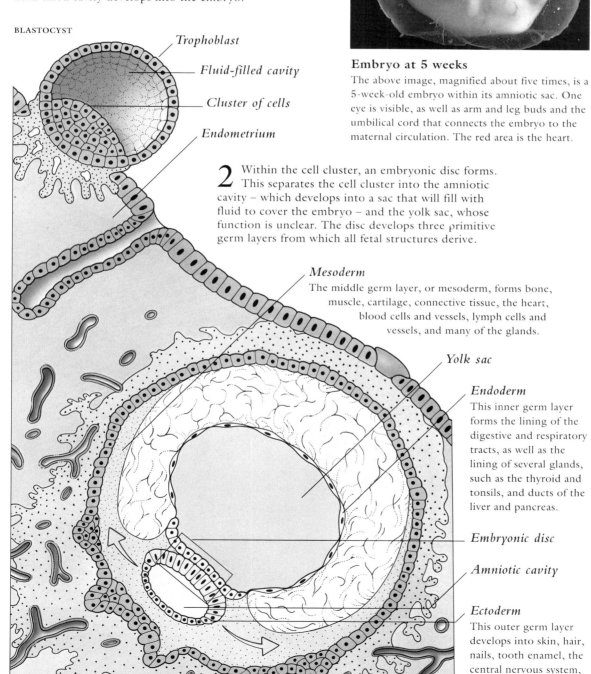

BLASTOCYST

Trophoblast

Fluid-filled cavity

Cluster of cells

Endometrium

Embryo at 5 weeks
The above image, magnified about five times, is a 5-week-old embryo within its amniotic sac. One eye is visible, as well as arm and leg buds and the umbilical cord that connects the embryo to the maternal circulation. The red area is the heart.

2 Within the cell cluster, an embryonic disc forms. This separates the cell cluster into the amniotic cavity – which develops into a sac that will fill with fluid to cover the embryo – and the yolk sac, whose function is unclear. The disc develops three primitive germ layers from which all fetal structures derive.

Mesoderm
The middle germ layer, or mesoderm, forms bone, muscle, cartilage, connective tissue, the heart, blood cells and vessels, lymph cells and vessels, and many of the glands.

Yolk sac

Endoderm
This inner germ layer forms the lining of the digestive and respiratory tracts, as well as the lining of several glands, such as the thyroid and tonsils, and ducts of the liver and pancreas.

Embryonic disc

Amniotic cavity

Ectoderm
This outer germ layer develops into skin, hair, nails, tooth enamel, the central nervous system, and parts of the eyes, ears, and nasal cavity.

THE GROWING EMBRYO

By the end of the third week, a neural tube has formed, which will become the spinal cord. Between the third and fourth week, the heart begins to beat, and the liver and lungs can be seen. By the eighth week, the embryo starts to "quicken", or move. It is now called a fetus.

WEEKS   ACTUAL SIZE

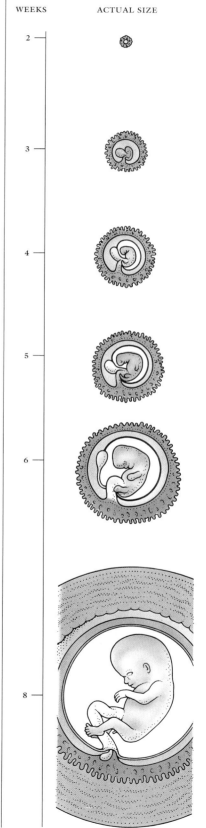

2

3

4

5

6

8

FETAL DEVELOPMENT

FROM THE EIGHTH WEEK OF PREGNANCY until childbirth, the unborn baby, now called a fetus, develops inside a sac within the uterus. The sac is filled with a clear fluid that cushions the delicate fetus against injury; called amniotic fluid, it is swallowed by the fetus, absorbed into its bloodstream, and excreted as urine. Oxygen and nutrients needed by the fetus are supplied from maternal blood through the placenta.

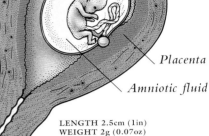

Placenta

Amniotic fluid

LENGTH 2.5cm (1in)
WEIGHT 2g (0.07oz)

THE GROWING FETUS

The major body organs of the fetus develop in the early months of pregnancy. During this phase, the fetus is most vulnerable to infectious organisms and toxic substances, such as alcohol and the virus that causes rubella (German measles). In later months, the fetus increases in size and complexity. By about week 32, the fetus turns into a head-down position and looks much as it will at birth.

8 weeks

The arms, legs, and major joints of the fetus are forming and it begins to move, although these movements will not be felt by the mother at this early stage. Toes and fingers are distinct but may still be joined by webs of skin. The fetal blood cells circulate within immature blood vessels.

12 weeks

Although its head is very large compared to the rest of its body, the fetus is recognizably a human being. Its major internal organs have developed, and tiny nails are growing on its fingers and toes. The external ears, the eyelids, and 32 permanent teeth buds have formed.

16 weeks

The fetus is growing rapidly and is able to move vigorously, although these movements are still not felt by the mother. External genital organs are visible, and a fine, downy hair, called lanugo hair, grows over its body.

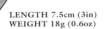

LENGTH 7.5cm (3in)
WEIGHT 18g (0.6oz)

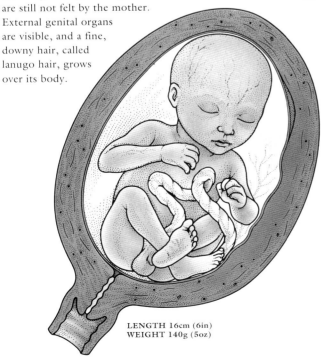

LENGTH 16cm (6in)
WEIGHT 140g (5oz)

LENGTH 51cm (20in)
WEIGHT 3.4kg (7.5lb)

40 weeks

The fetus is now mature and ready for life outside the uterus. Its skin is covered in a slightly greasy, white substance, called vernix, to ease its passage down the birth canal. A baby born before 37 weeks is termed premature, and may need to be placed in an incubator.

THE DEVELOPING PLACENTA

The placenta is a special organ that supplies the fetus with nutrients and oxygen, absorbs fetal waste products, and acts as a barrier against harmful substances. It derives from the trophoblast, the outer layer of the blastocyst (the mass of cells that implants in the uterine lining after fertilization). It begins to form as soon as implantation occurs and is well established by the tenth day. Placental hormones help maintain the endometrium so that the pregnancy continues.

1 Specialized cells of the embedded trophoblast extend into nearby uterine blood vessels. Blood from the mother flows from these blood vessels into spaces within the trophoblast.

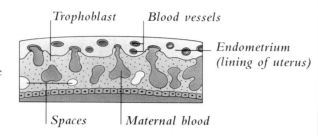

Trophoblast   *Blood vessels*

Endometrium (lining of uterus)

Spaces   *Maternal blood*

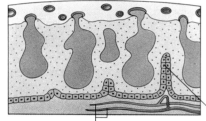

2 Other trophoblast cells extend finger-like projections, called chorionic villi, into the endometrium. These are surrounded by the spaces filled with maternal blood. Fetal blood vessels grow into the chorionic villi.

Chorionic villus

Fetal blood vessels

3 Maternal and fetal blood do not make direct contact in the placenta, but are separated by a barrier of cells. Oxygen, nutrients, and protective antibodies pass across the barrier to the fetus and waste products pass back to the placenta.

4 The placenta continues to develop as the fetus grows so that by the end of the pregnancy it is about 20cm (8in) wide and 2.5cm (1in) thick. It is attached to the centre of the baby's abdomen by the umbilical cord.

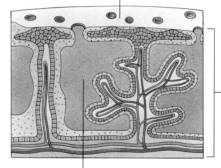

Endometrium

Maternal blood   *Placenta*

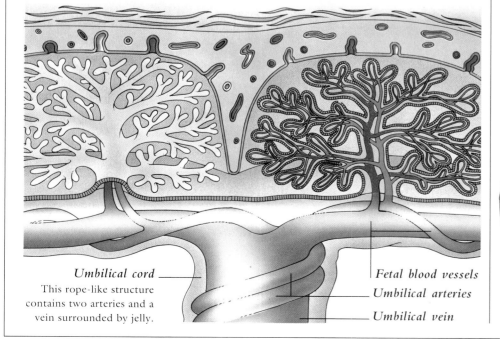

Umbilical cord
This rope-like structure contains two arteries and a vein surrounded by jelly.

Fetal blood vessels
Umbilical arteries
Umbilical vein

TRIMESTERS OF PREGNANCY

Pregnancy typically lasts 40 weeks from the first day of a woman's last menstrual period. By convention, the duration of pregnancy is divided into trimesters, each about 3 months long. During this time, a woman's body undergoes many changes to support the fetus and prepare for childbirth.

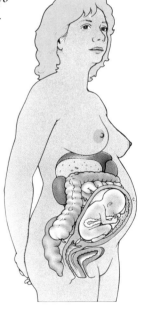

FIRST TRIMESTER

The woman's breasts become tender and begin to enlarge. Vaginal discharge sometimes increases, as does the need to urinate. Weight gain begins, and the areola surrounding the nipple darkens. Vomiting and nausea are common.

Areola
Stomach
Uterus
Embryo
Bladder

SECOND TRIMESTER

The woman begins to look noticeably pregnant as her uterus enlarges. Her heart rate increases as a result of circulatory changes. The fetus often begins to move at approximately 8 weeks, although most women feel the baby move only after 20 weeks of pregnancy.

THIRD TRIMESTER

The skin stretches over the abdomen, and very slight contractions are sometimes felt. The enlarged uterus presses on the bladder, which may cause slight incontinence. Fatigue is a common symptom, as is back pain, heartburn, or occasional breathlessness.

Compressed bladder

ANTENATAL TESTS

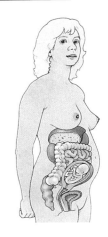

SOON AFTER A WOMAN KNOWS SHE IS PREGNANT, she should begin a series of regular visits to a doctor or midwife to check on her health and that of the growing fetus. Nowadays, this antenatal care includes not only routine tests, such as blood group analysis and blood pressure readings, but also several tests to identify any abnormality in the developing fetus. The recognition of problems at an early stage is desirable because it may allow for treatment. If an abnormality is severe, the parents may wish to consider counselling.

ULTRASOUND SCANNING

An obstetrician can obtain a clear view of the fetus by use of ultrasound scanning, which is a harmless and reliable method of creating an image. Scans are done at about 16 weeks to check on the baby's growth and position, and on the development of its main body parts and internal organs, such as the heart and lungs.

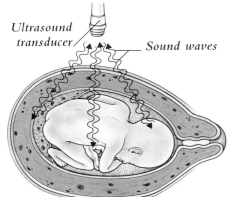

Ultrasound transducer
Sound waves

Method

High-frequency ultrasound waves penetrate body tissues but do not damage them. A transducer emits the waves as it is moved over the abdomen and detects them as they are reflected back from the fetus.

The image on the screen

Sound waves deciphered by a computer create an image of the moving fetus. The size of the fetus gives a reliable measure of its age, while the image of the internal organs allows for the early recognition of abnormalities that may need treatment or complicate delivery.

ULTRASOUND SCAN

ALPHAFETOPROTEIN TESTING

Alphafetoprotein is produced in the liver of the fetus, and then passes into the mother's bloodstream where it can be measured. Concentration above normal may suggest the possibility of twins or an abnormality such as spina bifida, in which vertebrae fail to close around the spinal cord.

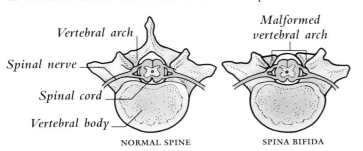

Vertebral arch
Malformed vertebral arch
Spinal nerve
Spinal cord
Vertebral body
NORMAL SPINE
SPINA BIFIDA

AMNIOCENTESIS

A membranous bag called the amniotic sac surrounds and protects the fetus. A sample of fluid taken from this sac contains fetal cells, which can be cultured to reveal fetal chromosomes, as well as substances that can be analyzed. Amniocentesis is most often carried out between 16 and 18 weeks of pregnancy.

Chromosome analysis

Fetal cells are grown in the laboratory and a chemical, colchicine, is added to stop division at a stage when they are most easily seen. The cells and the 23 pairs of chromosomes are checked. Four chromosomes are seen at right.

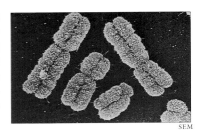

SEM

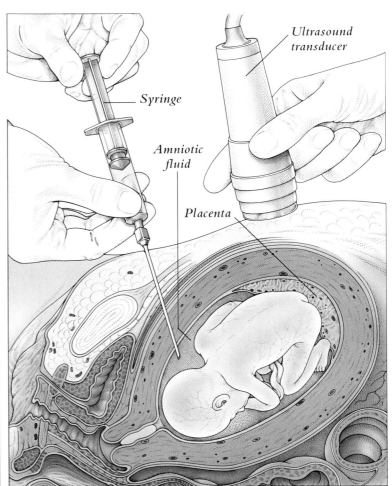

Syringe
Amniotic fluid
Ultrasound transducer
Placenta

CHORIONIC VILLUS SAMPLING

The chorion is the outermost of the two membrane layers of the amniotic sac surrounding the fetus. A tissue sample of the villi, which are tiny projections from the chorion, may be removed as early as the eighth week of pregnancy. Cells cultivated from the tissue sample may be used for chromosome analysis or gene testing. There is a slight risk of miscarriage.

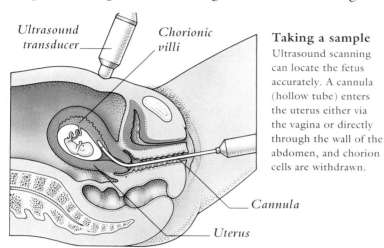

Ultrasound transducer *Chorionic villi*

Taking a sample
Ultrasound scanning can locate the fetus accurately. A cannula (hollow tube) enters the uterus either via the vagina or directly through the wall of the abdomen, and chorion cells are withdrawn.

Cannula

Uterus

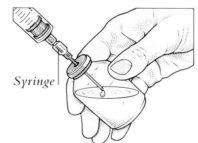

1 Chorion cells are transferred to a culture solution in order to provide them with nutrients as they multiply. For chromosome analysis, cell division is artificially halted at the optimum stage for viewing them under a microscope.

Syringe

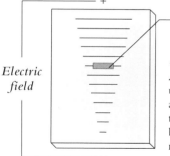

Piece of DNA for study

Electric field

2 For gene testing, DNA from the chorion cells is cut into fragments, using enzymes, and these are placed on a special gel. An electric current passed through the gel sorts the DNA strands by size. The strands are transferred to a membrane. A genetic probe is added.

3 The genetic probe consists of radioactively labelled DNA that will bind to DNA strands on the membrane if they contain a matching pattern. Binding makes dark bands appear on a film called an autoradiograph, which can be compared with reference patterns.

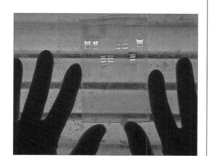

Autoradiograph analysis

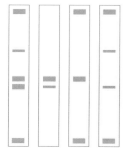

Results of a genetic analysis
Shown at left are the results of genetic probes carried out on four boys at risk of Duchenne-type muscular dystrophy. The pattern at far left is normal; the others are abnormal, with dark bands either missing or of a different size.

FETAL HEART MONITORING

During pregnancy and especially during labour, one of the most reliable indications of fetal health is the fetal heart rate. An electronic apparatus is often used to measure the heart rate (and the contractions of the uterus). Continuous heart monitoring during labour is usually reserved for babies who are thought to be at higher than average risk of developing complications.

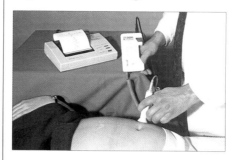

Doppler ultrasound
This technique, which may be used from about the 12th week of pregnancy, detects pulses of ultrasound that bounce off the fetus's heart; the waves are then converted into audible signals.

OTHER FETAL TESTS

If there is any indication that the fetus suffers from a blood disorder, a blood sample may be taken from the umbilical cord. If fetal problems cannot be diagnosed by other tests, fetoscopy, in which the fetus is viewed inside the uterus by means of an endoscope, may be done; the procedure carries a risk of miscarriage.

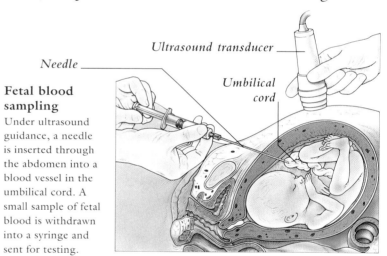

Ultrasound transducer

Needle

Umbilical cord

Fetal blood sampling
Under ultrasound guidance, a needle is inserted through the abdomen into a blood vessel in the umbilical cord. A small sample of fetal blood is withdrawn into a syringe and sent for testing.

SUMMARY OF ANTENATAL TESTS

TIMING	PROCEDURE AND REASON
BOOKING VISIT	Blood tests confirm blood group and check for anaemia; urine tests check for protein and sugar. Blood pressure, weight, and height are measured.
THROUGHOUT PREGNANCY	Blood pressure is measured and urine analyzed. The abdomen is palpated. Discomfort or warning signs, such as vaginal bleeding, are treated.
9–10 WEEKS	DNA analysis of fetal cells obtained by chorionic villus sampling assesses fetuses at risk of single-gene disorders, such as muscular dystrophy.
16–18 WEEKS	Ultrasound tests check growth and development. Amniocentesis or chorionic villus sampling may be performed in high-risk pregnancies.

ONSET *of* LABOUR

CHANGES OCCUR IN THE BODY during late pregnancy, signalling the approach of childbirth. The head of the fetus drops lower into the pelvis, and the expectant mother may experience loss of weight. As labour begins, the mucus plug sealing off the cervix is expelled as a blood-stained discharge known as "show". Uterine contractions become stronger and more regular. The membranous sac around the amniotic fluid ruptures, causing "breaking of the waters".

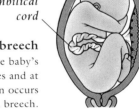

Twins
The presence of more than one fetus in the uterus is called a multiple pregnancy. Twinning is relatively common; it occurs in about one in every 80 pregnancies.

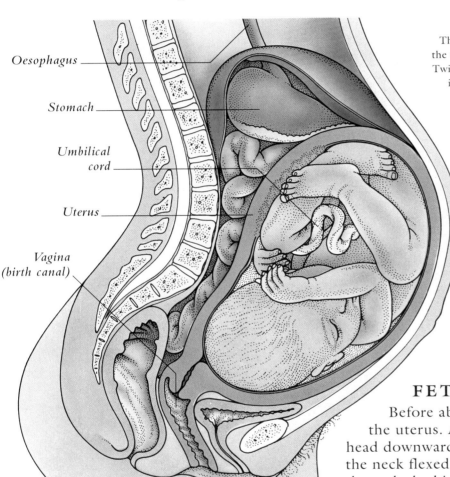

Oesophagus

Stomach

Umbilical cord

Uterus

Vagina (birth canal)

Frank breech
In this presentation, known as "frank" or "incomplete" breech, the baby's hips are flexed and the legs extend alongside the body. The feet lie beside the head.

Placenta

Umbilical cord

Complete breech
In "complete breech", the baby's legs are flexed at the knees and at the hips. This presentation occurs less commonly than frank breech.

FETAL POSITIONS
Before about 30 weeks, the fetus tends to turn in the uterus. After this time, the most usual position is head downward, facing toward the woman's back, with the neck flexed forward. Such a position makes passage through the birth canal easiest. About 3 per cent of full-term deliveries are breech, in which the baby's buttocks are delivered before the head. The incidence of breech delivery is much higher among premature babies.

CHANGES IN THE CERVIX
The cervix is a firm band of muscle and connective tissue that forms the lower end of the uterus. In late pregnancy, the cervix softens in readiness for childbirth. Braxton-Hicks uterine contractions, which are painless, gently help thin the cervix so that it merges with the uterus's lower segment.

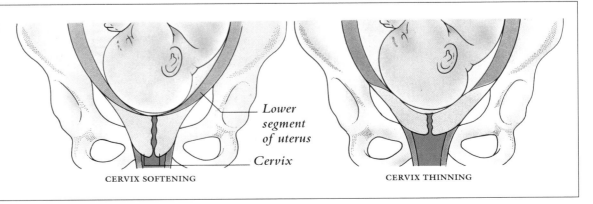

Lower segment of uterus

Cervix

CERVIX SOFTENING

CERVIX THINNING

CERVICAL DILATION

The first stage of labour begins with the onset of regular, painful contractions of the uterus that cause the cervix to dilate (widen) progressively. The cervix is fully dilated when its opening measures around 10cm (4in) in diameter, marking the onset of the second stage of labour. The amniotic membranes may rupture at any time after labour has started.

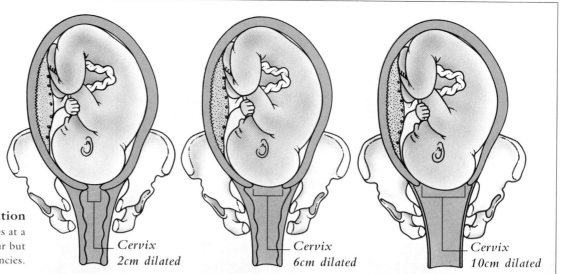

Progress of dilation

For a first baby, the cervix dilates at a rate of about 1cm (0.5in) per hour but more rapidly in subsequent pregnancies.

*Cervix
2cm dilated*

*Cervix
6cm dilated*

*Cervix
10cm dilated*

PELVIC SIZE AND SHAPE

The size and shape of the woman's pelvis are very important in determining the ease of childbirth. Any mismatch between the dimensions of the mother's pelvis and the baby's head, termed "disproportion", can obstruct the progress of labour.

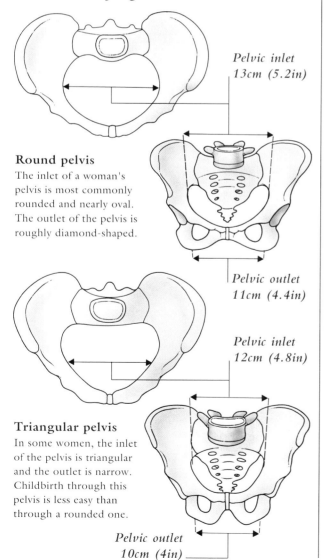

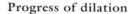

Round pelvis

The inlet of a woman's pelvis is most commonly rounded and nearly oval. The outlet of the pelvis is roughly diamond-shaped.

*Pelvic inlet
13cm (5.2in)*

*Pelvic outlet
11cm (4.4in)*

*Pelvic inlet
12cm (4.8in)*

Triangular pelvis

In some women, the inlet of the pelvis is triangular and the outlet is narrow. Childbirth through this pelvis is less easy than through a rounded one.

*Pelvic outlet
10cm (4in)*

ENGAGEMENT

During the last weeks of pregnancy, the baby's head descends into the cavity of the pelvis, a process called engagement. When this happens, many women feel the load "lightening" as descent of the baby's head takes pressure off the diaphragm, making breathing easier. Engagement usually takes place at around 36 weeks during a first pregnancy, but may not happen until the onset of labour during second and subsequent pregnancies.

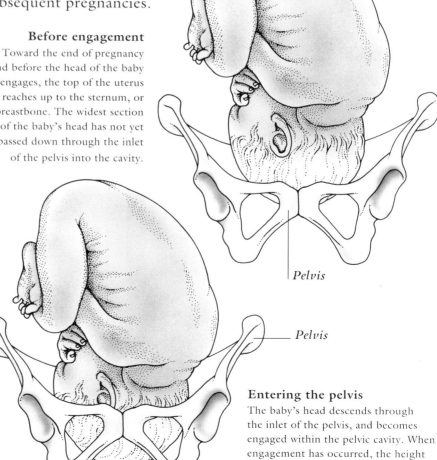

Before engagement

Toward the end of pregnancy and before the head of the baby engages, the top of the uterus reaches up to the sternum, or breastbone. The widest section of the baby's head has not yet passed down through the inlet of the pelvis into the cavity.

Pelvis

Pelvis

Entering the pelvis

The baby's head descends through the inlet of the pelvis, and becomes engaged within the pelvic cavity. When engagement has occurred, the height of the uterus drops and the baby's head rests against the uterine cervix.

DELIVERY *of the* BABY

DURING THE FIRST STAGE OF LABOUR, the opening of the cervix gradually widens. In the second stage, the woman feels a strong urge to push with each contraction until the baby is born. The third stage follows, lasting from delivery of the baby until the placenta is delivered. Some women experience relatively little pain during childbirth, others a great deal.

PROGRESS OF LABOUR

Labour progression is usually monitored by a midwife. The second stage lasts about 50 minutes for first babies and about 20 minutes for subsequent babies. The third stage usually lasts about 5 minutes. Drugs are given to the mother to reduce the risk of bleeding after delivery.

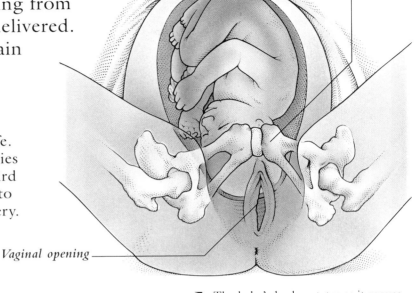

Pelvis

Vaginal opening

1 The baby's body rotates as it moves through the birth canal, while the muscles of the pelvic floor are pushed down. The perineum, which is the area around the vagina and the anus, bulges down, and the vaginal opening widens.

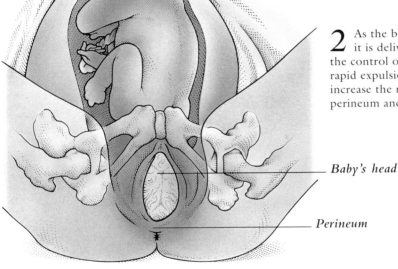

2 As the baby's head emerges, it is delivered slowly under the control of the midwife. Any rapid expulsion of the head could increase the risk of damage to the perineum and the baby's head.

Baby's head

Perineum

Umbilical cord

Baby's head

3 The baby's head usually emerges with the face toward the mother's anus. As the shoulders move down into the pelvis, the head then turns sideways so that the alignment of the baby's body is restored.

FETAL MONITORING

During labour, the condition of the fetus is monitored by measuring fetal heart rate (normally between 120 and 160 beats per minute, or BPM). Heart rate normally decreases when each contraction begins and should return to normal quickly. Prolonged deceleration may indicate a problem.

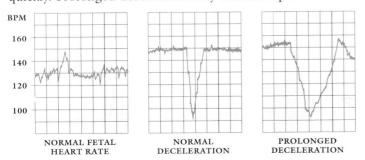

BPM

160

140

120

100

| NORMAL FETAL HEART RATE | NORMAL DECELERATION | PROLONGED DECELERATION |

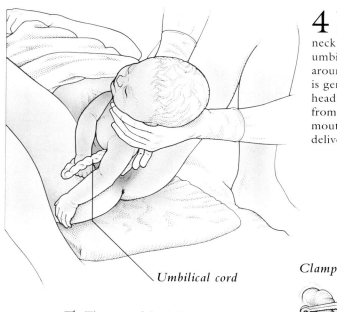

Umbilical cord

4 The midwife runs her finger along the baby's neck to check whether the umbilical cord is wrapped around it. If so, the cord is gently slipped over the head. After clearing fluid from the baby's nose and mouth, the midwife then delivers the shoulders.

PAIN RELIEF

Natural techniques, like relaxation and breathing, may help to relieve the pain of childbirth. Another safe method is a 50/50 mixture of nitrous oxide and air given via a hand-held mask at the start of each contraction. Pethidine injections are effective but should not be given near the time of delivery.

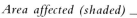

Clamp

Umbilical cord

5 The rest of the baby's body slides out easily with the next contraction. After the baby has been delivered, the midwife clamps the umbilical cord in two places and then cuts it in between the clamps. Cutting the cord does not hurt the baby.

Epidural anaesthesia
A hollow needle is inserted into the epidural space of the spinal canal, as shown left. A soft tube is fed through the needle and the needle is removed. Doses of local anaesthetic can be injected into the tube as necessary.

Area affected (shaded)

Area of numbness
An epidural effectively relieves pain by numbing the nerves that supply the pelvis as well as the lower abdomen. The injections reduce the mother's awareness of contractions.

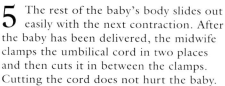

Clamp

Stump of umbilical cord

6 Using the Apgar score (see page 212), the baby's condition is evaluated. If all is well, he or she is usually given to the mother to hold. Meanwhile, contractions continue, causing the placenta to separate from the uterine wall.

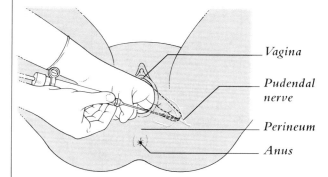

Vagina

Pudendal nerve

Perineum

Anus

Pudendal block
Injection of local anaesthetic via the vagina into the pudendal nerve can abolish stretching pain during the second stage of labour. However, it does not relieve the pain of contractions.

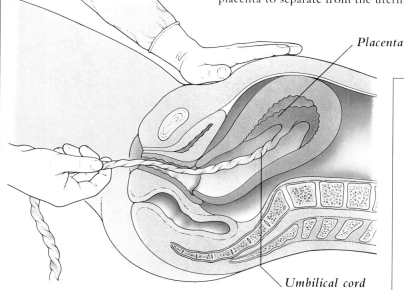

Placenta

Umbilical cord

7 When the placenta has separated from the wall of the uterus, the midwife gently starts to pull on the umbilical cord with one hand while pressing on the lower abdomen with the other. The placenta is eased out of the vagina.

MANAGING TWINS

Twins must be monitored closely during labour. After the first baby is delivered, the position of the second must be noted. If the second baby is lying in a head-down or breech position and is in good condition, it can be delivered normally. If lying transversely, an obstetrician may be able to turn the baby longitudinally.

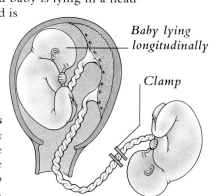

Baby lying longitudinally

Clamp

Delivery of twins
After delivery of the first twin, the cord must be clamped to prevent the second twin bleeding into the circulation of the first.

COMPLICATIONS *of* PREGNANCY *and* LABOUR

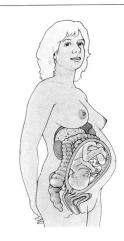

MOST WOMEN HAVE NORMAL PREGNANCIES and after 9 months have a healthy baby with relative ease. The minor discomforts that are often experienced are not a threat to the well-being of either the mother or child. However, not all pregnancies are straightforward and problems may occur; these may pose a serious threat to the health of the mother or her baby, and sometimes both.

EARLY PROBLEMS

If the fertilized egg implants outside the main cavity of the uterus, the pregnancy is known as ectopic. The cause is not always known, although it occurs most often in women who have used an intrauterine device or who have had pelvic infections or a previous ectopic pregnancy. Symptoms are pain, nausea, and vomiting.

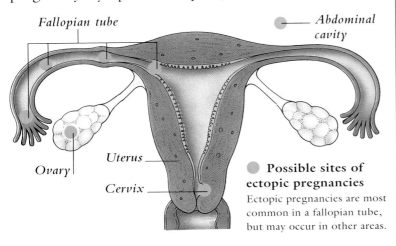

Fallopian tube

Abdominal cavity

Ovary

Uterus

Cervix

Possible sites of ectopic pregnancies
Ectopic pregnancies are most common in a fallopian tube, but may occur in other areas.

MISCARRIAGE

A miscarriage is the loss of a fetus before week 20 of a pregnancy. About 20 per cent of all pregnant women miscarry, and for many women this happens so early that they do not even know they are pregnant. The reason may be unknown, but common causes are fetal chromosomal abnormalities or developmental defects.

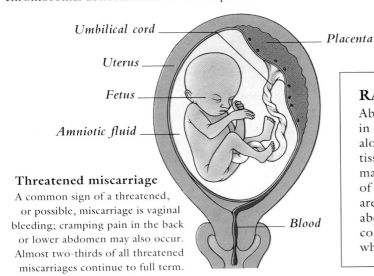

Umbilical cord

Placenta

Uterus

Fetus

Amniotic fluid

Threatened miscarriage
A common sign of a threatened, or possible, miscarriage is vaginal bleeding; cramping pain in the back or lower abdomen may also occur. Almost two-thirds of all threatened miscarriages continue to full term.

Blood

PLACENTAL PROBLEMS

A healthy placenta to nourish the fetus is essential for a normal pregnancy and a thriving baby. Very early in pregnancy, the placenta should develop in the upper wall of the uterus. Problems may occur if the placenta detaches or if it is abnormally low, which may lead to cervical obstruction, bleeding, or premature labour.

Placental abruption
In abruption, part of a normally positioned placenta detaches from the uterine wall. This often causes sudden abdominal pain. Bleeding at the site, which is not always apparent, may sometimes occur.

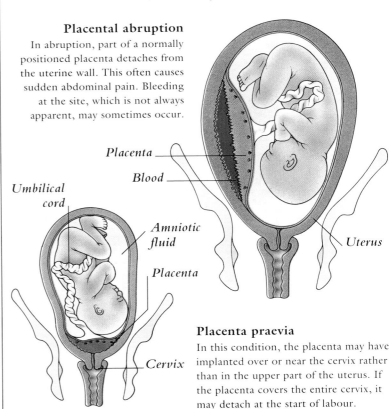

Placenta

Blood

Umbilical cord

Amniotic fluid

Placenta

Uterus

Cervix

Placenta praevia
In this condition, the placenta may have implanted over or near the cervix rather than in the upper part of the uterus. If the placenta covers the entire cervix, it may detach at the start of labour.

RAISED BLOOD PRESSURE

Abnormally raised blood pressure in the second half of pregnancy, along with oedema (fluid in the tissues) and protein in the urine, may indicate the serious condition of pre-eclampsia. Other symptoms are headaches, blurred vision, and abdominal pain. If untreated, this condition may cause eclampsia, in which dangerous seizures occur.

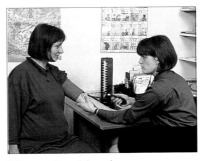

Measuring blood pressure

ASSISTED DELIVERY

An assisted delivery may be necessary if labour is not progressing satisfactorily. Forceps are not as common today as in the past, but they are useful for delivering a baby quickly – especially if the baby is in distress or the mother is exhausted or has bled excessively. An alternative procedure to forceps is vacuum extraction.

Forceps delivery

Obstetrical forceps consist of two curved metal blades designed to fit around the baby's head. The doctor pulls gently to guide the baby's head down into the vagina. Once the head has emerged, the forceps are removed, and delivery can then continue normally.

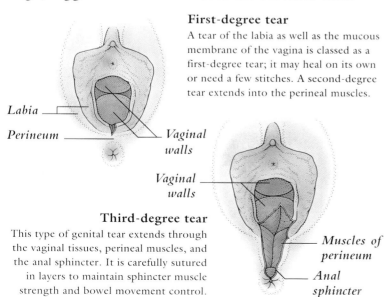

Forceps

Plastic cup

Vacuum extraction

A vacuum pump machine attaches to a suction cup made of metal, rubber, or plastic. The cup is placed on the baby's head. The pump is turned on, and, with each contraction, the doctor gently pulls the baby down the birth canal.

GENITAL TISSUE INJURIES

Injury to tissues of the genital tract is most common in women having their first child. The perineum, the area of tissue between the vagina and the anus, is most frequently torn. Tears vary in size from tiny splits to large, ragged tears. In rare cases the cervix is torn.

First-degree tear

A tear of the labia as well as the mucous membrane of the vagina is classed as a first-degree tear; it may heal on its own or need a few stitches. A second-degree tear extends into the perineal muscles.

Labia

Perineum

Vaginal walls

Vaginal walls

Third-degree tear

This type of genital tear extends through the vaginal tissues, perineal muscles, and the anal sphincter. It is carefully sutured in layers to maintain sphincter muscle strength and bowel movement control.

Muscles of perineum

Anal sphincter

OPERATION

CAESAREAN SECTION

In a caesarean, the baby is delivered through an incision in the abdomen. The operation may be pre-planned for multiple births or an abnormal fetal position, or if the mother has a vaginal infection or a scarred uterus as a result of previous caesareans. It is also performed as an emergency procedure during labour if the fetus becomes distressed. The operation takes about 40 to 60 minutes.

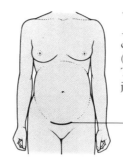

1 A general anaesthetic or an epidural is used. The woman's abdomen is cleaned with antiseptic, and a catheter (thin tube) is inserted into her bladder. The surgeon makes a horizontal incision just below the pubic hairline.

Incision

Skin and fatty tissue

2 The doctor carefully cuts through the fatty tissues and muscles of the abdominal wall. A retractor holds back the tissues, and an incision is made in the peritoneum, the thin membrane lining the abdominal cavity.

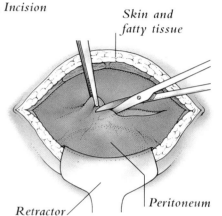

Retractor

Peritoneum

3 The doctor uses a retractor to hold back the bladder so that an incision can be made in the lower uterus down to the membranous amniotic sac. This protective sac encloses the baby.

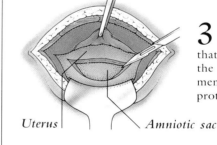

Uterus

Amniotic sac

4 The doctor ruptures the amniotic sac and inserts a hand below the baby's head or buttocks. The baby is gently removed from the uterus, and the cord is clamped and cut.

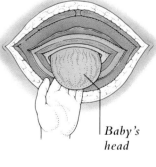

Baby's head

Stitches in uterus

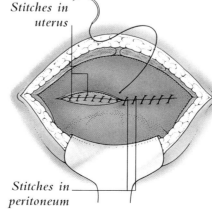

5 The uterus and abdominal layers are then closed with stitches. The incision in the skin is closed by metal clips (staples) or a long stitch. Stitches or staples are removed after 5 days, and the woman can go home.

Stitches in peritoneum

AFTER CHILDBIRTH

THE TIME FROM DELIVERY until most pregnancy changes have reverted to normal is called the postnatal period or puerperium. This lasts about 6 weeks, during which time minor discomforts such as vaginal soreness and constipation are common, but are usually overshadowed by the experience of having a new baby. Meanwhile, the newborn has to adapt to existence outside the protected environment of the uterus.

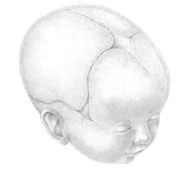

Fontanelles
Fontanelles are soft gaps between skull bones. By about 18 months, bones close over these spots.

THE NEWBORN BABY

A full-term baby weighs, on average, 3.5kg (7.7lb) and measures 51cm (20in) in length. During the first few days, the baby loses up to 10 per cent of its birthweight, but regains this by about the tenth day. At birth, the baby is usually covered with a greasy, whitish substance called vernix, which provides protection within the uterus. The vernix is wiped away shortly after birth.

Liver
Immaturity of the liver enzymes that break down the pigment bilirubin can cause temporary yellowing (jaundice).

Genitals
The external genitals of newborn boys and girls appear relatively large. Girls sometimes have a slight vaginal discharge.

Eyes
Newborn babies can see but tend to keep their eyes shut. The eyes are often greyish-blue at first, but change colour over the next few months.

Thymus
This lymph gland, which plays a role in the body's defences, is large at birth but shrinks over the next several years.

Intestines
The first faecal material excreted by the baby is a thick, sticky, greenish-black substance called meconium.

Skin
Slight skin peeling can occur in the first week. Minor rashes and skin blemishes are also common during the baby's early months.

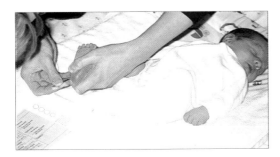

Heel-prick test
Within the first 10 days, the baby's heel is pricked to obtain a blood sample to test for phenylketonuria, a rare disorder that causes mental retardation, and for thyroid insufficiency. The blood may also checked for other types of disorder.

APGAR SCORE
Virginia Apgar, an American anaesthetist, devised an assessment for new babies. Heart rate, breathing, muscle tone, responsiveness, and colour are scored from 0 to 2 at 1 minute and 5 minutes after birth.

SIGN	SCORE: 0	SCORE: 1	SCORE: 2
HEART RATE	None	Below 100	Over 100
BREATHING	None	Slow or irregular; weak cry	Regular; strong cry
MUSCLE TONE	Limp	Some bending of limbs	Active movements
RESPONSE TO STIMULATION	None	Grimace or whimpering	Cry, sneeze, or cough
COLOUR	Pale; blue	Blue extremities	Pink

CHANGES IN CIRCULATION

Because the fetus obtains oxygen and nutrients from the placenta, its circulatory system (illustrated below) differs from that of a baby at birth. Special features of the fetal circulation are: the foramen ovale, a hole that allows blood to flow from the right atrium to the left atrium; the ductus arteriosus, a channel that bypasses the lungs; and the ductus venosus, a liver bypass.

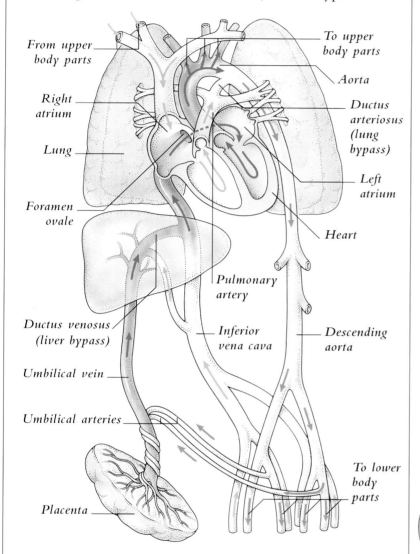

THE PUERPERIUM

During the puerperium, the mother's genital tract gradually reverts to its pre-pregnant state. As the placental site heals, tissue debris from the uterus is expelled in the form of a vaginal discharge called lochia. For the first week after childbirth, the lochia is bloodstained but then becomes cream-coloured. The vagina slowly shrinks back to its previous size.

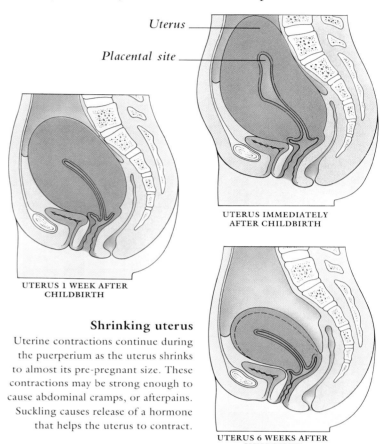

UTERUS 1 WEEK AFTER CHILDBIRTH

UTERUS IMMEDIATELY AFTER CHILDBIRTH

UTERUS 6 WEEKS AFTER CHILDBIRTH

Shrinking uterus

Uterine contractions continue during the puerperium as the uterus shrinks to almost its pre-pregnant size. These contractions may be strong enough to cause abdominal cramps, or afterpains. Suckling causes release of a hormone that helps the uterus to contract.

CERVIX OF NULLIPAROUS WOMAN

CERVIX AFTER GIVING BIRTH

The cervix

In nulliparous women (those who have never given birth), the cervical opening is nearly circular. Childbirth stretches and slightly tears the cervix. The cervical opening closes again, but does not regain its original appearance.

CIRCULATION AT BIRTH

At delivery, the lungs take over from the placenta. Lung blood flow increases while placental blood flow ceases. Pressure within the left heart chambers mounts, causing the foramen ovale to shut. The umbilical vessels, ductus arteriosus, and ductus venosus close, forming ligaments.

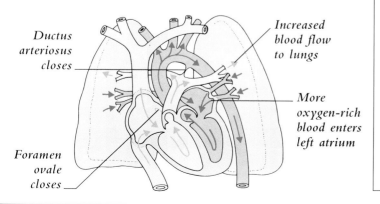

LACTATION

Breast size increases during pregnancy as glands develop for breastfeeding. Breast milk provides all the nourishment a newborn baby needs, and it also helps to protect against infection. The baby is able to suck immediately after birth; this stimulates the release of oxytocin, a pituitary hormone that promotes both milk flow and uterine contractions.

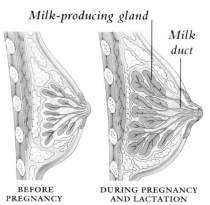

Milk-producing gland

Milk duct

BEFORE PREGNANCY

DURING PREGNANCY AND LACTATION

GROWTH *and* DEVELOPMENT

DURING THE EARLY YEARS, children develop basic physical skills such as walking and talking. While childhood progresses, agility improves and intellectual abilities increase. Growth is very rapid during infancy, then occurs at a fairly steady rate until growth rate speeds up again at puberty. During the pubertal years, the child becomes an adult, capable of sexual reproduction.

BONE GROWTH

Most of the long bones develop from cartilage by an orderly sequence of changes called ossification. The process starts before birth at zones called primary ossification centres in the bone shafts. After birth, secondary ossification centres develop near the bone ends. Growth ceases when ossification is complete.

Epiphyseal line
The epiphyseal growth plate ossifies during adolescence or early adult life, forming a dense epiphyseal line.

Growing ends
The shaft, or diaphysis, of a long bone is separated from the growing end, or epiphysis, of the bone by a zone near the bone's end called the epiphyseal plate. This plate is the principal site of bone elongation.

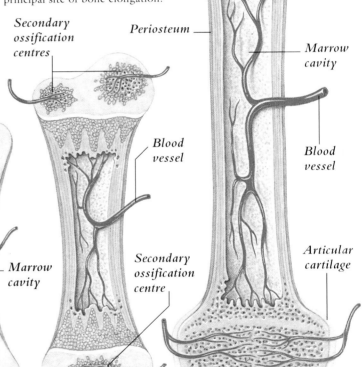

Diaphysis *Joint space* *Epiphyseal plate*

Epiphyses

Ossifying cartilage

Epiphyseal plate

Cartilage

Secondary ossification centres

Periosteum

Marrow cavity

Blood vessel

Blood vessel

NEWBORN   ABOUT 11 YEARS

Diaphysis

Bone

Marrow cavity

Secondary ossification centre

Epiphysis

Secondary ossification centre

Articular cartilage

Bone age
X-rays can reveal the maturity of a growing child because each bone ossifies at a predictable age and because cartilage, which is not as dense, shows up less clearly than bone does. The epiphyseal plates, other zones of cartilage growth, and joint spaces appear as gaps.

CHANGING BODY PROPORTIONS

Superimposing the body at different ages onto a grid divided into eight equal parts demonstrates the dramatic changes in body proportions that take place during childhood. In a newborn infant, the head is relatively large, representing about one-quarter of the baby's total length. As the child grows, the relative sizes of the head and trunk decrease and the limbs become longer. When final adult height is reached during adolescence, the head represents only about one-eighth of body length.

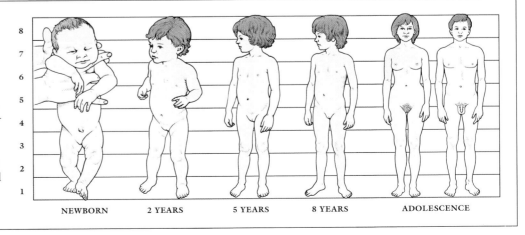

NEWBORN   2 YEARS   5 YEARS   8 YEARS   ADOLESCENCE

CHILD DEVELOPMENT

Babies are born able to see, hear, and perform reflex actions. During early childhood, basic skills of body movement, manipulation, and social behaviour are acquired, and language develops. Development takes place in well-recognized steps, called developmental "milestones", which occur at predictable ages. Each child, however, progresses at a slightly different rate.

DENTAL DEVELOPMENT

The first set of teeth, known as primary or deciduous teeth, erupts through the gums in a set pattern from about 8 months into the third year. The primary teeth become loose and fall out as the second, or permanent, teeth push through the gums; this starts to happen at about the age of 6 years. The set of 32 permanent teeth is complete only when the third molars, or wisdom teeth, appear in the late teens or early twenties.

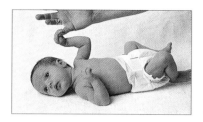

Neonatal grasp reflex
Newborn babies can perform certain automatic movements that are known as primitive reflexes. One example is the grasping of an object that is put firmly in the palm. Primitive reflexes disappear after a few months.

Rooting reflex
Lightly stroking the baby's face near the corner of the mouth will prompt the baby to turn his or her head to that side and also to open the mouth. This rooting reflex helps the baby locate the mother's nipple to start feeding.

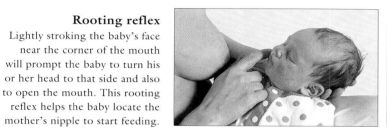

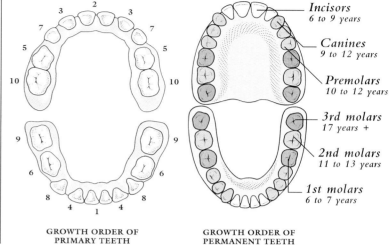

Incisors
6 to 9 years

Canines
9 to 12 years

Premolars
10 to 12 years

3rd molars
17 years +

2nd molars
11 to 13 years

1st molars
6 to 7 years

GROWTH ORDER OF PRIMARY TEETH

GROWTH ORDER OF PERMANENT TEETH

AGE	MOVEMENT		MANIPULATION		SOCIAL BEHAVIOUR	
1 MONTH		Lies with head to one side. Sleeps most of time when not being fed or handled.		Hands are normally closed at rest but grasp onto finger when palm is touched.		Watches mother's nearby face intently. Starts smiling at about 5 or 6 weeks.
6 MONTHS		Sits with support. Holds head and back straight. Turns head to look around.		Uses whole hand to grasp objects in palm. Passes objects between hands.		Takes everything to mouth. Turns quickly to sound of familiar voice across room.
9 MONTHS		Attempts to crawl on all fours. Stands holding onto support for a few moments.		Grasps between thumb and index finger. Pokes at small object with index finger.		Holds bottle or cup. Holds and chews solids. Babbles. Shouts to attract attention.
12 MONTHS		Walks with one or both hands held. Walks around furniture stepping sideways.		Deliberately drops toys, one by one, to the ground and watches them fall.		Holds out arms and feet to be dressed. Understands some simple commands.
18 MONTHS		Can get up and down stairs with a helping hand or holding rail. Throws ball.		Can build a tower of three or four cubes. Scribbles on paper with pencil or crayon.		Uses spoon well. Indicates need for toilet. Uses some words; understands many.
2 YEARS	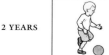	Runs around with ease. Can open doors. Kicks a ball without overbalancing.		Turns pages of book one at a time. Can build a tower six or seven cubes high.		Puts on shoes and socks. Makes simple sentences. Asks for food and drink.
3 YEARS		Can ride a tricycle and walk on tiptoe. Uses alternating feet to walk upstairs.		Can copy lines and circles. Able to copy a bridge made from three cubes.		Understands the idea of sharing. Plays with others. Tries to tidy up. Uses fork.
4 YEARS		Able to hop on one foot, and to run on tiptoe. Can climb up trees and ladders.		Copies some letters, such as X, V, H, T, and O. Can draw a man and a house.		Can dress and undress. Speech grammatical and completely intelligible.
5 YEARS		Able to skip on alternate feet. Runs lightly on toes. Can dance well to music.		Copies squares, triangles, many letters. Writes a few letters without prompting.		Washes and dries face. Uses knife. Knows birthday. Can act out stories in detail.

PUBERTY

At puberty, hormonal changes stimulate physical growth, alterations in behaviour, and the development of sex organs so that reproduction can occur. These changes are triggered when gonadotrophin-releasing hormone (GnRH) from the hypothalamus acts on the anterior pituitary gland.

HORMONES IN GIRLS

The pituitary gland releases follicle-stimulating hormone (FSH) and luteinizing hormone (LH), which stimulate the ovary to release eggs and to produce the two female sex hormones.

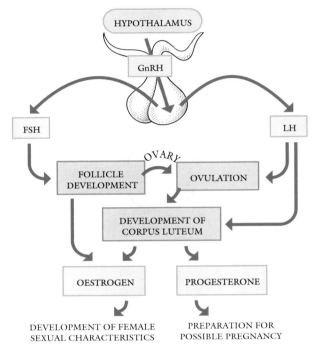

HORMONES IN BOYS

FSH and LH from the pituitary gland prompt cells of the testes to increase their secretion of testosterone, the male sex hormone, and also to start producing spermatozoa, or sperm.

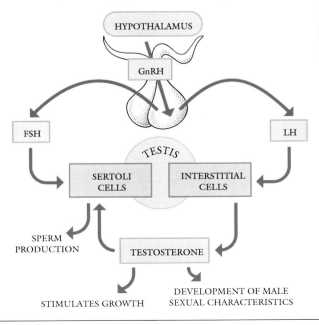

PUBERTAL DEVELOPMENT

The physical changes of puberty start at about age 10 or 11 years in girls, and about 12 or 13 years in boys, and sexual maturation is usually complete within about 3 or 4 years. In both sexes, puberty is accompanied by a rapid growth spurt and increase in weight, and by emotional and psychological changes. Because the growth spurt in boys begins later than it does in girls, boys have a longer period of steady growth, and thus usually attain a greater final adult height.

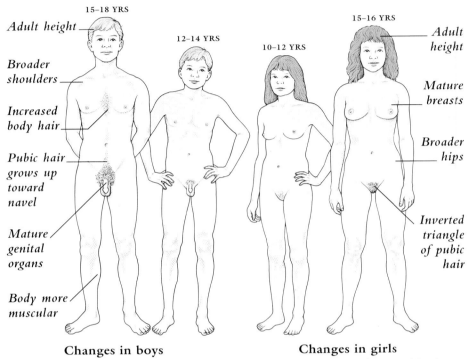

Changes in boys
The genital organs enlarge, pubic and underarm hair appear, facial and body hair increases, and muscle bulk increases. The voice deepens as the larynx enlarge.

Changes in girls
Budding of the breasts is followed by the growth of pubic and underarm hair, and by menstruation (which may be irregular at first). Fat is deposited around the hips.

SPERM PRODUCTION

The production of sperm takes place within the seminiferous tubules of the testes. Sperm develop through a complex series of events from cells called spermatogonia, which change first into spermatocytes, and then into spermatids. As the spermatids mature into sperm, they move away from supporting cells, called Sertoli cells, into the central cavity of the seminiferous tubule.

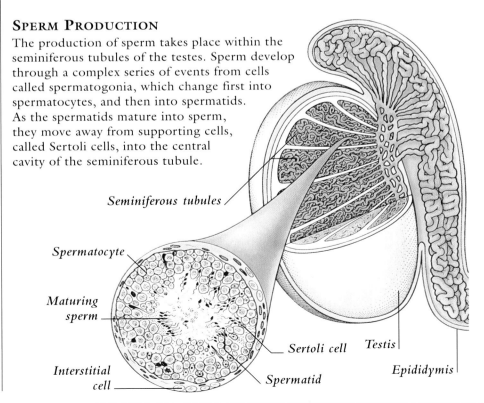

MENSTRUAL CYCLE

The principal sign that a girl has become sexually mature and is capable of reproduction is the onset of menstruation, a period of cyclical bleeding from the vagina. During each menstrual cycle, one or other of the two ovaries releases an egg, or ovum. Unless fertilization takes place, the uterine lining is shed about 2 weeks later during menstruation. The menstrual cycle is regulated by several hormones secreted by the pituitary gland and the ovaries.

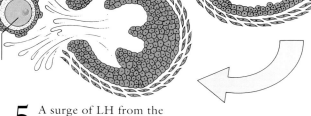

28-day cycle
The standard cycle is 28 days, but can range from 23 to 35 days. Bleeding lasts an average of 5 days, although this can vary from 1 to 8 days. In the standard cycle, ovulation occurs around day 14.

Menstruation

DAYS

1 FSH acts on the ovary to stimulate the growth of primary follicles (containing primary oöcytes). Usually, only one follicle reaches full maturity during each cycle.

→ *FSH*

Primary oöcyte

2 The developing oöycte enlarges, and the cells of the primary follicle multiply so that they form several layers around the oöcyte.

Primary follicle

Layers of follicular cells

3 As the follicle enlarges, a fluid-filled cavity forms and cells are pushed toward the rim of the follicle and around the oöcyte. The structure is now called a secondary follicle.

Primary oöcyte

Secondary follicle

Fluid-filled cavity

4 The mature follicle bulges toward the surface of the ovary and increases production of the hormone oestrogen.

Secondary oöcyte

Oestrogen

Corpus luteum

Progesterone

Corpus luteum

Oestrogen

→ *LH*

7 If fertilization does not take place, the corpus luteum breaks down during the second week after ovulation.

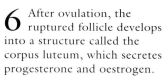

SEM x 72

6 After ovulation, the ruptured follicle develops into a structure called the corpus luteum, which secretes progesterone and oestrogen.

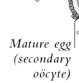

Mature egg (secondary oöcyte)

Ovulation

A mature egg (red) is released from the surface of the ovary at ovulation. The egg is surrounded by cells and fluid from the ruptured follicle.

5 A surge of LH from the pituitary gland causes the mature follicle to rupture and, release the egg from the ovary; this process is called ovulation.

CHANGES IN THE UTERUS

At the start of each menstrual cycle the uterine lining, or endometrium, is shed during menstruation. After each period of bleeding, the endometrium thickens to prepare the uterus for nurturing a fertilized egg and subsequent pregnancy. But if fertilization does not occur, the endometrium again breaks down and is shed – together with the unfertilized egg – and the cycle repeats itself.

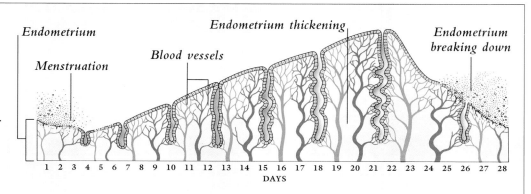

Endometrium

Endometrium thickening

Endometrium breaking down

Menstruation

Blood vessels

1 2 3 4 5 6 7 8 9 10 11 12 13 14 15 16 17 18 19 20 21 22 23 24 25 26 27 28
DAYS

The AGEING PROCESS

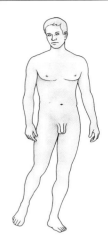

ALL LIVING CREATURES HAVE A NATURAL LIFESPAN. For humans this is around 85 years, although some people live much longer. The brain, the muscles and joints, the eyes and ears all decline with age, but in healthy people the changes are small until well past age 60. To maintain vigour, people should try to keep to their normal weight, take regular exercise, and avoid overconsumption of addictive substances such as tobacco and alcohol. Regular health screening allows early detection of problems when they are most effectively treated.

TISSUE CHANGES

Connective tissue, which consists mainly of collagen and elastin, is the body's main structural material. It forms the bulk of tendons and ligaments, and provides a framework for bones and muscles. As the body ages, tissues lose elasticity; the collagen fibres thicken and become stiff so that arteries harden, the muscles and joints are less flexible, and the skin becomes wrinkled.

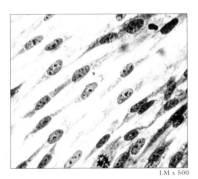

LM x 500

Young connective tissue
Dark, oval nuclei are arranged in a regular, pavement-like pattern throughout the structure, and pigment is evenly distributed.

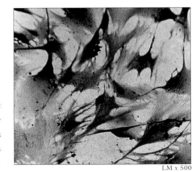

LM x 500

Ageing connective tissue
Tissue in older people has fewer cells; the irregular pattern makes the structure less flexible and less resilient after even minor injury.

SKIN

Older skin is thinner and more fragile, and the deep layers contain less elastic tissue. Blood vessels are also less elastic so that even minor injuries can cause bruising. The skin may be mottled with small, flat brown areas called lentigenes (from the Latin word for "lentils").

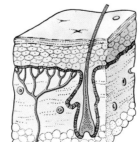

Young skin
A thick top layer and many elastic fibres in the deeper layers help to maintain the smoothness of young skin.

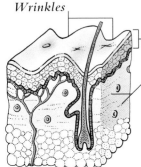

Wrinkles

Thinner outer layer

Fewer elastic fibres

Older skin
A thinner outer layer and fewer elastic fibres in the deeper layers result in skin that appears loose, with deeper creases and wrinkles.

THE NERVOUS SYSTEM

The number of brain cells declines from age 20, but the decline is more rapid in older people. Circulation of blood to the brain slows, and mental functions, such as memory, can become impaired. Nonetheless, many people remain mentally alert well past age 80.

HEARING

Ageing usually causes a loss of sensitivity to sounds, which may become duller or distorted so that speech becomes difficult to follow. Annual hearing tests for older people are recommended; hearing aids may restore the ability to understand speech.

Cochlear deterioration
Hearing loss in older people may be due to degeneration of the cochlea; repeated or prolonged exposure to loud noises hastens deterioration.

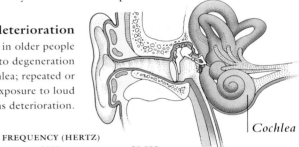

Cochlea

Hearing loss
As people get older, some hearing loss is inevitable. High-pitched sounds are the first that are difficult to detect; eventually, all frequencies are affected.

VISION

With age, vision may become impaired by structural changes that affect the eyes' ability to focus on nearby objects. Vision is sometimes affected by degeneration of the macula, the central area of the retina, or by a cataract (clouding of the lens).

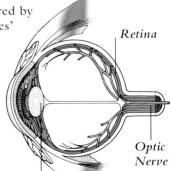

Retina

Optic Nerve

Changes in the lens
Loss of elastic tissue stiffens the lens so that it is unable to change shape and create a clear image on the retina. *Lens*

BONES, MUSCLES, AND JOINTS

The main, bulky structures of the body are affected by ageing in several ways. Bones become thinner and more brittle as a result of osteoporosis, the loss of collagen reduces muscle bulk and strength, and loss of cartilage makes joints painful, stiff, and distorted.

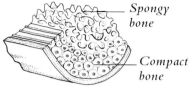

Spongy bone

Compact bone

Young bone
This type of bone has a thick, strong outer layer of dense, compact bone and an inner core of soft, spongy bone that is rich in blood vessels.

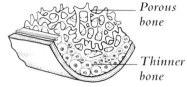

Porous bone

Thinner bone

Osteoporotic bone
Bone in older people has a thinner, outer layer that lacks strength. Inner spongy bone is more porous, and has fewer blood vessels and less calcium.

HEART AND CIRCULATION

Narrowing of the arteries by atherosclerosis and the consequent rise in blood pressure forces the heart to work harder. Like all muscles, the heart becomes less efficient and weaker with age. Heart valves become stiff, and the electrical conduction system that helps maintain a regular heart rhythm often becomes faulty.

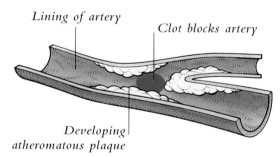

Lining of artery

Clot blocks artery

Developing atheromatous plaque

Atherosclerosis
The internal lining of the arteries thickens with cholesterol-rich atheroma in deposits called plaques. When the plaques become fissured, blood clots often form, which restricts blood flow.

LIVER AND KIDNEY FUNCTION

In youth, organs such as the liver and kidneys have a greater capacity than the body needs; they can easily compensate for any damage due to disease. With age, even a minor illness may cause failure. Raised blood pressure, atherosclerosis, alcohol, and the prolonged use of analgesic drugs can hasten natural decline.

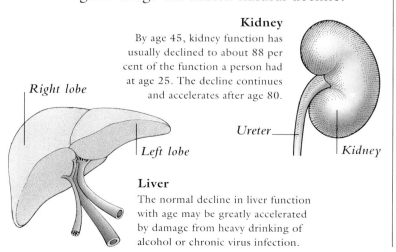

Kidney
By age 45, kidney function has usually declined to about 88 per cent of the function a person had at age 25. The decline continues and accelerates after age 80.

Right lobe

Left lobe

Ureter

Kidney

Liver
The normal decline in liver function with age may be greatly accelerated by damage from heavy drinking of alcohol or chronic virus infection.

MENOPAUSE

A gradual loss of ovarian function in women over several years causes variable symptoms, mostly due to a lack of oestrogen. Menstruation ceases, and some women have hot flushes, night sweats, a thinned and dry vagina that may cause discomfort during sexual intercourse, and urinary symptoms. Psychological difficulties may accompany these physical changes.

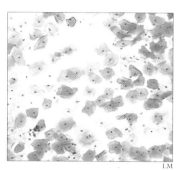

Premenopausal vaginal cells
Before the menopause, the vaginal lining is thick and well lubricated. A cervical smear usually reveals many large cells with small nuclei.

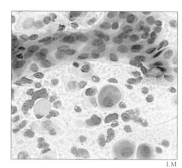

Postmenopausal vaginal cells
Declining levels of oestrogen cause the lining of the vagina to become thinner. The smear at right reveals fewer cells, which clump together, and larger nuclei.

HORMONE REPLACEMENT THERAPY

For many women, menopausal symptoms can be reversed by regular treatment with replacement oestrogens. These may be given as tablets, injections, implants, skin patches, creams, or suppositories. The choice of medication and method of delivery depend on whether the woman has had a hysterectomy, her general health, and her symptoms.

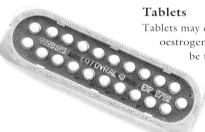

Tablets
Tablets may consist of oestrogen alone or oestrogen and progestogen. They may be taken every day or for 21 to 25 days every month.

Skin patches
Patches deliver the hormone through the skin into the bloodstream. They are usually applied to the abdomen, in a different position, every 3 to 4 days.

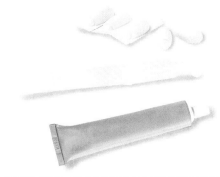

Creams and suppositories
To relieve dryness, a hormone-containing cream can be applied to the vaginal walls. Rectal or vaginal suppositories allow absorption of hormone into the bloodstream.

INHERITANCE

MOST INFORMATION PASSED ON IN GENES IS BASIC, such as the instruction to a fertilized egg to develop into a human embryo rather than another species. Genes also pass on more complex information about psychological and other personal features of parents, such as susceptibility to diseases and athletic ability. Genetics is the study of how genes are selected and packaged within the tiny volume of the newly fertilized ovum.

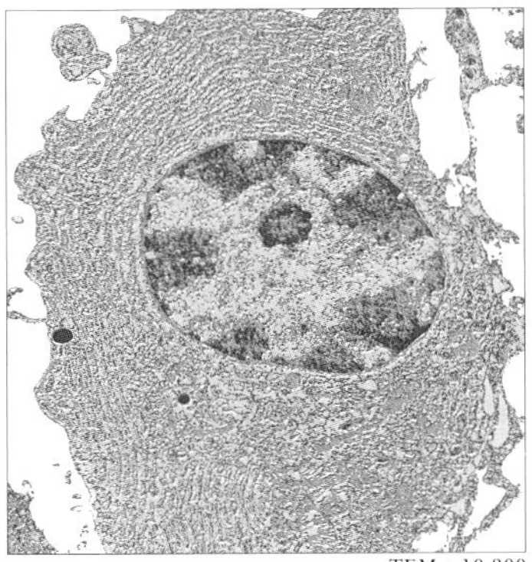

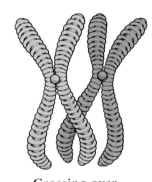

TEM x 10,800

Location of genes
Genes, which are tiny segments of chromosomes, are contained in the cell's nucleus (centre of image).

MEIOSIS: SEX CELL FORMATION

During meiosis, genes from both parents are exchanged so that each sperm or egg cell has a unique genetic mix. The cells then divide in two stages to produce four new sex cells: each has 23 chromosomes, half the number in all other human cells. When the sex cells (the male sperm and the female ovum) fuse at conception, the embryo ends up with a complete set of all 46 chromosomes, half from each parent.

1 Meiosis starts with duplication of each member of the 23 pairs of chromosomes (four pairs are seen here). Each of these "doubled-up" chromosomes, which is X-shaped, lines up with its partner.

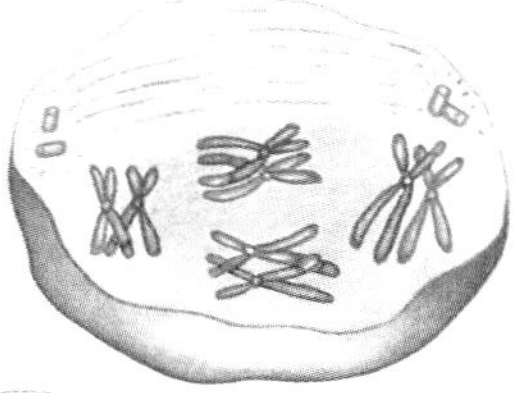

2 As pairs of chromosomes entwine, they exchange a random selection of DNA. Like shuffling a deck of cards, this process (known as crossing over) combines genes in a way that will never be repeated.

KEY

■ *Father's gene*

■ *Mother's gene*

Homologous chromosomes
The chromosomes in a pair are similar but not identical, and are called homologous.

3 The matching (homologous) pairs of chromosomes line up in the middle of the cell. Threads form a structure called the spindle between the poles of the cell.

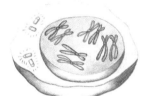

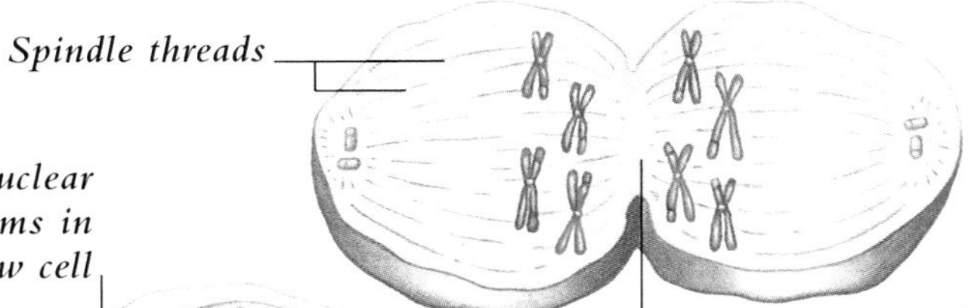

Crossing over
During this process, pairs of homologous chromosomes exchange corresponding genes (those located at the same point on each chromosome).

Spindle threads

A new nuclear membrane forms in each new cell

4 The threads of the spindle pull each of the "doubled-up" chromosomes in a pair to opposite sides. The cell begins to divide into two separate cells.

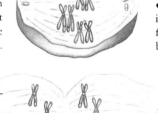

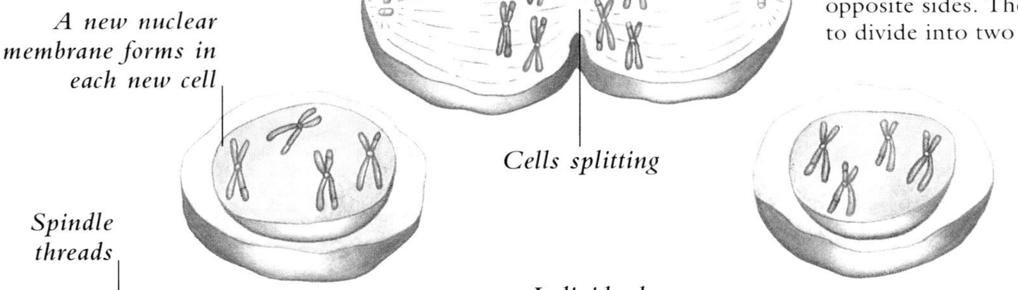

Cells splitting

5 Each new cell, complete with a new nuclear membrane, now has a "doubled-up" chromosome from each of the 23 pairs.

Spindle threads

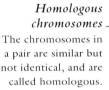

Individual chromosomes

6 Spindle threads form and the chromosomes line up at the centre of the cell. They separate to form individual chromosomes, which are pulled to opposite sides.

7 The two cells divide again. After division, each of the four new cells contains a unique set of 23 chromosomes that contain DNA from the original cell's 46 chromosomes.

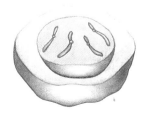
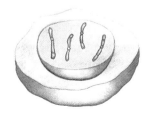
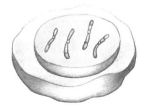
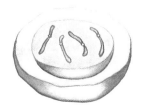
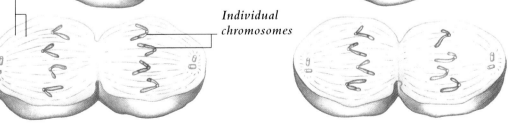

THE ROLE OF GENES

For most genes, the mix received from parents makes no difference since both genes code for the same chemical processes. For other functions or characteristics, two or more genes "compete" for the same quality, such as hair colour or height. The mix of these genes that a person receives helps to determine his or her individual traits.

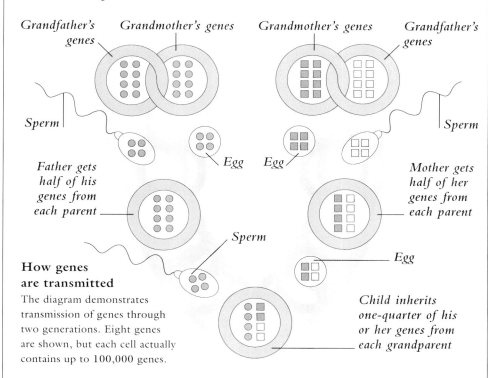

Grandfather's genes *Grandmother's genes* *Grandmother's genes* *Grandfather's genes*

Sperm *Sperm*

Egg *Egg*

Father gets half of his genes from each parent *Mother gets half of her genes from each parent*

Sperm *Egg*

How genes are transmitted

The diagram demonstrates transmission of genes through two generations. Eight genes are shown, but each cell actually contains up to 100,000 genes.

Child inherits one-quarter of his or her genes from each grandparent

PATTERNS OF HEREDITY

Sex, and some other traits, are determined by the 23rd pair of chromosomes. The other 22 pairs carry genes for most other traits. Some are determined by a single gene, such as eye colour, but most, such as intelligence, involve several genes on different chromosomes. Environmental factors also modify some characteristics, such as height.

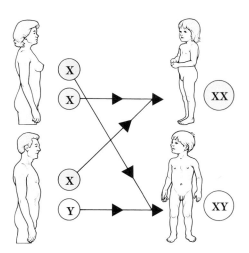

X **X** **XX**

X **Y** **XY**

Sex determination

Embryos with two X chromosomes – one from each parent – develop into females; those with a Y chromosome from the father and an X chromosome from the mother develop into males. The Y chromosome is much smaller than the X chromosome.

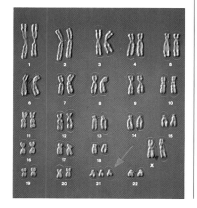

Chromosomal abnormalities

If sex cells with damaged chromosomes or the wrong number take part in fertilization, a miscarriage usually results, or a child may be handicapped. Down's syndrome is due to an extra chromosome 21 (see right).

DOMINANT AND RECESSIVE GENES

When several different genes are found at the same position on a pair of chromosomes, the cell takes instructions from only one, the so-called dominant gene. Its effects "mask" those of the other, recessive gene. For a recessive characteristic to be visible, a person must have two copies of the recessive gene.

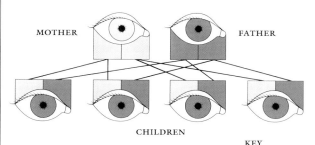

MOTHER FATHER

CHILDREN

KEY

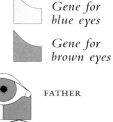

Genes for eye colour

The gene for brown eyes is dominant over the blue-eye gene. A child who inherits a brown-eye gene from either parent will have brown eyes.

Gene for blue eyes

Gene for brown eyes

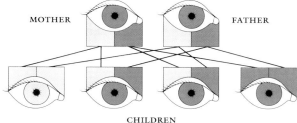

MOTHER FATHER

CHILDREN

Blue or brown eyes?

If both parents have one gene for brown eyes and one for blue (known as heterozygous), each child has a 1 in 4 chance of having blue eyes and a 3 in 4 chance of being brown-eyed.

SEX-LINKED INHERITANCE

Several important diseases, including haemophilia, are due to defective genes on the X chromosome. These genes are recessive, so a woman who inherits one normal and one diseased gene will often appear healthy but may carry the disease, while a man with one defective X chromosome develops the disease.

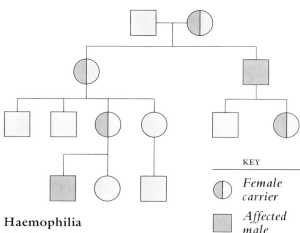

Haemophilia

Healthy men do not have the faulty gene and are not carriers. A daughter of an affected man will have one abnormal gene and pass the disease to half of her sons; half her daughters will be carriers.

KEY

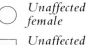

Female carrier

Affected male

Unaffected female

Unaffected male

GLOSSARY

Text terms in *boldface italics* refer to other items in the glossary.

A

Abscess
A walled cavity containing pus, surrounded by inflamed or dying tissue.

Accommodation
The process by which the eyes adjust to focus on nearby or distant objects.

Acoustic neuroma
A *tumour* on the *nerve* that connects the ear and brain.

Acquired immune deficiency syndrome
AIDS. An infection with the *human immunodeficiency virus* (HIV) that is spread by sexual intercourse or infected blood. AIDS results in the loss of resistance to infections and some *cancers*.

Acute
Medical conditions that begin abruptly and last for a short time. Contrasts with *chronic* conditions.

Adenoids
Masses of *lymphoid tissue* on each side of the back of the upper part of the throat.

Allergen
Any substance causing an allergic reaction in a person previously exposed to it.

Alveolus
See illustration above right.

Alzheimer's disease
A progressive *dementia* due to loss of nerve cells in the brain affecting more than 10 per cent of people over 65.

Amniocentesis
The process of withdrawing a sample of fluid from the *uterus* to obtain information about the health and genetic constitution of the *fetus*.

Anaemia
A disorder in which the amount of *haemoglobin* in the blood is reduced.

Aneurysm
A swelling of an *artery* caused by damage to or weakness in the vessel wall.

Angina
Pain or tightness in the centre of the chest brought on by exercise; caused by an inadequate blood supply to the heart muscle.

Angiography
See illustration below right.

Angioplasty
Any process used to widen the bore of an *artery* that is narrowed by disease. See also *Balloon angioplasty*.

Antibody
A soluble protein that attaches to body invaders, such as *bacteria*, and helps to destroy them.

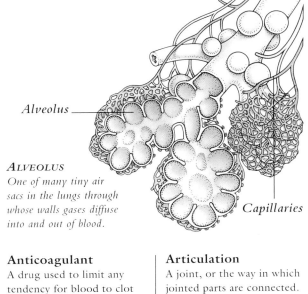

Alveolus — — *Capillaries*

ALVEOLUS
One of many tiny air sacs in the lungs through whose walls gases diffuse into and out of blood.

Anticoagulant
A drug used to limit any tendency for blood to clot within *arteries* or *veins*.

Aorta
See illustration below left.

Aortic valve
A triple-cusped valve at the origin of the *aorta* that allows blood to leave the left ventricle of the heart but prevents backward flow.

Appendix
The worm-like structure attached to the initial part of the large intestine. It has no known function.

Aqueous humour
The fluid filling the front chamber of the eye between the back of the *cornea* and front of the iris and *lens*.

Arrhythmia
An irregular heartbeat, due to a defect in the electrical impulses or pathways that control contractions.

Arteriole
A small terminal branch of an *artery* leading to even smaller *capillaries*, which make the link to the *veins*.

Artery
An elastic, muscular-walled tube that transports blood away from the heart to all other parts of the body.

Arthritis
Inflammation in a joint, causing varying degrees of pain, swelling, redness, and restriction of movement.

Articulation
A joint, or the way in which jointed parts are connected.

Asthma
A disease featuring variable narrowing of the air tubes so that breathing becomes intermittently difficult.

Atherosclerosis
A degenerative disease of *arteries* in which raised plaques of fatty material limit blood flow and cause local *blood clotting*.

Atria
The thin-walled upper chambers of the heart.

Atrial fibrillation
A disorder in which the *atria* beat very rapidly.

Atrial septal defect
A hole in the wall (the septum) between the upper two chambers of the heart.

ANGIOGRAM

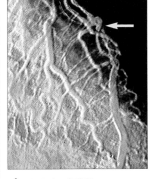

ANGIOGRAPHY
*A method of imaging blood vessels in which X-rays are taken after a **contrast medium** has been injected. Shown above is a narrowed **coronary** artery (arrow).*

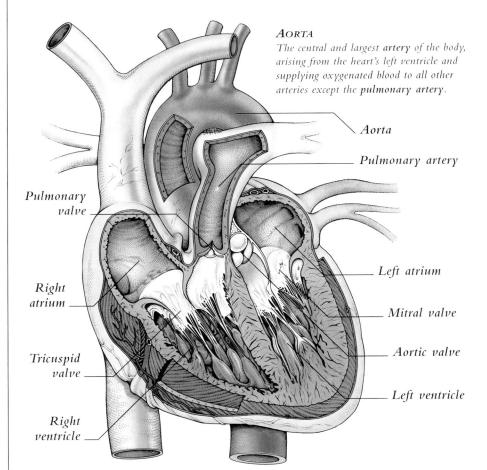

AORTA
*The central and largest **artery** of the body, arising from the heart's left ventricle and supplying oxygenated blood to all other arteries except the **pulmonary** artery.*

Aorta

Pulmonary artery

Pulmonary valve

Right atrium

Tricuspid valve

Right ventricle

Left atrium

Mitral valve

Aortic valve

Left ventricle

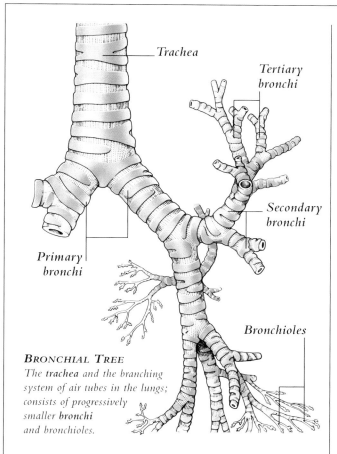

Trachea

Tertiary bronchi

Secondary bronchi

Primary bronchi

Bronchioles

BRONCHIAL TREE
The trachea and the branching system of air tubes in the lungs; consists of progressively smaller bronchi and bronchioles.

Autoimmune disease
A disease caused by a defect in the immune system, which fails to recognize body tissues as "self".

Autonomic nervous system
The part of the nervous system that controls unconscious functions, such as heartbeat and breathing.

Axon
The long, fibre-like process of a nerve cell that conducts nerve impulses to or from the cell body; bundles of many axons form *nerves*.

B

Bacterium
A type of microorganism consisting of one cell. Only a few of the many different species cause disease.

Balloon angioplasty
The use of a catheter with an inflatable balloon tip to widen an *artery*.

Basal ganglia
Paired masses of nerve cell bodies, or nuclei, lying deep in the brain; concerned with control of movement.

Benign
Mild and with no tendency to spread; contrasts with a *malignant* condition.

Beta-blocker
A drug that blocks the action of adrenaline, thus slowing the pulse and reducing blood pressure.

Bile
A greenish-brown fluid produced by the *liver* and stored in the *gallbladder*; helps the digestion of fats.

Biliary system
The network of bile vessels formed by the ducts from the *liver* and the *gallbladder*, and the gallbladder itself.

Biopsy
A sample of tissue from any part of the body suspected of disease that is taken for *microscopic* examination.

Blood clot
A meshwork of the protein *fibrin*, *platelets*, and blood cells that forms when a blood vessel is damaged.

Boil
An inflamed, pus-filled area of skin, which is usually an infected *hair follicle*.

Bolus
A chewed-up quantity of food ready to be swallowed; also, a drug dose injected into the bloodstream.

Bone marrow
The fatty tissue within bone cavities, which may be red or yellow. Red bone marrow produces *red blood cells*.

Bradycardia
A slow heart rate. This is normal in athletes but may signal disorders in others.

Brain stem
The lower part of the brain; houses the centres that control vital functions such as breathing and heartbeat.

Breech delivery
A buttock-first birth; carries a slightly higher risk to the fetus than a head-first birth.

Bronchial tree
See illustration at left.

Bronchitis
Inflammation of the lining of the breathing tubes, resulting in a cough that produces large amounts of sputum (phlegm).

Bronchus
One of the larger air tubes in the lungs. Each lung has a main bronchus that divides into smaller branches.

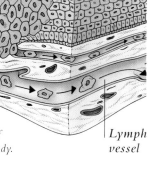

Epidermis of the skin

Cluster of cancer cells

Lymph vessel

CANCER
A localized growth from uncontrolled cell reproduction, which can spread (if untreated) to other parts of the body.

C

Calcium-channel blocker
A drug that limits movement of dissolved calcium across cell membranes; used to treat high blood pressure and heart irregularity.

Cancer
See illustration above.

Capillary
One of the tiny blood vessels that link the smallest *arteries* and smallest *veins*.

Carcinoma
A *cancer* of a surface layer (epithelium). Carcinomas commonly occur in the skin, the breast, the large intestine, the linings of the air tubes, the *prostate gland*, and the *uterus*.

Carpal tunnel syndrome
See illustration below.

Cartilage
A tough, fibrous connective tissue, also known as gristle.

Central nervous system
The brain and spinal cord; receives and analyzes sensory data, and then initiates a response.

Cerebellum
The region of the brain located behind the *brain stem*. It is concerned with balance and the control of fine movement.

Cerebrospinal fluid
A watery fluid that bathes the brain and spinal cord.

Cerebrum
The largest part of the brain, which is made up of two hemispheres. It contains the nerve centres for thought, personality, the senses, and voluntary movement.

Chlamydia
Small bacteria causing the eye disease trachoma and *pelvic inflammatory disease*.

Cholecystitis
Inflammation of the *gallbladder*; commonly the result of obstructed outflow of *bile* by a *gallstone*.

Cholecystography
X-ray of the *gallbladder* after a *contrast medium* has been introduced into it.

Cholestasis
A slowing or cessation of the flow of *bile* in the *liver*.

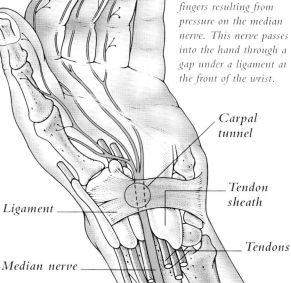

CARPAL TUNNEL SYNDROME
Numbness and pain in the thumb and middle fingers resulting from pressure on the median nerve. This nerve passes into the hand through a gap under a ligament at the front of the wrist.

Carpal tunnel

Tendon sheath

Ligament

Tendons

Median nerve

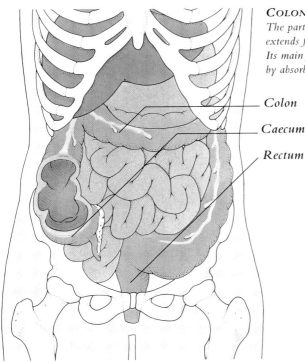

COLON
The part of the large intestine that extends from the caecum to the rectum. Its main function is to conserve water by absorbing it from the bowel contents.

— Colon

— Caecum

— Rectum

Chorionic villus sampling
Removal of a small piece of tissue from the *placenta* for *chromosome* or *gene* analysis; allows for early detection of fetal abnormalities.

Chromosome
See illustration below.

Chronic
Persistent medical conditions that usually cause some long-term change in the body; contrasts with *acute*.

Cirrhosis
Replacement of healthy *liver* tissue by fine fibrous tissue, resulting in hardening and impairment of function; may be caused by excessive consumption of alcohol.

Cochlea
The coiled structure in the inner ear that contains the organ of Corti, which converts sound vibrations into nerve impulses for transmission to the brain.

Collagen
An important structural protein that is present in bones, *tendons*, *ligaments*, and other connective tissues. Collagen fibres are twisted into bundles.

Colon
See illustration above left.

Congenital
Present at birth. Congenital disorders may be hereditary or may result from diseases or injuries that occur during fetal life or the birth itself.

Contrast medium
A substance through which X-rays are unable to pass.

Cornea
The transparent dome at the front of the eyeball that is the eye's main focusing lens.

Coronary
A term meaning "crown". Refers to the *arteries* that encircle and supply the heart with blood.

Corpus callosum
The wide curved band of about 20 million nerve fibres that connects the two hemispheres of the *cerebrum*.

Corticosteroid
A drug that simulates the natural steroid *hormones* of the outer zone (cortex) of the adrenal glands.

Cranial nerves
The 12 pairs of *nerves* that emerge from the brain and *brain stem*. They include the nerves for smell, sight, eye movement, facial movement and sensation, hearing, taste, and head movement.

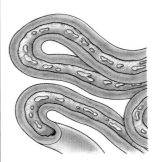

CROHN'S DISEASE
An inflammatory disease that affects the gastrointestinal tract. Symptoms may include pain, fever, and diarrhoea.

Crohn's disease
See illustration above.

Cyst
A walled cavity, usually spherical, filled with secreted fluid or semi-solid matter. Usually *benign*.

Cystadenoma
A harmless, *cyst*-like growth of glandular tissue.

Cystitis
An inflammation of the urinary bladder, caused by infection. Produces frequent, painful urination and sometimes incontinence.

D

Defibrillation
A strong pulse of electric current that is applied to the heart to restore its normal rhythm. Commonly used if the heart is in a state of rapid, ineffectual twitching, such as after a heart attack.

Dementia
The loss of mental powers and *memory* as a result of degenerative brain disease or narrowed *arteries* supplying blood to the brain.

Dermis
See illustration below.

Dialysis
The separation of dissolved substances using membranes through which only small molecules can pass. Dialysis is the basis of artificial *kidney* machines.

Diaphragm
The dome-shaped muscular sheet that separates the chest from the abdomen. When the muscle contracts the dome flattens, increasing the volume of the chest.

Diastole
The period in the heart cycle when the ventricles are relaxed and the heart is filling with blood.

Digestive system
The mouth, *pharynx*, *oesophagus*, stomach, and intestines. Associated organs are the *pancreas*, *liver*, and the *gallbladder* and its ducts.

Diverticular disease
See illustration above right.

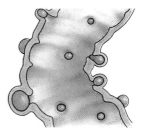

DIVERTICULAR DISEASE
The presence of diverticula, small sacs that are created by protrusion of the intestine's inner lining through the wall.

Dopamine
A chemical messenger (neurotransmitter) in the brain that is involved in the control of body movement. Dopamine is related to the substance levodopa, which is used to treat people who have *Parkinson's disease*.

Down's syndrome
A genetic disorder in which a person's cells contain an extra *chromosome* 21. People with Down's syndrome have a characteristic appearance and always some degree of mental impairment.

Duodenum
The C-shaped first part of the small intestine, about 25cm (10in) long, into which the stomach empties. Ducts from the *gallbladder*, *liver*, and *pancreas* all enter the duodenum.

Dura mater
A tough membrane, the outer of the three layers of the *meninges* that cover the brain and the spinal cord. The dura mater lies over the arachnoid and the pia mater.

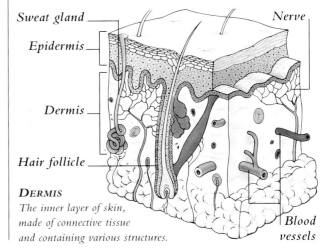

Sweat gland

Epidermis

Dermis

Hair follicle

Nerve

Blood vessels

DERMIS
The inner layer of skin, made of connective tissue and containing various structures.

CHROMOSOME
A thread-like structure, present in all nucleated body cells, that carries the genetic code for the formation of the body. A normal human body cell has 46 chromosomes arranged in 23 pairs.

SEM

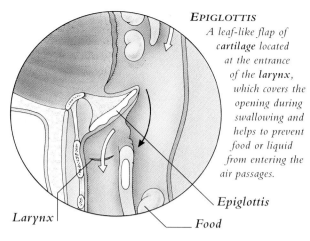

EPIGLOTTIS
A leaf-like flap of cartilage located at the entrance of the larynx, which covers the opening during swallowing and helps to prevent food or liquid from entering the air passages.

Larynx

Epiglottis

Food

E

Eardrum
The membrane separating the outer ear from the *middle ear* that vibrates in response to sound.

Ectopic pregnancy
Implantation of the fertilized egg in a site other than the uterine lining.

Electrocardiography
Recording and study of the electrical changes associated with heartbeat.

Electroencephalography
Recording and study of the electrical signals produced by the brain.

Embolus
Any material, such as *blood clots*, air bubbles, *bone marrow*, or *tumour* cells, carried in the bloodstream.

Embryo
The developing baby from conception until the eighth week of pregnancy.

Endocarditis
Inflammation of the inner lining of the heart wall or a heart valve.

Endorphin
A morphine-like substance produced by the body in times of pain and stress.

Enzyme
A protein that acts as a catalyst to accelerate a chemical reaction.

Epidermis
The outer layer of the skin; its cells flatten and become scale-like toward the surface.

Epiglottis
See illustration above.

Epilepsy
A disorder featuring episodes of unregulated electrical discharge throughout the brain or in a specific area.

Eustachian tube
The tube connecting the back of the nose to the cavity of the *middle ear* that equalizes air pressure.

F

Fallopian tube
One of two open-ended tubes along which an egg travels to the *uterus*, after release from an *ovary*.

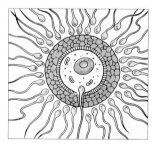

FERTILIZATION
The union of a sperm and an egg after sexual intercourse, artificial insemination, or in a laboratory test tube.

Fertilization
See illustration above.

Fetus
See illustration at right.

Fever
A body temperature that registers above 37°C (97.6°F), measured in the mouth, or 37.7°C (99.8°F), measured in the rectum.

Fibrin
An insoluble protein that is converted from the blood protein fibrinogen to form a fibrous network – a stage in the creation of a *blood clot*.

Fibroid
A *benign* tumour of fibrous and muscular tissue growing in the wall of the *uterus* usually in women over 30. Fibroids are often multiple and may cause pain.

Fistula
An abnormal channel between any part of the interior of the body and the surface of the skin or between two internal organs

G

Gallbladder
The small, fig-shaped bag lying under the *liver*, into which *bile* secreted by the *liver* passes to be stored.

Gallstone
An oval or faceted mass of cholesterol, calcium, and *bile* that forms in the *gallbladder*. Gallstones vary in size and are commoner in women than in men.

Gastric juice
A mixture produced by the cells of the stomach that contains hydrochloric acid, and digestive *enzymes*.

Gastritis
Inflammation of the stomach lining from any cause, such as infection, alcohol, or irritating food.

Gastrointestinal tract
The muscular tube that consists of the mouth, *pharynx*, *oesophagus*, stomach, and intestines.

Gene
A distinct section of a *chromosome* that is the basic unit of inheritance. Each gene contains the code that governs the manufacture of a specific protein.

Glaucoma
A rise in the pressure in the fluids within the eye that, if untreated, causes internal damage and affects vision.

Glial cell
A nerve cell that provides support for *neurons*.

Glue ear
A disorder in which sticky fluid accumulates in the *middle ear* and impedes the movement of the *ossicles*.

Gonorrhoea
See illustration above.

Gout
A metabolic disorder causing attacks of *arthritis*, usually in a single joint.

Grey matter
The regions of the brain and spinal cord that are composed mainly of *neuron* cell bodies as opposed to their projecting fibres, which form white matter.

TEM x 7500

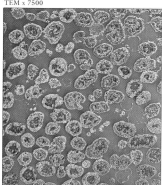

GONORRHOEA
A sexually transmitted disease that may cause pelvic inflammation in women and narrowing of the urine outlet tube in men. If untreated, the disease may spread to other parts of the body. Shown at left is a colony of the bacteria causing the disease, Neisseria gonorrhoeae.

H

Haematoma
Accumulated blood within any part of the body, caused by a ruptured blood vessel; may be minor or fatal.

Haemoglobin
The protein that fills *red blood cells* and combines with oxygen so that it can be carried from the lungs to all parts of the body.

Haemophilia
An inherited bleeding disorder that is caused by shortage of a particular blood protein.

Haemorrhage
The escape of blood from a blood vessel, usually as a result of injury.

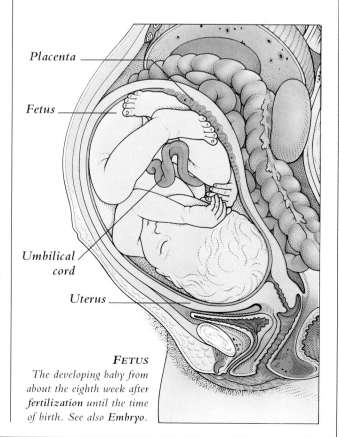

Placenta

Fetus

Umbilical cord

Uterus

FETUS
The developing baby from about the eighth week after fertilization until the time of birth. See also Embryo.

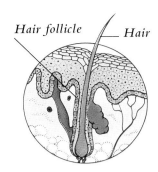

HAIR FOLLICLE
A pit on the surface of the skin from which a hair grows.

Haemorrhoids
Ballooning of veins in the lining of the anus (external haemorrhoids) or in the lower part of the rectum (internal haemorrhoids).

Hair follicle
See illustration above.

Heart-lung machine
A pump and oxygenator that performs the functions of the heart and the lungs during surgical operations.

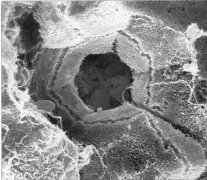

SEM x 1550

Heart valves
Four structures of the heart that allow passage of blood in one direction only.

Hemiplegia
Paralysis of one half of the body, from damage to the motor areas located in the opposite side of the brain, or to the nerve tracts that connect these motor areas to the spinal cord.

Hepatitis
Inflammation of the *liver*, usually as a result of a viral infection, alcohol, or toxic substances. The symptoms include *fever* and *jaundice*.

Hepatocyte
See illustration above.

Hiatal hernia
Sliding upward of part of the stomach through the opening in the *diaphragm*.

Hippocampus
A structure in the brain concerned with learning and long-term *memory*.

Homeostasis
Active processes by which an organism maintains a constant internal state despite external changes.

Hormones
Chemical substances released into the bloodstream from endocrine glands and some tissues. Hormones act on specific receptor sites in other parts of the body.

Human immunodeficiency virus
HIV – the cause of AIDS. HIV destroys certain cells of the immune system, thereby seriously undermining the efficiency of the system.

HEPATOCYTE
A liver cell that manufactures bile. Shown here in brown are hepatocytes surrounding a channel filled with blood.

Hypothalamus
A small structure located at the base of the brain where the nervous and hormonal systems of the body interact.

I–J

Ileum
The final part of the small intestine; it completes the absorption of nutrients.

Immune deficiency
Any failure of the function of the immune system from causes such as AIDS, cancer treatment, or ageing.

Immunosuppressant
A drug that interferes with immune system activity.

Interferon
A protein substance produced by cells to provide a defence against viral infections and some *cancers*.

In vitro fertilization
Fertilization of an egg in a laboratory container by the addition of sperm.

Irritable bowel syndrome
Recurrent abdominal discomfort, excessive gas, and intermittent diarrhoea.

Jaundice
Yellowing of the skin and whites of the eyes due to deposition of *bile* pigment, usually from *liver* disease.

K

Kaposi's sarcoma
A slow-growing *tumour* of blood vessels that affects many people with AIDS. It is characterized by firm, bluish-brown scattered nodules on the skin.

Keratin
A hard protein found in hair and nails and in the outer layers of the skin.

Kidney
One of two reddish-brown, bean-shaped structures at the back of the abdominal cavity; the kidneys filter blood and remove wastes.

Killer T cells
White blood cells that can destroy damaged, infected, or *malignant* body cells.

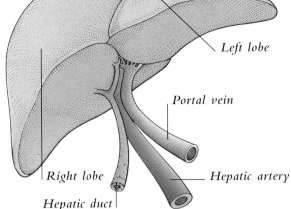

LIVER
The large organ in the upper right abdomen that performs vital chemical functions, including processing of nutrients from the intestines; synthesis of sugars, proteins and fats; detoxification of poisons; and conversion of waste to urea.

Kupffer cells
Cells lining the *capillaries* of the *liver* to scavenge old *red blood cells*, *bacteria*, and other foreign material.

L

Laparoscopy
Visual inspection of the interior of the abdomen through a narrow optical and illuminating device, often using a video camera.

Laparotomy
An exploratory operation of the abdomen to discover the cause of an illness.

Larynx
The structure in the neck at the top of the *trachea*, known as the voice box, that contains the vocal cords.

Lens
The internal lens of the eye, also called the crystalline lens. It adjusts fine focus by alterations in curvature. The eye also has an outer lens, called the *cornea*.

Leukaemia
A group of blood disorders in which abnormal *white blood cells* proliferate in the bone marrow, crowding out other healthy cells.

Ligament
See illustration below.

Limbic system
A part of the brain that plays a role in automatic body functions, emotions, and the sense of smell.

Liver
See illustration above.

LIGAMENT
A band of tissue consisting of collagen – a tough, fibrous, elastic protein. Ligaments support bones, mainly in and around joints.

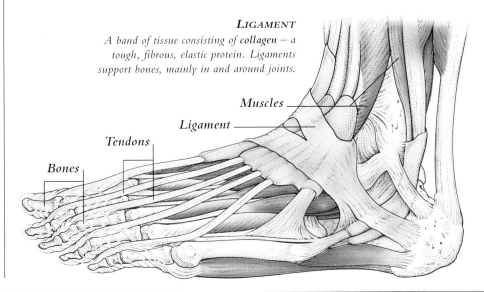

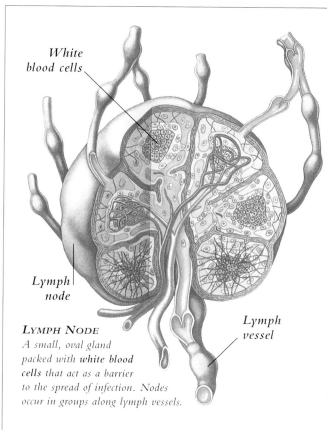

White blood cells

Lymph node

LYMPH NODE
A small, oval gland packed with white blood cells that act as a barrier to the spread of infection. Nodes occur in groups along lymph vessels.

Lymph vessel

Lobe
A rounded projection or subdivision forming part of a larger structure such as the brain, lung, or *liver*.

Lymphatic system
An extensive network of transparent lymph vessels and *lymph nodes*. It returns excess tissue fluid to the circulation and helps combat infections and *tumour* cells.

Lymph node
See illustration above.

Lymphocyte
Small *white blood cells* that are part of the immune system; they protect against *virus* infections and *cancer*.

Lymphoid tissue
A tissue rich in *lymphocytes* found in *lymph nodes*, the *spleen*, *adenoids*, and *tonsils*.

M

Macula
Any small, flat, coloured spot on the skin; also the central region of the *retina*.

Malignant
Tending to become worse and to result in death unless effectively treated; malignant is the opposite of *benign*.

Mammography
X-ray screening of the breasts, using low-radiation X-rays; used to detect breast *cancer* at an early stage.

Mastectomy
Surgical removal of all or part of the breast. It is usually performed to treat breast *cancer* and often followed by radiotherapy.

Mastitis
Inflammation of the breast, usually due to an infection acquired during breast-feeding when *bacteria* may enter through cracks in the nipples. Symptoms include *fever*, redness, hardening, and tenderness of the breast.

Medulla
The inner part of an organ, such as the *kidneys*, or adrenal glands. Also refers to the part of the *brain stem* lying immediately above the start of the spinal cord, just in front of the *cerebellum*.

Meiosis
The stage in the formation of sperm and egg cells when chromosomal material is randomly redistributed and the number of *chromosomes* is reduced to 23 instead of the usual 46 found in the other body cells.

Memory
The data store for recent and remote experience. Short-term memory stores are small and the contents are soon lost. Long-term memory stores are larger.

Meninges
The three membrane layers that surround the brain and spinal cord. It consists of the pia mater, the arachnoid, and the *dura mater*.

Meningitis
Inflammation of the *meninges*, commonly as a result of a *virus* infection.

Meniscectomy
Surgical removal of a torn or displaced *cartilage (meniscus)* from the knee joint; usually carried out with the use of a fibreoptic viewing tube, which is inserted into the joint, and a TV monitor.

Meniscus
A crescent-shaped pad of *cartilage* found in the knee and some other joints.

Menopause
The end of the reproductive period in a woman when the *ovaries* have ceased their production of eggs and menstruation has stopped.

Metabolism
The sum of all the physical and chemical processes that take place in the body.

Metastasis
The spread or transfer of any disease, but especially *cancer*, from its original site to another site, where the disease process continues.

Microscopy
See illustration below.

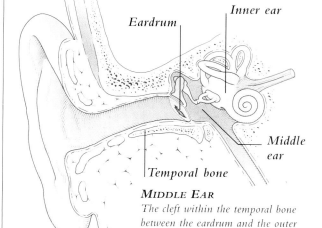

Eardrum

Inner ear

Middle ear

Temporal bone

MIDDLE EAR
The cleft within the temporal bone between the eardrum and the outer wall of the inner ear.

Middle ear
See illustration above.

Migraine
The effects of narrowing and then widening of some of the *arteries* of the scalp and brain, usually on one side. Symptoms include visual disturbances, nausea, and severe headache.

Miscarriage
A spontaneous ending of a pregnancy before the *fetus* is mature enough to survive outside the *uterus*.

Mitochondria
A class of microscopic cell organ containing genetic material and concerned with provision of energy for the various cell functions.

Mitosis
The process of division of a cell nucleus to produce two daughter cells, each with the identical genetic make-up of the parent cell.

Mitral valve
The valve on the left side of the heart lying between the upper and lower chambers.

Mole
Any *congenital* blemish, birthmark, growth, or pigmented spot – flat, raised, and/or hairy – on the skin.

Motor cortex
The part of the surface layer of each hemisphere of the *cerebrum* in which voluntary movement is initiated. The motor cortex can be mapped into areas that are linked to particular parts of the body.

Motor neuron
A nerve cell that carries impulses to muscles to cause movement.

Motor neuron disease
A rare disorder in which motor *neurons* suffer progressive destruction, resulting in corresponding loss of movement.

Mucocele
A *cyst*-like abnormal sac filled with mucus that arises from a *mucous membrane*.

Mucolytic
A drug that makes sputum (phlegm) less sticky and easier to cough up.

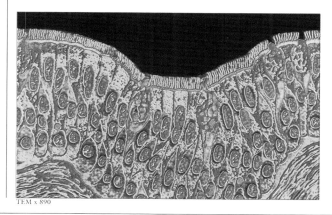

TEM x 890

MICROSCOPY
Examination by a microscope, usually to make a diagnosis. Simple techniques use focused light rays and magnifying lenses; in order to achieve higher magnifications, beams of electrons are used. Shown here is a type of electron microscope picture of the tissue lining the trachea.

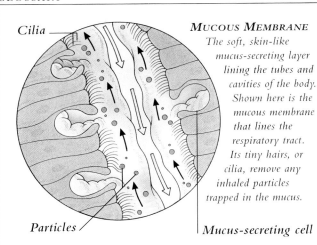

Cilia

Particles

MUCOUS MEMBRANE
The soft, skin-like mucus-secreting layer lining the tubes and cavities of the body. Shown here is the mucous membrane that lines the respiratory tract. Its tiny hairs, or cilia, remove any inhaled particles trapped in the mucus.

Mucus-secreting cell

Mucous membrane
See illustration above.

Muscular dystrophy
One of several hereditary muscle disorders featuring gradual, progressive muscle degeneration and weakening.

Myocardium
The special muscle of the heart, in which the fibres make up a network that will contract spontaneously.

Myofibril
Cylindrical elements within muscle cells (fibres). These, in turn, consist of thinner filaments, which move to produce muscle contraction.

N

Nephron
The *kidney's* filtering and reabsorption unit, consisting of a filtration capsule, also known as glomerulus, and a series of tubules. Each kidney contains about a million nephrons.

Nerve
The filamentous projections of individual *neurons* (nerve cells) held together by a fibrous sheath. Nerves carry electrical impulses to and from the brain and spinal cord and other body parts.

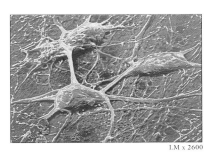

NEURON
A single nerve cell whose function is to transmit electrical impulses. Shown at left are three neurons found in the cerebral cortex, the outer layer of the brain.

LM x 2600

Neuron
See illustration below.

Nociceptor
A *nerve* ending that responds to painful stimuli.

Non-invasive
Any medical procedure that does not involve penetration of the skin or an entry into the body through any of the natural openings

O

Oesophagitis
Inflammation of the *oesophagus*, often from reflux of stomach acid into the oesophagus.

Oesophagus
The muscular tube that extends from the *pharynx* (throat) to the stomach, down which food is carried.

Oestrogen
A female *sex hormone* that stimulates the development of secondary sexual characteristics and prepares the uterine lining for an implanted fertilized egg.

Olfactory nerve
One of two *nerves* of smell that run from the roof of the nose directly into the underside of the brain.

Optic nerve
One of the two nerves of vision. Each has about one million nerve fibres running from the *retina* to the brain, carrying visual information.

Ossicle
One of three tiny bones of the *middle ear* that convey vibrations from the eardrum to the inner ear.

Osteoarthritis
A degenerative joint disease that features damage to the *cartilage*-covered, bearing surfaces in the joint.

Osteomalacia
Bone softening as a result of defective mineralization, usually because of poor calcium absorption from vitamin D deficiency.

Osteon
The rod-shaped unit, also called a haversian system, that is the building block of cortical (hard) bone.

Osteoporosis
Loss of bone substance due to bone being reabsorbed faster than it is formed. Bones become brittle and easily fractured.

Osteosarcoma
A highly *malignant* form of bone *cancer* mainly affecting adolescents. It develops most often near the knee.

Otitis media
Inflammation in the *middle ear* cavity, often caused by infection that has spread from the nose or throat.

Otosclerosis
A hereditary bone disease in which the foot of the inner *ossicle* becomes fused to the surrounding bone.

Ovary
One of two structures, lying on each side of the *uterus*, that produce eggs and female *sex hormones*.

Ovulation
See illustration at right.

Ovum
The egg cell; if *fertilization* occurs, the ovum develops into an *embryo*.

P

Pacemaker
See illustration at right.

Paget's disease
A disease that causes bone to become weaker, thicker, and distorted.

Pancreas
A gland situated behind the stomach that secretes digestive *enzymes* and *hormones* that regulate blood glucose levels.

Pancreatitis
Inflammation of the *pancreas* causing severe upper abdominal pain.

Paralysis
Loss of movement of part of the body due to a *nerve* or a muscle disorder.

Paraplegia
Paralysis of the lower limbs, usually from injury or disease to the spinal cord or brain.

Parasympathetic nervous system
One of the two divisions of the *autonomic nervous system*; it maintains and restores energy, for example by slowing the heart rate.

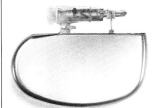

PACEMAKER
An electronic device implanted in the chest that delivers short pulses of electricity to stimulate or regulate the heartbeat.

Parathyroid glands
Two pairs of glands located behind the thyroid gland that help control the level of calcium in blood.

Parietal
A term referring to the wall of a body cavity.

Parkinson's disease
A neurological disorder that features involuntary tremor, slowness of movements, muscle rigidity, tottering steps, and small handwriting. The intellect is not affected.

Parotid glands
The largest pair of *salivary glands* that are situated, one on each side, over the angles of the jaw below and in front of the ears.

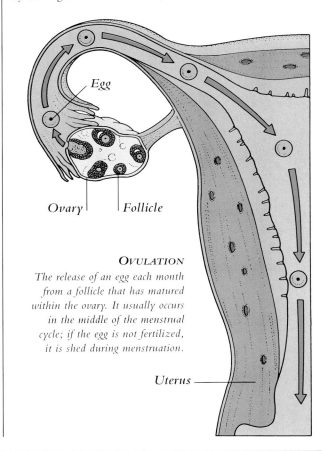

Egg

Ovary | Follicle

OVULATION
The release of an egg each month from a follicle that has matured within the ovary. It usually occurs in the middle of the menstrual cycle; if the egg is not fertilized, it is shed during menstruation.

Uterus

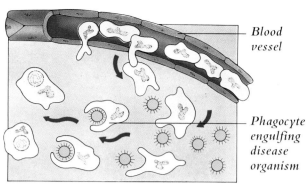

PHAGOCYTE
An amoeba-like cell of the immune system that can surround, kill, and digest disease organisms and scavenge foreign material.

Blood vessel

Phagocyte engulfing disease organism

Pelvic inflammatory disease
Persistent infection of the internal reproductive organs of the female. It may not have any obvious cause, but often occurs after a sexually transmitted disease.

Pelvis
The basin-like ring of bones to which the lower *spine* is attached and with which the thigh bones articulate. The term is also used to refer to the soft tissue contents.

Peptic ulcer
Erosion of the membrane lining of the *oesophagus*, stomach, or *duodenum* from excess stomach acid and digestive *enzymes*.

Pericarditis
Inflammation of the membranous *pericardium* that surrounds the heart. It may cause pain and the accumulation of fluid, called a pericardial effusion.

Pericardium
The tough, fibrous sac, consisting of two layers, that encloses the heart and the roots of the major blood vessels that emerge from it.

Periosteum
The tough tissue that surrounds bone and from which new bone can be formed; contains blood vessels and *nerves*.

Peripheral nervous system
All the *nerves* and their coverings that fan out from the brain and spinal cord, linking them with the rest of the body; consists of *cranial nerves* and *spinal nerves*.

Peristalsis
A coordinated succession of contractions and relaxations of the muscular wall of a tubular structure, such as the intestines; causes the contents to move along.

Peritoneum
A double-layered membrane that lines the inner wall of the abdomen; covers the abdominal organs and secretes fluid that lubricates their movement.

Peritonitis
Inflammation of the *peritoneum* due to bacteria, bile, pancreatic enzymes, or chemicals; sometimes the cause may be unknown.

Phagocyte
See illustration at left.

Pharynx
See illustration at right.

Pituitary gland
A pea-sized gland hanging from the underside of the brain; secretes *hormones* that help to control many other glands in the body.

Placenta
See illustration below.

Plasma
The fluid part of blood from which all cells have been removed; contains proteins, salts, and various nutrients that regulate blood volume.

Platelet
A fragment of large cells, called megakaryocytes, present in large numbers in the blood and necessary for normal *blood clotting*.

Pleura
A double-layered membrane, the inner layer of which covers the lung and the outer layer of which lines the chest cavity. A layer of fluid lubricates and enables movement between the two.

Pleural effusion
Accumulation of excessive fluid between the layers of the *pleura*, which separates them and compresses the underlying lung.

Pleurisy
Inflammation of the *pleura*, usually from a lung infection such as *pneumonia*; may lead to adhesion between the pleural membranes.

Plexus
A network of interwoven *nerves* or blood vessels.

Pneumoconiosis
Any lung-scarring disorder due to inhalation of mineral dust; scarring causes the lungs to be less efficient in supplying oxygen to blood.

Pneumocystis pneumonia
A lung infection with the microorganism *Pneumocystis carinii*; occurs mainly in *immune deficiency disorders*.

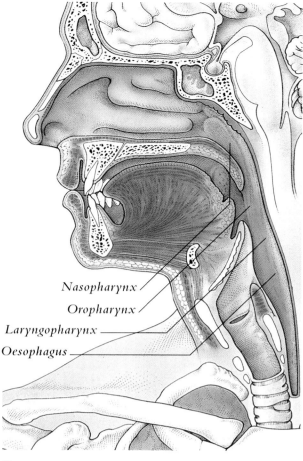

PHARYNX
The passage leading down from the back of the nose and the mouth to the oesophagus; it consists of the nasopharynx, the oropharynx, and the laryngopharynx.

Nasopharynx

Oropharynx

Laryngopharynx

Oesophagus

Pneumonia
Inflammation of the smaller air passages and *alveoli* of the lungs due to infection or contact with inhaled irritants or toxic material.

Pneumothorax
The presence of air in the space between the two layers of the *pleura*, causing the collapse of the lung.

Primary
A term describing a disorder that has originated in the affected structure.

Progesterone
A female *sex hormone* secreted by the *ovaries* and the *placenta*; prepares the uterine lining to receive and retain a fertilized egg.

Prostaglandins
A group of fatty acids made naturally in the body that act much like *hormones*.

Prosthesis
See illustration at right.

Prostate gland
The structure at the base of the bladder that secretes some of the fluid in semen.

Psoriasis
A common skin disease that features thickened patches of red, inflamed skin.

Pulmonary artery
The *artery* conveying blood from the heart to the lungs for reoxygenating.

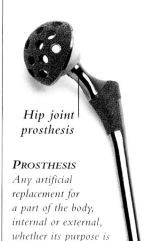

Hip joint prosthesis

PROSTHESIS
Any artificial replacement for a part of the body, internal or external, whether its purpose is functional or cosmetic.

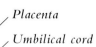

Placenta

Umbilical cord

PLACENTA
The disc-shaped organ that forms in the uterus during pregnancy. It links the blood supplies of the mother and baby via the umbilical cord.

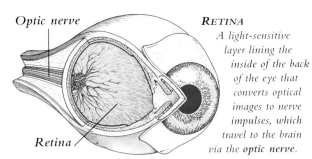

Optic nerve

Retina

RETINA
A light-sensitive layer lining the inside of the back of the eye that converts optical images to nerve impulses, which travel to the brain via the optic nerve.

Pulse
Rhythmic expansion and contraction of an *artery* as blood is forced through it.

Pus
A yellowish or green fluid that forms at the site of a bacterial infection; contains *bacteria*, dead *white blood cells*, and damaged tissue.

Q–R

Quadriplegia
Paralysis of both arms, both legs, and the trunk, usually caused by severe spinal cord damage in the neck region.

Red blood cells
Small, biconcave discs with no nuclei that are filled with *haemoglobin*. Each cubic millimetre of blood contains about five million red cells.

Respiration
The process by which oxygen is conveyed to body cells and carbon dioxide is removed from the cells.

Reticular formation
Nerve cells scattered throughout the *brain stem* that are concerned with alertness and direction of attention to external events.

Retina
See illustration above.

Rheumatoid arthritis
A disorder that causes joint deformity and destruction.

Rubella
A mild viral infection, also known as German measles; if it affects a woman in early pregnancy, it can cause serious harm to the *fetus*.

S

Saccharide
The basic unit that makes up carbohydrates.

Saliva
A watery fluid secreted into the mouth by the *salivary glands* to aid in chewing, tasting, and digestion.

Salivary glands
See illustration below.

Sarcoma
A *cancer* that arises from connective tissue (such as bone), muscle, fibrous tissue, or blood vessels.

Sciatica
Pain caused by pressure on the sciatic nerve; usually felt in the buttock and thigh.

Secondary
A term describing a disorder that follows or results from another disorder (called the *primary* disorder).

Septal defect
An abnormal opening in the central heart wall that allows blood to flow from the right side to the left or vice versa.

Sex hormones
Steroid substances that bring about the development of bodily sex characteristics. Sex hormones also regulate sperm and egg production and the menstrual cycle.

Sinoatrial node
A cluster of specialized muscle cells in the right *atrium* that acts as the heart's natural pacemaker.

Sinus bradycardia
An abnormally slow, but regular, heart rate resulting from a low rate of pacing by the *sinoatrial node*.

Sphincter
A muscle ring, or local thickening of the muscle coat, surrounding an opening in the body.

Spinal fusion
A surgical operation to fuse the bodies of two or more adjacent *vertebrae* in order to stabilize the *spine*.

Spinal nerves
The 31 pairs of combined motor and sensory *nerves* that emerge from and enter the *spinal cord*.

Spine
See illustration at right.

Spleen
A lymphatic organ on the left of the abdominal cavity that removes and destroys worn-out *red blood cells* and helps to fight infection.

Stapedectomy
An operation to relieve deafness due to *otosclerosis*.

Steroid drug
A drug that simulates the actions of the natural *corticosteroids* or the *sex hormones* of the body.

Stroke
Damage to the brain by deprivation of its full blood supply or leakage of blood from a ruptured vessel; may impair movement, sensation, vision, or speech.

Subarachnoid haemorrhage
Bleeding from a ruptured *artery* or *aneurysm* lying under the arachnoid layer of the *meninges*.

Subdural haemorrhage
Bleeding between the *dura mater* and the arachnoid layers of the *meninges*.

Sublingual glands
The pair of *salivary glands* in the floor of the mouth.

Submandibular glands
The pair of *salivary glands* that lie immediately under the jawbone near its angle.

Suture
A surgical stitch used to close a wound or incision.

Sympathetic nervous system
One of the two divisions f the *autonomic nervous system*; prepares the body for action, for example by constricting the intestinal and skin blood vessels, widening eye pupils, and increasing heart rate.

Synapse
The junction between two nerve cells, or between a nerve cell and a muscle fibre or a gland. Chemical messengers are passed across a synapse to produce a response in a target cell.

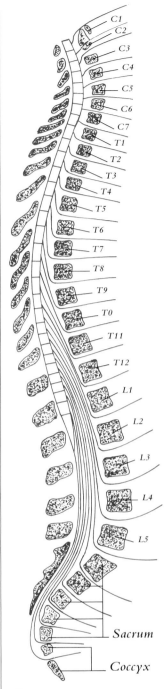

C1
C2
C3
C4
C5
C6
C7
T1
T2
T3
T4
T5
T6
T7
T8
T9
T0
T11
T12
L1
L2
L3
L4
L5

Sacrum

Coccyx

SPINE
The column of 33 ring-like bones, called vertebrae, that divides into seven cervical, 12 thoracic, five lumbar vertebrae, and the fused vertebrae of the sacrum and coccyx.

Synovial joint
A mobile joint lined with a membrane that produces a clear, lubricating fluid.

Syphilis
A sexually transmitted or *congenital* infection that, if untreated, passes through three stages and can involve serious damage to the nervous system. *Congenital* syphilis is now very rare.

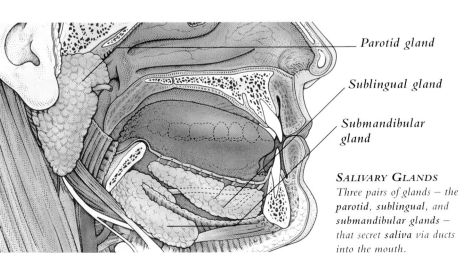

Parotid gland

Sublingual gland

Submandibular gland

SALIVARY GLANDS
Three pairs of glands – the parotid, sublingual, and submandibular glands – that secret saliva via ducts into the mouth.

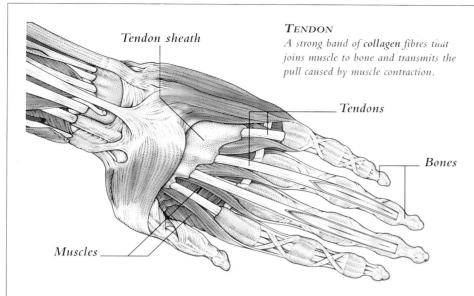

Tendon sheath

TENDON
*A strong band of **collagen** fibres that joins muscle to bone and transmits the pull caused by muscle contraction.*

Tendons

Bones

Muscles

T

Taste bud
A spherical nest of receptor cells found mainly on the tongue; each responds most strongly to either sweet, salty, sour, or bitter flavours.

Tendinitis
Inflammation of a *tendon*, causing pain and tenderness, usually from injury.

Tendon
See illustration above.

Tenosynovitis
Inflammation of the inner lining of a *tendon* sheath, usually from excessive friction due to overuse.

Testis
One of a pair of the sperm-producing male sex glands, suspended in the scrotum.

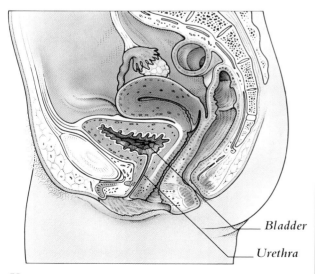

URETHRA
*The tube that carries **urine** from the bladder to the exterior; much longer in the male than the female.*

Bladder

Urethra

Testosterone
The principal *sex hormone* produced in the *testis* and in small amounts in the adrenal cortex and *ovary*.

Thalamus
A mass of *grey matter* that lies deep within the brain. It receives and coordinates sensory information.

Thorax
The part of the trunk between the neck and the abdomen that contains the heart and the lungs.

Thrombolytic drug
A drug that dissolves *blood clots* and restores blood flow in blocked *arteries*.

Thrombus
A *blood clot* that is usually a result of damage to the blood vessel lining.

Tonsils
Oval masses of *lymphoid tissue* on the back of the throat on either side of the soft palate; help protect against childhood infections.

Trachea
The windpipe. A muscular tube lined with a *mucous membrane* and reinforced by about 20 rings of *cartilage*.

Transient ischaemic attack
A "mini-stroke" that passes completely in 24 hours. Such an attack can imply danger of a full *stroke*.

Tumour
A *benign* or *malignant* swelling, especially a mass of cells resulting from uncontrolled multiplication.

U

Umbilical cord
The structure that connects the *placenta* and the *fetus*; provides the immunological, nutritional, and hormonal link with the mother.

Urea
A waste product of the breakdown of proteins and the nitrogen-containing component of *urine*.

Urethra
See illustration at left.

Urethritis
Inflammation of the lining of the *urethra*, which is usually caused by a sexually transmitted disease.

Urinary tract
The waste system that forms and excretes *urine*; made up of the *kidneys*, ureters, bladder, and *urethra*.

Urine
Fluid containing wastes produced by the *kidneys*.

Uterus
The hollow muscular organ in which the *fetus* grows and is nourished until birth.

V

Vagina
The passage from the *uterus* to the external genitals that stretches to accommodate the erect penis during sexual intercourse and to allow the passage of a baby.

Vagus nerves
The tenth pair of *cranial nerves*; help to control automatic functions such as heartbeat and digestion.

Vas deferens
One of a pair of tubes that lead from the *testis* carrying sperm, which mix with fluid before entering the *urethra*.

Vasectomy
See illustration above right.

Vein
A thin-walled blood vessel that returns blood at low pressure to the heart.

Vena cava
One of the two large *veins* in the body that empty into the heart's right atrium.

Vertebra
One of the 33 bones of the vertebral column (*spine*).

Virus
See illustration at right.

Vitreous body
A gel in the main cavity of the eye between the back of the *lens* and the *retina*.

Vocal cord
One of two sheets of *mucous membrane* stretched across the inside of the *larynx* that vibrate to produce voice sounds when air passes between them.

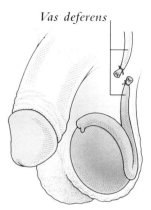

Vas deferens

VASECTOMY
*A surgical procedure for male sterilization in which each **vas deferens** is cut and tied.*

W–Z

Wart
A contagious, harmless skin growth that is caused by the human papilloma *virus*.

White blood cell
Any of the colourless blood cells that play various roles in the immune system.

X chromosome
A sex *chromosome*. Body cells of females have two X chromosomes.

Y chromosome
A sex *chromosome*. Its presence is necessary for the development of male characteristics. Body cells of males have one Y and one X *chromosome*.

Zygote
The cell produced when an egg is fertilized by a sperm; contains genetic material for a new person.

TEM x 117,000

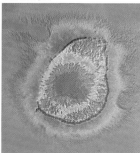

VIRUS
A small infectious agent capable of invading and damaging body cells and reproducing within them. Shown here is a herpes simplex virus; herpes can cause mouth or genital infections.

INDEX

U–V

W–Z

PICTURE CREDITS

c centre; l left ; r right; b bottom; t top; bla bottom left above; cla centre left above; bra bottom right above

Biophoto Associates: 11br, 13tr, 14tl, 21tr, 37bla, bl, 57c, cr, 72tr, 77crb, 101tr, 104tr, 109bra, br, 168bla, bl, 181tl, 190bl, 197cl, 214cl. Courtesy Dr Leonard Hayflick, University of California, San Francisco, School of Medicine: 218cl, cla. HNE Healthcare: 205tr; Life Science Images/Ron Boardman: 37tl, 40t. Living Technology: 171bl. National Medical Slide Bank: 45bl, 131tl, 193c. Northwick Park Hospital: 170c, bc, 173bla, bl. Institute of Orthopaedics, University College, London: 34tr. Barry Richards, St Petersburg, Florida: 114bl. Reynolds Medical Ltd: 116bl. Audio Visual Department, St Mary's Hospital Medical School: 164cl, 188c. Science Photo Library: 34tc, cr, 81crb, 107t, 131cl, 138bl, 166br, 191tl, cl, 192cr, 219tc, cr; John Durham: 2tr, 13br, 26; Professors Motta, Correr & Nottola/University "La Sapienza", Rome: 2bc, 17tr, 23cr, 94;

Bill Longcore: 3bc, 16c, 19tl; Professor P. Motta, Department of Anatomy, University "La Sapienza", Rome: 3cr, 14bl, 23bl, 33tl, bl, 49, 54cl, 134c, 151tr, 160tl, 161tl, 162tr, 174, 179bl, 226cl; Alfred Pasieka: 3cl, tc, 9tl, 199cl, 220tr, 227bc; Secchi-Lecaque/Roussel-UCLAF/CNRI: 6br, 65br, 87br, 228bl; Sandoz/D. Zagury/Petit Format: 7tl, 127bl; CNRI: 9bl, crb, cla, 12tr, 14br, 27cl, 39bc, 45cl, 62tr, 69bc, 84bl, 108br, 110bl, 123cl, 128cl, 130c, 140tr, 142bc, 161br, 167cl, 171tl, 172tl, 175cl, 180br, 183cl, 194tr, br, 195tl, 197tl, 204cl, 221bc, 222br; Mehau Kulyk: 9clb, 36tc, 84br; GCa/CNRI: 9tr, 37tr, 83tl; Tim Beddow: 9cra, 81bc, br; Petit Format/Nestle/Steiner: 9br, 68tr; J. C. Revy: 11tr, 58; Francis Leroy, Biocosmos: 11tl, 122; Don Fawcett: 12tl, 64tr, 100; Hossler/Custom Medical Stock Photo: 12bl; Astrid & Hanns Frieder Michler: 13cl, 86tc, 145tr, 182; Andrew Syred: 13bl; M.I. Walker: 14tr 195tr; Dr Gopal Murti: 20bl; David Scharf: 22tr, 135cl, 147bl; Biology Media: 23br; Dr P. Marazzi: 25cl, clb, cr; Scott Camazine: 33br, 82br; Eric Grave:

33cl; GJLP/CNRI: 35cl, 47bl; BSIP, LECA: 35bl; Biophoto Associates: 37cl, 66bl, 144bc, 204cr, 209tr, 224bl; Department of Clinical Radiology, Salisbury District Hospital: 44br; Princess Margaret Rose Orthopaedic Hospital: 46tr, 47cr; Manfred Kage: 59tr, 63bc, 179cr; Hank Morgan: 63tr; Petit Format/C. Edelmann: 66br; Dr M. Phelps & Dr John Mazziotta/Neurology: 79bla; Dr John Mazziotta: 79bl; Professor P. Motta/A. Caggiati/University "La Sapienza", Rome: 89tl; Dr G. Oran Bredberg: 89bl; Omikron: 90tr; Stanford Eye Clinic: 91bc; Professor Tony Wright, Institute of Laryngology & Otology: 92tc; GEC Research/Hammersmith Hospital Medical School: 92bc; Western Ophthalmic Hospital: 93c; Alexander Tsiaras: 93bl; Martin Dohrn/Royal College of Surgeons: 105c; Lungagrafix: 105cr; Frieder Michler: 107bl; Philippe Plailly: 107br; Cardiothoracic Centre, Freeman Hospital, Newcastle-upon-Tyne: 113cl, c; Adam Hart-Davis: 117bl; NIBSC: 131bl, 133tr, 231br; Jim Stevenson: 132tr; Barry Dowsett: 143br,

164br; Morendun Animal Health: 148bl, 172cl, 225tr; Cecil H. Fox: 150; John Burbidge: 166tc; King's College School of Medicine: 188bra; SIU: 192bl; NIH: 195cl; Petit Format/Nestle: 201tc; Petit Format/CSI: 200bl; Peter Menzel: 205bc; Mark Clarke: 212bl; Mark Clarke and Chris Priest: 210br; Professor P. Motta & J. van Blerkom: 217cr. C. James Webb: 154tr.

Every effort has been made to trace the copyright holders, and Dorling Kindersley apologises in advance in case any omission has occurred. If any omission does come to light, the company will be pleased to insert the appropriate acknowledgement in any subsequent editions of this book.

ACKNOWLEDGEMENTS

Additional editorial help: Edda Bohnsack, Edward Bunting, Will Hodgkinson, Sarah Miller, Seán O'Connell, and Michael Williams.
Additional medical and scientific help: Philip Fulford, Editor, *Journal of Bone and Joint Surgery*.